Smoking Kills

This paperback edition published in 2014 by
Signal Books Limited
36 Minster Road
Oxford
OX4 1LY
www.signalbooks.co.uk

The author and publishers gratefully acknowledge the assistance of
the Medical Research Council. The comments and views described
in this book are solely those of the author and subject, and not of the
Medical Research Council.

ISBN 978-1-909930-04-9

Production: Devdan Sen
Cover Design: Devdan Sen
Cover Images: courtesy Nick and Cathy Doll
Photographs: courtesy Nick and Cathy Doll and Clinical Trials
        Service Unit, University of Oxford
Printed in India

Smoking Kills

The Revolutionary Life of Richard Doll

Conrad Keating

Signal Books
Oxford

Contents

Part Three 1969-1984
THE ACADEMIC REVOLUTION
Oxford and the Wider World

Contents

To my parents

Preface & Acknowledgements

The first time I met Richard Doll he cried; but this was not because he had just discovered how little I knew about medicine. Rather it was an emotional response to the memory of what he had seen on the Jarrow Hunger March over sixty years before when at first hand he experienced the waste and despair of the 1930s. As a writer I thought, "He's vulnerable, he's emotional; a biography could provide a unique narrative window into the life and times of a great scientist." All I needed to do was some excavating, some digging. As with anyone starting out on a biography, there was a sense of curiosity mixed with optimism.

Yet for those who knew and worked with him, Doll was far from being an open book. His heart was certainly in the right place, but it was accustomed to being subordinated to his intellect. In nearly every way Doll embodied Charles Darwin's definition of a value-free experimenter. "A scientific man ought to have no wishes, no affections—a mere heart of stone." He was not an enigma, but while his friends described him as "gentle and kind", his emotional detachment and what some perceived as his "unconscious intimidation" led to him being both feared and respected. What was certainly true was that he had an unusual ability to camouflage his emotions. This made the writing of his biography a far more difficult task than I had first imagined. Every biography is partly fictional in that it is impossible to know or write a complete life, and the story is necessarily partial and selective. Even so, it must follow the documented record and the obligations to history; it cannot be made up.

I decided on the title *Smoking Kills: The Revolutionary Life of Richard Doll* because smoking forms the main thread of Richard Doll's story as a scientist. One of his great intuitive skills was the ability to see patterns and he did this in an enduring way when he explained the epidemic of lung cancer. In 1950 British men had the highest lung cancer rates in the world and by 1970 almost half of all male deaths in middle age and an increasing number of female deaths in middle age in Britain were being caused by smoking. Since 1970, when the media truly got behind the public health campaign, Britain has seen the greatest decline in tobacco-related deaths

in the world. Doll's careful statistical science marked the Big Bang in thinking, and today in Britain two-thirds of all smokers wished they had never
started the habit. Doll changed the health of the nation and caused a revolution in medicine.

While Doll was born into a conventional bourgeois family in the
1930s, he was also a political revolutionary and he wanted the overthrow
of Stanley Baldwin's government. He remained a Marxist and communist
for over a quarter of a century and his politics gave him clarity, pointing
him in the direction of the greatest good for the greatest number: preventive medicine. He ushered in a new era in medicine, shaped by the
intellectual ascendancy of medical statistics, a revolution built substantially on Doll's scientific contribution.

Any history of modern Britain should contain something of Doll's
life. I did not want to fit him into a prescribed straitjacket, but I wanted
to walk with him through the history of twentieth-century Britain.
Because it was all there: his birth in the same year the *Titanic* was
launched, his life in the aftermath of the First World War, his politics, the
Jarrow March, Dunkirk, the greatest ever advance in the history of
medical science, the rise of the new epidemiology, the Cold War, the
Agnostic Adoption Society, the end of his communist dream—and,
above all, how he exposed the true hazards of smoking. All these subjects
had to be investigated if I was to get an understanding of Richard Doll the
man. As so many physicians around the world say that they were inspired
by Doll, I wanted to find out what inspired him to dedicate his life to the
prevention of cancer.

Nothing in life is flawless, and while Doll achieved the accolade of
being described by the *British Medical Journal* as "perhaps Britain's most
distinguished doctor", some of his work has been criticised. His pioneering work on the dangers of asbestos, the most lethal of all industrial
carcinogens, has been rewritten by the environmental lobby. His
humanitarian beliefs compelled him to establish the Agnostic Adoption
Society in the 1960s yet his decisions taken as chairman led him to be vil-
ified as a racist by the *New Statesman*. To some he will be remembered
as the most influential Regius Professor of Medicine at Oxford

University ever, yet he was initially cold-shouldered by the city's medical establishment. And even in death the forces of evil gathered in posthumous attack. Doll's passion was work. He never retired and continued his scientific experiments into his 93rd year. In some ways it was for Doll as it had been for Goethe: "There has been nothing but toil and care. It has been the perpetual rolling of a stone, which I have always had to raise anew."

The last time I saw Richard Doll was the first time his exemplary good manners failed him. It was the last week of his life and he knew it. While I was reading through the mass of cards and letters from well-wishers that covered his hospital bedside locker he looked at me and said, "What are you looking for now? You're always digging around my life." Of course, it must be a question those who achieve world-renown often ask themselves: "Who would I trust to meddle with my immortality?" I admired Richard Doll, but I had to do the digging, I had to find the man. He would have respected me less if I had not.

Acknowledgements

During the epic journey of researching and writing this biography I interviewed 191 people: too numerous to name individually, but for their generosity and kindness, I will forever be in their debt. However, there are four people without whom this book would not exist. First is Richard Doll for his full co-operation in telling the story of his life, even though he knew it would uncover some uncomfortable truths. His willingness to answer questions that revealed my ignorance of medical science, statistics and literature only rarely caused him to look at his watch or fix me with a perplexed gaze. But he gave me the strength to do what I had never done before, while knowing, that he would not be alive to see the finished product—in fact insisting that this would be the case. Secondly, I thank my friend Rory Collins for introducing me to his colleague Richard Peto, Doll's scientific protégé. Richard Peto gave my work scientific guidance and the institutional support which allowed me the opportunity to devote myself wholeheartedly to writing, liberated from any other consideration. Lastly, this book would not have been possible without the help and encouragement of my friend Richard Ramage. His incisive intellect and feel for the English language have informed me as a writer and honed any skills that I may have. Without these four individuals I would still be floundering in a vast sea of papers, scribbles and uncertainty.

And how could I have prevailed without those small crumbs of encouragement that made my heart swell? As when the historian Charles Webster said to me one morning on Broad Street in Oxford: "You're a good writer, Richard Doll's lucky to get you." Or when I received a phone call on a long winter afternoon from someone who remembered working with Doll on a hospital ship in the Mediterranean in 1941. What is certain is that the human intellect is more moved by affirmatives than by negatives. While writing this book I received my fair share of negatives, but it is the affirmatives that I wish to list here.

I would like to thank the Wellcome Trust and the Wellcome Unit for the History of Medicine for supporting me from the beginning, and I would like to extend my appreciation to Green Templeton College for their goodwill. For much of the twenty-first century I have hibernated in libraries to such an extent that I am now addicted to their atmospheres of tranquillity and relaxed creativity. The final long stretch of writing was done in the Taylor Bodleian Slavonic and Modern Greek Library at 47 Wellington Square, where the staff were truly magnificent in their professionalism and encouragement. All books need a good editor and Polly Pattullo's dedication to detail gave this one the cohesion that it previously lacked. Many people read the book before the final draft but the wisdom and advice of Georgina Ferry and Leo Kinlen have been invaluable. As indeed has been the institutional and financial support of Jude Eades and Leszek Borysiewicz at the Medical Research Council. Finally, I am eternally grateful to the staff [whom Joan Doll referred to as "Richard Peto's slaves"] of the Clinical Trials Statistical Unit for their technical expertise, perspicacious statistical guidance and for putting up with me for so long. Of course, any mistakes that readers uncover are entirely of my own making.

Conrad Keating
Oxford July 2009

"Death in old age is inevitable but death before old age is not. In previous centuries seventy years used to be regarded as humanity's allotted span of life and only about one in five lived to such an age. Nowadays, however, for non-smokers in Western countries, the situation is reversed; only about one in five will die before seventy and the non-smoker death rates are still decreasing, offering the promise, at least in developed countries, of a world where death before seventy is uncommon. But, for this promise to be properly realised, ways must be found to limit the vast damage being done by tobacco and to bring home, to not only the many millions of people in developed countries but also the far larger populations elsewhere, the extent to which those who continue to smoke are shortening their expectation of life by so doing."

Richard Doll, 1994

Introduction

Millions of people are alive today who would otherwise be dead had Richard Doll not made his enduring contribution to medical science. In the second quarter of the twentieth century, routine official mortality statistics showed an unprecedented rise in death from cancer of the lung. By the late 1940s, Britain had the highest lung cancer rates in the world, and the reasons for this were completely unknown.[1] In 1948, eighty per cent of men smoked, and an increasing proportion of women. During the twentieth century, some 100 million people were killed by smoking; in the present century, if current patterns continue, the figure could be nearer to one billion.

Medicine entered a new era with the discovery of penicillin and the other antibiotics that rapidly followed. Even tuberculosis, that most feared of infections, could be controlled. By 1950, the fundamental change in the balance of disease could be seen in those indisputable facts—vital statistics. For the first time the number of deaths from lung cancer (13,000) exceeded those from tuberculosis.[2] But as the fear of infectious diseases began to recede, a new preoccupation with non-infectious diseases such as cancer, heart attacks and strokes began to engage medical researchers—though not yet society at large.

Tobacco is much the largest external cause of premature death in developed countries, and Richard Doll did more than any other physician to identify this hazard. In 2004 he completed a fifty-year follow-up of the prospective study of smoking and mortality among British male doctors that he had started in 1951, one year after publishing his 1950 case-control study showing that smoking was "a factor, and an important factor"[3] in the production of lung cancer. The early results from his fifty-year prospective study revealed, for the first time, the full range of diseases caused by smoking, and the later results first revealed the full hazards of lifelong smoking, and the benefits of quitting. It showed that half of all smokers were eventually killed by the habit, but, importantly, it also showed that stopping smoking works remarkably well.[4]

His achievements were such that Sir Robert May, the president of the Royal Society, wrote in 2001: "It is not too much to say that Richard Doll has done more to change our general understanding of cancer epidemiology than any other individual."[5] Doll's contribution to global public health was described by Sir Paul Nurse, director general of the Imperial Cancer Research Fund, as transcending "the boundaries of professional medicine into the general community of mankind".[6]

While, throughout Doll's professional life, assessments of his character would oscillate wildly (some would describe him as "warm and friendly", others as "a bit of a cold fish, difficult to get to know"), he was revered for his intellectual integrity, clarity of thought and pursuit of the truth. Over his long life—he died at the age of 92—he was at different times described, by a colleague as "a workaholic, uneasy if he isn't working"; in the *British Medical Journal* as "perhaps Britain's most distinguished doctor"; by one of England's most famous solicitors as "the most impressive expert witness I've ever seen"; and by his first collaborator in medical research as "the leading epidemiologist of our time".

A prophet of uncomfortable truths in the 1950s, his devotion to scientific inquiry and the resulting benefits to the health of the global community came at some considerable cost. One would be fortunate to live through ten decades and not encounter either scandal or tragedy; Doll encountered both. He was a driven scientist, dispassionate when faced with the evidence, and he was also courageous, taking on the vested interests of the tobacco industry, big business, the uninformed (including the politicians), and an equivocal medical profession.

It was Doll who carried out the first epidemiological study in Britain into the cause of lung cancer in collaboration with his great mentor, the father of medical statistics, Sir Austin Bradford Hill. Now looked upon as a watershed, its publication on 30 September 1950 was greeted with a combination of apathy, disbelief and scientific condemnation. It was not generally accepted by medical or statistical scientists, and certainly not by the UK Ministry of Health's standing advisory committee on cancer and radiotherapy.[7] Predictably the tobacco industry tried to discredit the study's findings, and instigated a campaign to undermine Doll and Hill scientifically using their own statistician, Geoffrey Todd. More damaging for the pioneering scientists was the vehement attack upon them by RA Fisher, the chain-smoking mathematical genius and the world's leading theoretical statistician. Even this savage onslaught[8] from such a giant analytical brain was successfully demolished, and some believe that Fisher recanted on his death bed,[9] but was not allowed the time to accept publicly the validity of the Doll and Hill hypothesis. The two men dealt thoughtfully and reliably with the many objections raised to their conclusions about smoking and lung cancer, and in so doing ushered in the modern era of cancer epidemiology.

Doll's contributions to epidemiological research included descriptive studies of global incidence of cancer; ecological analyses of external factors in relation to cancer in different populations; pioneering studies of ionised radiation and chemical health hazards at work; and statistical analyses of carcinogenesis as a multi-stage process. In the late 1950s and 1960s, Doll helped demonstrate the prevention of cancer by showing each type of cancer that is relatively common in one population is relatively uncommon in another, indicating that wherever that particular disease is common it need not be.[10]

Doll developed the tools of epidemiological inquiry and then by example taught a generation of younger medical scientists and physicians to apply these techniques across the whole field of medicine. Through his own work and that arising from his discoveries and leadership—again in collaboration with Hill—he pioneered the randomised controlled medical trial. This objective evaluation of data, accurately measuring the effectiveness of medical procedures, is one of the major medical advances of the twentieth century. Beginning his career in research in 1946, Doll was still producing original work in his 93rd year; he published more than 500 scientific papers, and established a "Doll philosophy"[11] based on rigorous scientific documentation. By his own admission it was "through a series of fortunate accidents" that he became an epidemiologist, but once the decision had been made, he became one of the truly great medical investigators of modern times.

So what were the emotional and intellectual developments that established him as a uniquely revolutionary doctor? What sets him apart? What made the world recognise that his work really did matter? His two formative interests were "mathematics and public health medicine", but would these intellectual rails of ideas have been sufficient to enable him to make such an enduring contribution to medical knowledge? Did his 25 years as an active communist give a political dimension to his science?[12] Or, was it his 52-year marriage to Joan Faulkner, the most powerful woman in the Medical Research Council, which afforded him the time to concentrate and work with such dedication for the benefit of humankind?

Sir Liam Donaldson, the chief medical officer for England, wrote that Doll was "without doubt a towering figure of twentieth-century public health. Millions are alive today because of him and his inspiration continues to fire action to combat tobacco use right across the world."[13] Celebrated as one of the nation's most dispassionate scientists, a trusted arbiter of controversial issues by national governments, Doll enjoyed international respect for his work.

The story this book tells has three principal narrative strands. First, there is the life of Doll himself, how the age imprinted itself on him and how he lived through one of the most tumultuous periods of human history. Secondly, there is the development of the discipline he championed from a subsidiary branch of medicine, concerned primarily with infectious diseases, into a vital and burgeoning medical science. Finally, there is the changing nature of society itself and the diseases of modernity, primarily cancer. In following these three strands I have covered a period that begins with the late Edwardian era and Great War and ends with the anxieties and uncertainties of the new millennium.

Richard Doll was witness to the greatest ever advance in medical knowledge as well as unimaginable acts of human cruelty on an industrial scale. The story, in the main, follows a chronological pattern, but the chapters on asbestos and Alice Stewart are thematic as the subjects transcend time. In the pages that follow I have in part attempted to put Doll at the centre of this extraordinary history, and to make this book a testament to the equally extraordinary contribution he made to his world. "History," according to EH Carr, "is how you tell the story."

Part One 1912-1945

The Political Revolution
Politics and Society

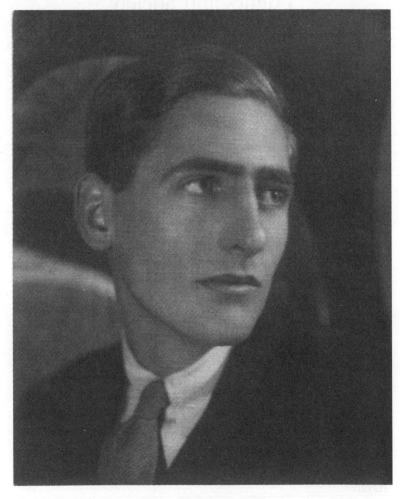

The young idealist, 1933

Chapter 1

The Early Years

"If only the geologists would let me alone, I could do very well, but those dreadful hammers! I hear a clink of them at the end of every cadence of the Bible verses."

John Ruskin

William Richard Shaboe Doll was born at 15 Park Road, Hampton Hill, in Middlesex, an outer suburb of London on 28 October 1912 into an Edwardian middle-class family, a mix of the conventional and the artistic. His father, Henry William Doll, was a physician and surgeon. His mother, Amy Kathleen May Doll (née Shaboe) was a celebrated classical pianist. A graduate of the Guildhall School of Music and a contemporary of Myra Hess, she played with both Sir Henry Wood and Sir Thomas Beecham. Throughout the first year of his life, she continued to play professionally but this unswerving dedication came at a price. Later, Richard became jealous and remembered accompanying his mother, lying under the piano, hitting the floor with his fists in a rhythm of abandonment as she practised rhapsodically for her public performances. To the vulnerable child, this devotion created an unbridgeable void and prevented him, by his own admission, from ever forming a bond of love with his mother. Before Richard's second birthday the First World War intervened, and his father, William, a medical doctor, immediately joined the war effort, and whenever possible—while not entertaining the troops at patriotic concerts—Kathleen joined him on his army attachments.

As a consequence much of Richard's early life was spent in the care of his maternal grandmother, Amy Agnes Shaboe, an affectionate and enlightened woman. He was often sent down to Bournemouth and looked after by her in Ferndown in the New Forest, where his godfather Aubrey Lewis lived—"a very generous, fine man," according to Doll. He stayed with Lewis quite often because Amy Shaboe, who had fallen on hard times, lived in part of Lewis's home, in what we might call a granny flat.

In 1919 his world was turned upside down with the arrival of a brother, Christopher. Many years later he would confess that the only thing they had in common was their parents, and the new sibling did create a fault line within the family. For Doll his father became the most important influence in his life. "Early on, my father was absent, but he was always a very important figure for me after the war. I felt close to him, not to my mother." In 1917 William Doll had been invalided out of the army and returned to general practice in Kensington, a wealthy area of west London.

In the 1930s the poverty in which many Londoners lived would have a radicalising effect upon Doll, but his childhood was lived in a protected oasis. The family home at 42 Montpellier Square, Knightsbridge, was a magnificent eighteenth-century house, set in leafy seclusion in one of the capital's most select areas. The family had a chauffeur, and Doll's playground was Hyde Park and the Natural History Museum. Only very rarely were the barriers of social exclusivity compromised. Doll remembered: "I know I got into trouble when I was young for playing games with 'street children'; it was thought that they were not the sort of friends for me to have."

Who can tell what subterranean emotions influenced a family almost a century ago, as documented evidence of their inner lives does not exist? What we do know is that Kathleen gave up her career as a professional musician after her husband came out of the army, and the maternal devotion, so missing from Doll's early life, was manifestly present for Christopher. "She was a real sweetie, my mother, and she played for two hours every night, and in the top room of Montpellier Square I would lean over the balcony and listen to her playing, mostly Chopin, I just listened night after night," he remembered. "At that age it wasn't so worrying, but as I got older I suddenly realised that she gave up her life, completely, for my father, and then suddenly he became ill."[1]

William Doll was diagnosed with multiple sclerosis in 1925, the early onslaught of the disease being so severe that he was incapacitated for a year. William, himself one of ten children, had had to make his own way in the world, but suffering from such a debilitating and progressive disease, he knew there was a limited amount of time in which to provide for his family. His practice was not for the wealthy; rather his large panel was mostly the servants of the people in the big houses. While the family did not suffer any material deprivations, for Christopher the deprivations lay elsewhere. "He was, from my point of view, sad. I was born in 1919, and by 1925 he'd got this terrible disease and was in bed for a year, and then he came back again and worked for ten years, and then gave up [and became] an invalid in the chair. I knew him pretty much as an old man all of my life. And that was one of the reasons why I believe Richard took up medicine, because of the multiple sclerosis—there wasn't a lot known about it—and I think he thought, 'I might be able to do something for my father.'"

The catastrophe cast a shadow over the family, and may have influenced Doll's future as a scientist, but he considered his childhood "a very happy one". Family life—in the traumatic aftermath of the First World War—still reflected order and certainty, and the enchantment of this continuity was strong enough to persuade the teenage Doll to later stand as a Liberal candidate in a Westminster School election (he won, much to the displeasure of the Conservative-voting headmaster). It would not be long, however, before the allure of Liberalism would desert the young idealist as it would also leave the British electorate.

Doll's conventional middle-class childhood was tempered by the absence of unconditional motherly love although after Kathleen's career as a professional musician ended she must have cared for him deeply. Within the extended family, there were also the grandmothers. His paternal grandmother was a respected and frequent presence. According to Doll, she was a little woman who ran a big household with complete authority and efficiency, and all of her children loved her. But he did not have much personal connection with her. "I wasn't in a 'cuddling relationship' with her." The most influential woman in Doll's childhood was "Granny" (Amy Shaboe), a woman whose social and ethical mores dated from the middle decades of the nineteenth century. She had been a "mother equivalent" for him, and her death in 1931 had a profound effect: "I was in Germany, on a walking tour of the Black Forest with Bill Deakin. I was there when she died and I burst into tears, and I remember the Germans we were staying with in the hostel saying, 'Isn't it a bit exaggerated? You don't cry when your grandmother dies.' But she was emotionally my mother, and I did cry."

When, at the age of seven, Doll had his first day at Gibbs's Preparatory

School at 134 Sloane Street, it was "Granny" who took him to school for his first year. Indeed, her dedication to his pre-school education may have been a formative influence in his fascination with mathematics. "It was my grandmother who taught me my tables so I arrived at school knowing my twelve times tables and other children didn't know their two times tables. I can clearly remember saying to my grandmother, 'Let's do the thirteen times table!' She was shocked and said, 'There's no such thing.' I was terribly disappointed, but I worked it out for myself some time later."

In 1924, at the age of twelve, he stood on the threshold of a new challenge, a place at Westminster School, a quintessential establishment institution. His world was expanding, and he wanted to find his place within it.

Westminster School had been a conveyor belt for the production of the British elite since the twelfth century. Its architectural splendour and medieval grounds are around the corner from the House of Commons. The school's chapel is the flying-buttressed Westminster Abbey. It was, and still is, one of the most celebrated public schools in England.

Even by the standards of the mid-1920s the school had some anachronistic customs. All the boys had to carry an umbrella and those under five feet four inches tall wore an Eton collar (a deep circular collar worn outside the lapels of a top coat). When that height was reached, the accepted symbolism demanded a winged collar. Until 1939, all the boys wore top hats.

Doll went to Westminster in April 1925 when Ramsay MacDonald was the first Labour prime minister, and when Britain was on the eve of a devastating economic struggle that changed the political landscape of the country. Two years later, he took the school certificate, became a King's scholar and a weekly boarder. Intelligent, athletic (he excelled at cricket[2]) and clubbable, Doll had made the transition into his new environment seamlessly.

Despite the umbrellas and top hats, somewhere in the twenty years between the two world wars lie the roots of Westminster as a liberal school. The careers of other old boys such as John Gielgud, Angus Wilson and Tony Benn suggest some aspects of a qualitative change—from tradition, conformity, classics, narrowness of vision, towards the arts, independence of mind and action, internationalism, or at least political interest of a national and European kind.[3]

> When I was a boarder, the headmaster allowed me to go out after dinner and I went to the first meeting of Oswald Mosley's New Party. The school encouraged you to go and do a wide variety of activities in the afternoons. As a King's scholar you had the right to go into the House of Commons gallery at any time, ahead of the queue. I remember on one occasion I saw James Maxton, of the Independent Labour Party, being thrown out. He was a fine representative of the real left. I had great respect for him, he was an honest man who stuck to his beliefs, and wouldn't bend.[4]

In 1926, however, the routine tranquillity of his daily bus ride to school was interrupted by the General Strike, the greatest revolt of organised labour in British history. The terrible cycle of industrial decline, unemployment, and social bitterness led to the worst explosion of class conflict that Britain had yet known. Prime Minister Stanley Baldwin called for "Peace in our Time, O Lord"[5] but in the greatest industry in the land, coal-mining, tension remained high, with a background of wage cuts, dismissals and falling living standards for mining families. In April 1926 the government refused to renew a subsidy to the mining industry. On 2 May Baldwin broke off negotiations with the Trades Union Congress delegation. Almost by accident, the unions lurched into a general strike. On the first morning of the General Strike, Britain awoke to silence: no buses, no trains, no hum of human industry. Three million men and women had not turned up for work.

For the following nine days, Britain was at a virtual standstill. There was an "odd pale unnatural atmosphere", observed Virginia Woolf. Tanks patrolled the streets and troops were bivouacked in Kensington Gardens ready to defend the King and parliament against a feared socialist revolution. In practice, the General Strike was peaceful enough. There was no violence directed against the many "blacklegs" (including some Westminster boys who drove buses and trams)[6] or the other participants in strike-breaking activities.

Still only fourteen, Doll had not yet developed the communist philosophy that was to dominate his life in the 1930s. For him, the identification of religion with middle-class values, with the family, the community and a safe form of patriotism was still discernible. So too was the link of religion with the empire, notable through youth movements such as the Boy Scouts and the Church Brigade. As a consequence Doll became involved with the Children's Special Service Mission, and fell under the seductive spell of fundamentalist Christians. He was entering a period of his life where he sought an identity and meaning. As a teenager he did not look to science for salvation; his first experiment was with religion. "I believed all the things that I was told then. You do as a twelve year old, and I thought what they said about the Christian religion was right. And I got quite involved with them. My parents sent me away on holiday with them; they provided skiing camps and other camps in the Easter holidays where we played games, cricket and hockey, which I enjoyed."[7]

The mission's camps were staffed by undergraduates, and for the sport-loving teenager, whose brother was too young to play games, and whose father was too incapacitated, the Christian fundamentalists provided earthly liberation. In the beginning, the only sacrifice—and it did not seem burdensome—"was listening to a sermon and a prayer meeting for about three-quarters of an hour in the evening."[8]

Gradually he came under the influence of the evangelical teaching and, on occasion, went preaching in pursuit of converts. Richard Doll never suffered a clinical depression in his life, but at sixteen he was deeply unhappy as he faced the dilemma of fully accepting religion or refuting it. He chose the latter, and suffered the consequences. "It was the most unhappy period of my life, when I was in conflict as to whether I believed it or not, and then gradually giving it up. The housemaster of College House—where all the King's scholars were—was the Reverend AGGC Pentreath; he was a very evangelical type, and when I broke away it made our relationship difficult."[9] The rebarbative Pentreath was a strong spiritual influence on Doll, and when his disciple rejected Christian teachings, he refused to promote the heretic to the position of prefect. It was an injustice in Doll's eyes and he never forgot it. "I was not given the position that I thought I ought to have had, not being made a prefect upset me—it was part of the conflict with religion and giving up what the housemaster believed in."[10]

Now that he was emancipated from the religious strictures of the fundamentalist Christians, his social conscience turned towards politics, addressing inequality "on earth" and not "as it is in heaven". By the end of the 1920s in Britain it was impossible not to see that poverty destroyed both souls and bodies, and that ill health was part of a wider structural problem with capitalism. More than anything else it was the growing numbers of unemployed, and the political initiatives to end their suffering, that pulled Doll away from prayer towards party political action.

In old age, eighty years after encountering the first moral dilemma of his life—losing his faith—he was able to view his teenage immersion in religion as a rite of passage. "I had this confusion which is not uncommon, and it was to do with finding your place in the world, and where you stand, in relation to other people. I was seeking a role in life."[11] In fact, his one memory of the daily sermons in Westminster Abbey was one of philosophical rejection. "I can remember only one thing and that was the man who said 'You can't do two things at once.' And I thought that was nonsense—of course you can—I was determined. And for the rest of my life I've demonstrated I can, and indeed I have done."[12]

Another strand in Doll's political development was the effect of reading exhaustively about the First World War, inspired by his father's participation in the conflict. It led to a horror of warfare. Under the proselytising influence of Dick Shepherd, a campaigning clergyman and influential pacifist thinker, Doll became a pacifist. "I didn't observe the two-minute silence that was then invoked to commemorate the dead of the First World War. I thought it was hypocritical while Britain was preparing for the next war. I was wrong—it was a genuine expression of sympathy for relatives who had died and recognition of their sacrifice."[13] His attitude changed completely in the 1930s when the politically sentient recognised that there was no alternative to fighting fascism.

In October 1921 the Young Communist League of Great Britain was formed and Doll joined it as a schoolboy; he remained an active communist until May 1957. As Doll's devotion to the Communist Party began so young and lasted so long, there has been much speculation as to how he first became impassioned by the cause. A fellow King's scholar at

Westminster was Kim Philby, the Cambridge spy; however, Doll's embrace of "democratic communism" came from his wish to fight social injustice. He had come to believe that only communists cared enough about things. "I joined the Young Communist League because it had a solution for the problem of the three million unemployed. I read a lot about politics, but there was no one person who got me to join a party. Kim Philby was one year ahead of me as a King's scholar; he was very quiet and reclusive—we didn't discuss politics much."[14]

Richard Doll was the most outstanding mathematician at Westminster School, and he had matured into a tall, athletic, blonde-haired and blue-eyed intellectual. But he had yet to display the leadership qualities that distinguished his service in the Second World War; nor had he developed the single-mindedness that would underpin his scientific achievements. He did possess a coherent set of political beliefs, derived from the Young Communist League, which he held with conviction, and a sense of public service. Ultimately the young idealist found the freedom to pursue his two formative interests—mathematics and public health medicine—but one of the greatest medical scientists of the twentieth century was almost lost to the colonial service.

> At various times I thought, as one does at the end of one's school days, as to what you're going to do, and I did think of becoming an Indian civil servant. I was enthused, as I think many boys were at the time, by Kipling's stories. And a colonial civil servant, particularly an Indian civil servant, seemed to be the height of ambition, if one could dedicate oneself to looking after several million people. It seemed to be a great career, but I was quite rapidly talked out of that by my parents. Then I thought of becoming a forester, but that was all based on the novels I read. Essentially, I wanted to do mathematics—I wanted to go to university and read mathematics.[15]

Doll's father had the biggest influence on his choice of career. At one time he thought his son would excel as a barrister, and at another because of his mathematical prowess he even advised him to become an actuary. In reality, this was a chimera—what he really wanted Doll to do was follow in his own footsteps and study medicine in one of the great

London teaching hospitals. Yet Doll had established a reputation as a gifted mathematician: it seemed that he had found something he was born to do. "I had studied the sciences, biology, physics, and chemistry, because I didn't want to rule out medicine entirely. But I really concentrated on mathematics, I loved mathematics, and I determined to make it my life."[16]

An immutable aspect of Doll's character—and one that was already evident at Westminster—was his abhorrence of nepotism. The school had numerous closed scholarships set aside for their students at Trinity College, Cambridge, and Christ Church, Oxford—and Doll's academic standing meant that one of these sinecures could be his for the asking. This was anathema to the young Doll. He recognised that going to Cambridge would be a financial struggle for his family so he decided to sit the examination for an open scholarship, in open competition.

> So I went up to Caius Cambridge, and took the scholarship examination in mathematics. And I did all right on the first three days, but on the third night some "friends" who had gone up the year before and were at Trinity took me out to dinner at Trinity College where I was treated to three pints of Trinity Audit ale—eight per cent alcohol, which was quite strong stuff. Anyway, the fourth day of the paper was not very good and the examiners rang my father and said they would have given me the scholarship on the first three days, but they couldn't on the fourth. So, would I accept an exhibition? Well, I was so annoyed with myself, I said to father, "I will not go to Cambridge and read mathematics—I'll do what you want me to. I'll go to London and read medicine instead."[17]

It was a decision he never regretted. Indeed, if it had not been for the combined influence of his father and the Audit ale, British medicine would have lost one of its longest-serving and most prodigious scientists. If he had got the scholarship, would he have studied mathematics? "Oh, yes," said Doll. "I loved doing mathematics. I was good at mathematics, but I wasn't a genius, and all the really important things in mathematics were developed by people in their twenties and I just wasn't in that class. And I would have ended up being a teacher. In those days, mathematics wasn't needed in industry—now it's very different—perhaps I would have ended up an actuary!"[18]

In an interview in 2003 Doll looked back on that turning point in his career, and made an admission that adds a new perspective to the story:

> There was one other factor which discouraged me from going to Cambridge, which I've never told anybody. And that was that I knew I would be subject to the pressure of fundamentalist Christians. I had got really entangled with them when I was seventeen and I had broken away from it completely; but I knew that there would be a lot of people at Cambridge that would put pressure on me to get involved with the movement in Cambridge and I didn't want to have that pressure. So that was a second reason why I decided to do medicine instead, and to avoid going to Cambridge.[19]

At least one of Doll's friends also wondered what might have become of the communist-minded mathematician in Cambridge in the 1930s.[20] Philby had not been among his circle at Westminster, but they shared a similar political world view that would have inevitably led them to join forces. Might Doll have become "the fifth man" in the ring of British spies who passed information to the Soviet Union during the Second World War and into the 1950s? Undeniably, Doll would have found the communist student group known as the Cambridge Apostles intellectually companionable but he would have been ill at ease with their sexuality.

By 1930 his dedication to the communist ideal was total, and his desire to be a "good communist" had an almost religious devotion. But before he could fully adhere to its rigid doctrines he first had to erase all vestiges of established religion from his past. The opportunity to exorcise it came when his brother, Christopher, became a teenager and doubted whether he possessed the high moral standards demanded by the Anglican Church. He explained that:

> Richard had been confirmed in Westminster Abbey, but when I reached fourteen, I said to myself, "I don't like this." I told my mother, "I don't want to be confirmed," and she asked why and I said I didn't think I could go through life being completely honest and virtuous

about things and that I'd rather wait until I was about eighteen or nineteen. When Richard heard about this he became very annoyed that he had been confirmed when he was fourteen and decided to become "unconfirmed". He wanted it removed. So he wrote to the Archbishop of Canterbury, saying "I wish not to be confirmed any more."[21]

Implausibly, he got a reply. "I got a letter back which said the only way for me to be unconfirmed was if he excommunicated me, and he wasn't prepared to do that. He advised me to talk to a vicar and thought that I would then feel more comfortable with church teachings. But, alas, that once I was confirmed, that was it—I couldn't be unconfirmed."[22]

In July 1931 Doll left Westminster School.* It was only a five-minute walk across the River Thames to St Thomas's Hospital where he would spend the next six years of his life. Leaving one part of his life behind him, he said, "Thank God, I haven't got to write any more essays." How wrong that prophecy would be.

---

* According to the Westminster School archivist, Rita Boswell, "I have had a good hunt for records concerning Richard Doll and am sorry to say that there are none, not even a photograph that I can identify which is extremely disappointing for such a distinguished man." Interestingly, Doll later became a school governor between 1967 and 1977.

Chapter 2

The Politics of Persuasion

"The future belongs to science."

Sir William Osler

St Thomas's Hospital opened up the universe a little more for Richard Doll. In the iconography of London medicine, University College Hospital was seen as the most intellectual,[1] St George's as the most snobbish, and St Thomas's as most associated with privilege. Doll's father had been a student at Guy's and advised his son that the obvious benefits of St Thomas's would make it a compelling choice. "He said if I was going to spend six years of my life in London it would be much more pleasant to spend it by the river than at Guy's, and of course it's one of the most interesting parts of London, and walking on the Embankment after lunch was a delight."[2]

The hospital in the 1930s was very different to the white-tiled edifice that stands there today. Architecturally, it was made up of five magnificent Victorian blocks fronted by a riverside terrace (even at the most unsocial hours the hospital had an enchantment). John Crofton was part of that celebrated 1930s intake of students: "I can remember being called to attend to patients in the middle of the night and seeing the tugs chugging up and down the river and the Houses of Parliament opposite—it really was a wonderful location."[3]

If opinions about the hospital's geographical situation were unequivocal, the same could not be said about the sociology of its student body. The distinguished Oxford physician John Ledingham—whose mother, Mrs Una Ledingham, consultant physician and strident anti-feminist, was a legendary figure on the wards of the Royal Free—was a generation younger than Doll. Nevertheless, he was conscious of the values that it had come to represent.

Doll went to the worst of all medical schools; it was the acme of the most right-wing privilege. "You can't go to Thomas's, boy. There's no intellect there, just privilege." That was what my father said. Even so, when Doll was there it produced Hugh de Wardner, Tony Dornhorst, John Crofton, and Ivor Mills. Pretty good for a medical school that picked you because you went to Eton or could run one hundred metres fast. So the old privilege could sometimes produce the goods.[4]

Dornhorst, who was widely seen as the most academically gifted student of his generation, did not totally share Ledingham's view. "Like other London hospitals it was choosy about its admissions and on the whole drew from a privileged class, but it doesn't follow that it wasn't an effective teaching hospital, and in fact it was, quite clearly. It certainly had a Cambridge bias, and it was more difficult for London graduates to get house jobs, and most of the staff came from Cambridge."[5]

In general, the world of 1930s London medicine was a remarkable place—fiercely hierarchical, chauvinistic, competitive and traditional. Very few of the London teaching hospitals took women. (Joan Faulkner, who would later become Doll's wife, discovered that her first job after qualifying at the Royal Free at the age of 22 was to wait for the consultant's car to drop him at the hospital entrance and pin a carnation to his buttonhole.)

St Thomas's, of course, had been Florence Nightingale's hospital and her presence was still palpable for Doll's generation. Women doctors may have been a rarity, but there were powerful women on the wards who were respected, and even feared. John Crofton remembered: "The nursing was revered at St Thomas's. In my time the matron was revered and feared and when she came down the corridor even the consultants were terrified. The nursing staff were all excellent and knew a great deal about each patient; of course you felt Nightingale's ghost was hovering above you all the time."[6] Doll too was conscious of the sacrifice and achievement of the remarkable women who represented an alluring example of a caring profession. "The nurses were actually called 'nightingales', and my goodness they did have to slave. The matron in my time was just like a general in the army, she was a real queen."[7]

Outside the immediate hospital environment, it was the endemic poverty of the period that most affected Doll and fellow students such as Jerry Morris, John Pemberton, and Archie Cochrane—who, as teachers, would later go on to change our understanding of non-infectious disease. If the social exclusivity of Knightsbridge and Westminster School had already converted Doll into a communist, the corrosive squalor under which many of his patients lived reaffirmed his political commitment to public health medicine. The young idealist soon recognised the effects of poverty on health when, as part of his medical training, he had to deliver twenty babies, half in people's homes. Lambeth had some of the worst slums in London, and Doll became convinced that addressing social deprivation, the effects of malnutrition and people's living conditions was crucial to improving the nation's health.

> Doing these domiciliary deliveries, my goodness, you did see how people were living then. But, of course, by that time I had also developed a concern about the effects of poverty generally on health. I was also struck by the way the consultants would discharge men from hospital with, for example, a peptic ulcer and say, "You have got to go on a diet of fish, eggs and milk," without paying the slightest attention or consideration as to whether [the patient] could afford these items. No inquiry was made about the home conditions, and this rather upset me.[8]

It was the recognition of the injustice of the inequalities in health caused so largely by poverty that stimulated many of Doll's generation to devote their careers to social medicine, and by the 1930s a few doctors were beginning to write about social conditions and health. The association between poverty, overcrowding and infectious disease had, of course, been known to medical officers of health since the appointment of Dr William Henry Duncan (1805-63) to Liverpool in 1847 and before. The sanitary movement of the late nineteenth century, guided by pioneers such as Edwin Chadwick, had brought about great improvements in health. In the 1930s some clinicians and some working in the field of nutrition began to believe that a good deal of ill health, not just infectious disease, was environmental in origin. Some were also coming to realise that political and economic action was needed to change these conditions.[9]

In the early 1930s there were more than three million unemployed in Britain, concentrated mainly in the then great industrial heartlands of Scotland, south Wales and the north-east. One long-term effect of this "social evil" was addressed by the British Medical Association nutrition committee report[10] published as a special supplement in the *British Medical Journal* of 25 November 1933. It consisted mainly of tables of model diets, with their minimal costs, for the range of families and individuals, for "health and working capacity". This article had a politicising effect on John Pemberton, then a medical student at University College Hospital, and it inspired him to write an article, "Malnutrition in England" for the University College Hospital magazine. The aim of the article was to show that "a large section of the community at the present time is not able to buy the amount of food necessary for maintaining health and activity."[11]

Compelled to take some action against the moral paradox of hunger in the midst of plenty, Doll came under the influence of Dame Janet Vaughan (1899-1993), a haematologist, radiobiologist and socialist who was fundamental to the planning of the national blood transfusion service, and the charismatic Bill Le Gros Clark who in 1934 founded and led the Committee against Malnutrition. Doll wrote:

> I was greatly influenced by Bill Le Gros Clark, he was a wonderful man. He had lost his sight and right hand in the last week of the First World War. But he had always wanted to be a scientist and he didn't allow that to stop him, and he ran the committee, and I was very involved with it, especially the effect of malnutrition on children. So quite a lot of my colleagues by this time were very concerned with the effect of social conditions on health and we had all, of course, become active socialists by then.[12]

John Crofton was not a socialist. He had entered St Thomas's after studying at Cambridge, where he had captained his college at rugby. Yet the social conditions he encountered in Lambeth sometimes made him feel embarrassed to have a meal to eat in the evening. "There was such awful poverty then, I began to feel that this is politically important; I started voting Labour, but Doll was much more sophisticated politically. I didn't take political action, as he did."[13]

With the emergence of fascism during the Spanish Civil War, left-wing London medicine was in political ferment with meetings and publications supporting the Republic. In solidarity, Doll helped organise the St Thomas's Socialist Society as part of London's Inter-Hospitals' Socialist Society. Its existence greatly antagonised the dean, Professor LS Dudgeon, who declared, "There's no such thing as a St Thomas's Socialist Society" feeling that it would alienate the wealthy people whose contributions were essential for the upkeep of the hospital. While agreeing to make the existence of the society less visible to the hospital's benefactors, Doll stood up to the admonishment, saying, "Well I'm sorry, but we've got one."[14]

As the society's organising officer Doll began to meet other politically like-minded medics in London. One of them was Joan Faulkner. Yet when they first met, she was already married to Hugh Faulkner, the medical propagandist, who became influential in the development of the general practitioners' service. For Joan and Richard, their initial relationship was not one of reciprocal love: as she was already married he did not allow her to enter his heart or mind, while she initially thought him "a callow youth".[15]

The small "c" that described the political conservatism of 1930s London medicine was a great deal larger than it is today. The dean of St Thomas's resistance to left-wing pressure groups was replicated across the London teaching hospitals. At University College Hospital, for example, Jerry Morris and John Pemberton, both young housemen decided to invite a group of fellow doctors to discuss medico-political subjects. Unlike Doll, they were not in the Communist Party—in fact Morris was hostile to it, but both men were members of the Independent Labour Party. They called the new group the Hippocratic Society to disguise its left-wing tendencies and held some memorable meetings. "The great JBS Haldane was one of our speakers. Other left-wing intellectual giants who influenced many of us at that time were Lancelot Hogben, Bertrand Russell and Bernard Shaw."[16]

By now Doll had become a campaigning member of the Communist Party although he always referred to himself as a "democratic communist". At the age of 21 he visited the Soviet Union, a trip made possible by a gift of £100 from Aubrey Lewis, his godfather. Lewis had become extremely wealthy by zealously following the dictum of "save half of everything you earn". A good capitalist, he ended up owning a large margarine factory. Doll was advised never to reveal to his godfather what he had spent the windfall on.

Sailing from Westminster Pier on a ship whose passengers included the political theorist Harold Laski, Doll shared a cabin with a memorable companion. A Russian, who had emigrated before the 1917 Revolution, he had subsequently worked in New York City as a cobbler. Unfortunately, his shop was in a basement, giving him a clear view up the skirts of all the women who passed by on the pavement above. This became so sexually disturbing to the émigré that he decided the only answer to his growing sense of insanity was castration, and the person to perform it—himself! Doll seemingly registered an expression close to disbelief, which provoked the Russian to stand and shout, "I'll show you!" Still at the pre-clinical stage of his training, and truly wanting to end the tale of erotic tragedy, he punctuated the tension with a "No. No thank you. No."

When the ship arrived in the Soviet Union, the stage-managed tour included visits to the Bolshevik Park of Culture and Rest, enlightened state-funded nursery schools and factories full of happy workers. Stalin's grip on society was by then total and omnipresent. For Doll, as for many of that generation, the allure of Russian communism was inexorably linked with the fight against fascism. But perhaps more than the illusion of creating a heaven on earth in Russia, it was George Orwell's dystopian portrayal of totalitarianism as "the jackboot in your face forever" that made him an implacable opponent of fascism.

His detestation was not merely philosophical. As a medical student, Doll visited Nazi Germany and saw how deeply antisemitic propaganda had corrupted medical teaching.* In a lecture on radiotherapy in Frankfurt, the SS radiologist Professor Dr Hans Holfelder showed students in attendance a slide in which cancer cells were portrayed as Jews.

> We were told that the radiotherapist was a keen Nazi and he would expect us all to stand up and say "Heil Hitler" in response when he came in, which of course we didn't. But he came in and "Heil Hitler"-ed and then, in the course of the lecture, he showed slides in which the X-ray beams were illustrated as Nazi storm troopers and the cancer cells had all got Jewish emblems on them. So, we didn't require many experiences of that sort to realise there was something evil that had to be eliminated from the world.[17]

As a supporter of the Popular Front against fascism, Doll was immediately antipathetic to those pro-Nazi students enthusiastic about Hitler's Germany. His defence of the Jews led to a bizarre incident in Frankfurt involving anatomical development and eugenics. "I was drinking with some of the medical students in a café and criticising the way the Jews were being treated—this led immediately to being told that I must be a Jew myself, which I denied that I was, which in fact I'm not. It sounds ridiculous now, but I was made to stand up on a table whilst they measured my ankles, because apparently thick ankles were one of the physical signs of being a Jew. I haven't got thick ankles, so they had to drop the idea that I was Jewish."[18]

Doll's dedication to the cause of a universal and free health service had begun in the 1930s, and it was the Socialist Medical Association (SMA), founded in 1930 and affiliated to the Labour Party the following year, which was the organisation used in the battle for the nation's health. The association emphasised preventive rather than curative medicine; its members also believed that medical practice, when allowed to work coop-

---

* Physicians joined the Nazi party in large numbers while about sixty per cent of all biologists and some eighty per cent of all professors of anthropology were members.

eratively and without economic barriers to the care of all patients, in itself provided a model for socialism. The way in which a socialised service was set up was therefore of equal importance with the care being delivered.

In 1936 communists were allowed to join the SMA and Doll then came under the influence of visionary individuals like David Stark Murray, Christopher Addison, the first minister of health, and in particular Somerville Hastings. A high-powered ear, nose and throat surgeon, Hastings, unlike other specialist consultants, invited revolutionary students and nurses to his home in Harley Street for drinks (despite being a teetotaller) and persuaded them, by example, to work together, irrespective of faction. For those like Doll who were members of the SMA, Hastings, who later became a Labour MP, was known as the father of the National Health Service, advancing the goal of providing equal opportunity for equal treatment "regardless of financial means, age, sex, employment or vocation, area or residence, or insurance qualifications".

As a communist, Doll also made speeches advocating the building of 400,000 new homes to eradicate the squalor that caused disease and ill health. Scientifically, he realised that it could prove difficult in some areas to plot an exact linear correlation between the eradication of social deprivation and an irreversible improvement in health.[19]

There is no better example of the blind revolt of deprivation in modern British history than the Jarrow Hunger March of 1936. Two hundred unemployed men began the long march to London to protest about their appalling social conditions. Doll, with his friend Trevor Gibbens, volunteered to offer medical care for the unemployed crusaders. Joining them at Pontefract, the medical students treated the exhausted, lame and distressed walkers. One evening, as the men were resting and having food, Doll observed the pathos and compassion of the human condition. "I noticed that one of the men was taking the ham out of his sandwich and putting it in an envelope. When I asked what he was doing, he said, 'I'm sending it to my family—they haven't eaten fresh meat for six weeks.'"[20]

In the same year John Boyd Orr published his classic book *Food, Health and Income,* which demonstrated that about half the population were not getting enough nutrition for full growth and health.[21] The age was one of high rates of unemployment and low rates of benefits. It is little wonder that the epithet of the "hungry thirties" captured the spirit of the time.

The Spanish Civil War was another landmark of the decade, and it attracted a remarkable vintage of British doctors who volunteered to support the Republican cause against General Franco. Throughout the three years of the conflict, beginning in 1936, humanitarian aid flowed into Spain from Britain. Ambulance drivers, nurses and doctors sympathetic to the International Brigade saw the conflict as a fascist attack on democracy, and one that had to be confronted. At a meeting in Trafalgar Square in 1938, the Republican politician La Pasionaria made the fateful prophecy: "Bombs on Barcelona and Madrid today, will be bombs on London tomorrow."

From London left-wing medicine, Len Chrome, Alex Tudor Hart, Reginald Saxton and Archie Cochrane were just some of the people Doll knew who volunteered to fight fascism. Doll did not seriously think of going himself: he had yet to qualify and, dependent on his parents, he did not want his political commitments to financially burden them. But he showed his support of the Republican cause by energetically raising money for Medical Aid for Spain, and taking part in protest marches. For the first three years at medical school he lived at home, then, aged 22, needing more independence he moved into lodgings with other medical students in Lambeth.

In 1934, knowing that his multiple sclerosis would inevitably disable him, William Doll had decided to take his family on a year-long world tour. Immersed as he was in his studies, Doll left St Thomas's for only a few weeks to accompany his brother on the *Mauretania*, bound for New York, where they would rendezvous with their parents. On the homeward journey he was one of the few young, available men on board. This was exceptionally good luck because he became friendly with an all-female dance troupe, bound for a series of performances in the West End. On his return to London, parties were organised by his all-male colleagues to which Doll invited his glamorous new friends. "Yes, I was extremely popular with the other medical students at the time."[22]

This alluring episode took on even greater significance for Doll when, on one occasion, he was walking in London with the dancers' Hungarian choreographer. They were looking for a chemist and walking from Leicester Square towards Charing Cross. Unsure of the best direction to go, Doll said, "whichever way we turn will be the wrong way." "No, it won't," came the reply, "whichever way we turn will be the right way. Because there is no alternative, so it's the right thing we've done—there's no possibility of having done anything else. So you might as well assume that it is correct."[23] This truism stayed with Doll all of his life. What it came to mean, was that he had no regrets. From that encounter, he believed that once action has been taken, you base your next action on the previous one. If you say you're going to do something, you do it, and you pursue it with single-minded determination.

When Doll's contemporary and friend John Pemberton had entered University College London in 1930 his main interests were "medicine, left-wing politics and girls".[24] The same combination became irresistible for Doll. The 1930s was a relatively promiscuous time for him. "Not amongst all the classes, but the 1930s was a sexually liberated era—to a lesser extent than the 1960s—it's just that people didn't talk about it so much." Sexually, Doll saw himself as relatively immature, not having romantic relationships with women until he was eighteen, while the first true female friend he had was Joan Faulkner.

As a young man he was handsome, and this brought some unwanted male attention especially in the years after he left school. Inevitably, he had a lot of men friends and there were many male-only activities; however, rather than having any sexual desire for them, he thought of young men as members of a hunting pack. But on one occasion an older man tried to seduce him at the family's house and he had to shout for his father's chauffeur to come and rescue him. Ideologically and erotically, he would have preferred to socialise with like-minded left-wing women, but invariably he had adventures with debutantes whom he found politically off-putting if sexually attractive.

Before his marriage to Joan Faulkner, Doll had several relationships that would prove "completely incompatible", while one love affair in particular became so intense that it led to his engagement. Doll met a young Spanish girl called Dolores through Geoffrey Lea, a friend from Westminster School, who was engaged to Dolores's sister, and Doll followed his example. The relationship must have been passionate for Doll in his 93rd year could still recite the closing sentence of each letter to her: "*Con un millón de besos del que siempre te quiere* (with a million kisses from he who loves you forever) but my forever lasted about six weeks." When he told his parents about the engagement one said, "Christ" and the other, "God". After the evangelical Christianity of his school days Doll had now become vehemently anti-religious, and the thought of his children being brought up Catholic was unthinkable, and so the relationship ended. The vicissitudes of romantic love were further complicated when set within the prejudiced world of medicine. In 1937, the year he qualified, Doll became involved with one of St Thomas's "nightingales". It was a very clandestine affair: nurses were strictly regulated, and if found out she would have been immediately expelled.

A recurrent motif in Doll's early life was his dedication to sport and team games. Physically, he had been a late developer and was rather small as a child—this may have been because he had celiac disease, a condition that went undiagnosed until he became ill at the age of 47—but as a teenager he grew to be almost six feet tall. His annual walking tours in the German mountains had given him sufficient skill as a skater that he was appropriated into playing for the London Medical Schools' ice-hockey team. But the great love of his sporting life was cricket, which was forged in the bucolic setting of Cecil and Vi Brown's Georgian house in the village of Lyminster in Sussex, with its expansive lawns and its own private cricket ground. Their son Jim Brown was one of Doll's greatest friends from Westminster, and it was there that the Triflers cricket team[25] played throughout the 1930s, during most of which Doll was its treasurer and wicket keeper. A good cricketer, he was still playing a straight bat while warden of Green College Oxford in the 1980s, on one occasion keeping wicket for the staff against the students.

At St Thomas's, Richard Bayliss, who would go on to become, among other things, the Queen's physician, was three years junior to Doll; but he could, even then, recognise his contemporary's genuine qualities of leadership. "We could all see that he was unusually intellectually bright, and he had got that quietness that so many clever people have. He was very unbombastic and very lacking in noise and thrust at medical school, you could see that Doll was going to go to the top of something."[26]

With his interest in mathematics Doll had been looking for ways to apply it to medicine. Reading RA Fisher's classic book *Statistical Methods for Research Workers*, he grew to understand how science could influence his work. Fisher was a giant in statistical theory; the book was extremely complex and the only part Doll could understand was the use of the Chi-squared test (a theory of probability distribution). At about the same time one of Doll's tutors had drawn his attention to a new treatment for undescended testes in boys by giving pituitary extracts that helped bring down the testes. Doll remembered:

> He prescribed this for an outpatient and referred to a paper where its beneficial effects were reported. I read the paper and the results were based on very small numbers. I did a Chi-squared test and came to the conclusion that the results could have turned out by chance six times out of ten. I then wrote an article on the use of the Chi-squared test in the *St Thomas's Hospital Gazette* illustrating it by this example, which I don't suppose was very much appreciated by [the person] who'd told me about this wonderful new treatment.[27]

This was one of the earliest uses of the Chi-squared test, itself a modern development in statistical analysis. Doll's 1937 article is little-known yet significant in the history of British medical research both as an indicator of Doll's future career in epidemiology, and as a philosophical manifesto for the use of statistics in evaluating the efficacy of medical interventions. In the opening paragraph he stressed the need to get the facts absolutely right and present them correctly. "Statistics is essentially a practical science; its methods have been elaborated for the benefit of all scientific workers, physicians equally with economists and mathematicians. Were physicians to abide more strictly to the rules of statistics they would find it very much easier to assess the values of their methods of treatments."[28]

This is prototypical Doll, showing a religious zeal for science. He did not write the article intending to suggest that gonadotropic treatment is valueless; it was chosen because it provided a very good example of the misuse of statistics. To avoid confusion and bring clarity to the results of clinical investigations Doll advanced a thesis that became one of the guiding principles of modern clinical medicine:

> To facilitate this, a qualified statistician should be available to co-operate with clinical workers at any centre of research. Not only would he be able to help in evaluating the results obtained, but he could also help beforehand in designing the experiment to suit the conditions. Advantage would accrue to the medical profession, for they would have to waste less time in disproving ill-founded claims, and to the general public, for they would be less liable to suffer from the continued use of a useless remedy.[29]

Sixty-eight years after the publication of this research paper, a former research student of Doll's believed that "If he hadn't existed, epidemiology would not be the same today."[30]

For Doll's generation at St Thomas's, especially for those who were not freemasons, the most pressing difficulty was securing a job. In 1937 Doll took two sets of exams, the first in January, and then his MBBS in July. This enabled him to apply for house jobs, and he became casualty officer and house physician at St Thomas's. To some extent, he had been forgiven by the hospital hierarchy as this post was only given to promising students. The post lasted for one year, with six months in casualty giving anaesthetics, followed by a further six months working with Sir Leslie Tidy, the endocrinologist. At the end of February 1938 Doll visited the heads of the different departments to see if they had an opening that he might apply for. This unsuccessful trawl took him to the Brompton Chest Hospital, and the celebrated neurology unit at Queen Square.

Then, out of the employment gloom came financial liberation. The London Clinic, an expensive private nursing home in Wimpole Street, wanted round-the-clock medical care for its patients. "It was a private clinic and they wanted a doctor there on duty the whole time. There was no work to be done, but they still wanted a qualified doctor there. I shared the job with a colleague called Dunlop, who did the job during the day and me at night. This allowed time to do voluntary research—that was the only way then." In parallel with this private work, in 1939 Doll was house physician at the Royal Postgraduate Medical School, Hammersmith, and was supervised by Paul Wood, a cardiologist at the Hammersmith Hospital, in carrying out some research into heart disease due to Vitamin B1 deficiency, which was not successful. While doing this work Doll became intrigued by research on blood coagulation by Professor Gwyn MacFarlane, and together with another volunteer he carried out some fascinating experiments under MacFarlane's inspiring influence. "I became very interested in the mechanism of blood clotting and did some experiments with him and other people: but that job ultimately went to another volunteer. It appeared that the clotting agents varied with emotion and mine seemed to vary according to relationships with girls."

Having demonstrated an early aptitude for research, Doll began to think about a career as a neurosurgeon. His audacious plan was to bring together neurology, neurosurgery and psychiatry, to seek a greater understanding of how the mind worked. His father's condition may have had a direct influence on his thinking as he was intending to research the aetiology of multiple sclerosis. Working in a voluntary capacity with a neurologist at St Thomas's, Doll became aware of the pioneering use of electro-encephalography and wrote an article about the process in the *St Thomas's Hospital Gazette*.[31]

Already discernible at the time—and it became a determining factor in his career in medicine—was the allergic response of the medical hierarchy to Doll's political beliefs. Philip D'Arcy Hart, an inspirational figure for many young London doctors dedicated to social medicine, knew Doll in those years. "I can remember him at meetings and beginning a speech with the words 'As a communist'. Well, this labelled him."[32]

By the autumn of 1938 it was clear that war with Germany was inevitable. Chamberlain's policy after Munich was holed below the water-line. For Tony Dornhorst, it was a time of *realpolitik* and he came to understand Doll's view of the world:

> The outstanding question that was affecting the student community in those years was the threat of German aggression and [the fact] that the government was constantly underestimating it. And we felt, whatever our view of communist Russia, that it provided the only firm opposition to Germany, and most of us I think were in favour of the United Front [and] quite a number of students did join the Communist Party.[33]

Morally and philosophically Doll was ready for the conflict; the only problem was how best to make himself useful to the war effort. Conscious of the catastrophic mortality levels suffered by soldiers from head wounds in the First World War, Doll believed that neurosurgery was the field in which he could be of most use medically. At the time there were very few neurosurgeons in Britain, so he wrote to the War Office asking them to support him financially while he trained in the embryonic subject, and informing them that they would need a large number of neurosurgeons in the very near future.

> It wasn't an encouraging reply, only three lines long, saying something like: "Dear Dr Doll, If you want to help in arresting Nazism join the Army and we'll tell you what we want you to do." That marked the end of my association with Freud and neurosurgery—beneficially for me because I wouldn't have been a very good physician or surgeon either. I followed the advice of the War Office and joined the supplementary reserve in 1938.[34]

The following summer, Doll was awarded his membership of the Royal College of Physicians (MRCP) on the eve of war.

Chapter 3
Doctor at War

"As a wartime soldier I have learned to respect the regular army. Its traditions, its experience and its sacrifice were the leaven that saved England."

Raymond Williams

A week before the declaration of war on 3 September 1939, Richard Doll was called up and sent to Preston in Lancashire to be medical officer to a regular battalion, the 1st Loyals. On 6 September he became part of the British Expeditionary Force (BEF), the elite of the British Army, dispatched to France, with the belief that such a coalition of military strength might dissuade Hitler from making any attempt at invasion.

While a medical student Doll had published work on the efficacy of medical treatments using mathematical techniques. It was to be some years before the intellectual ascendancy of statistics was to become essentially the story of his life. However, while in Preston, during the first days with his battalion, Doll sought permission to conduct an experiment into how best to prevent infection of wounds.

When I joined the 1st Loyals as their medical officer, sulphonamides had not long been in use and the question had not been asked whether it would be of value to give them prophylactically to soldiers with open wounds rather than to wait and see if they became infected. As a regimental medical officer I had only a very small supply of suitable tablets and I submitted a request for more, with the proposal that I would give them to alternate soldiers before evacuating them to the nearest field ambulance, keeping a record of those I had and had not treated for later comparison of the rate at which their wounds had healed. In retrospect, it was hardly a practical project, but it was not for that reason that my request was refused. I was sent for by our divisional ADMS (army director of medical services, the head of the medical services for the division, and a full colonel) who berated me soundly. Either it was a good idea

31

to give wounded soldiers sulphonamides prophylactically at the earliest opportunity in which case I should give sulphonamides to all of them, or it was not, in which case I should not waste His Majesty's money. I obviously agreed, but when I asked whether or not it was a good idea I was told that was my job to decide, not his, and I was sharply dismissed![1]

Over the following nine months Doll built up tremendous respect for the British regular soldier, for his discipline under the most frightening conditions, combined with his humour and loyalty. His view of the officer class was more equivocal, as he saw some occupying their positions of authority by virtue of class rather than by talent or ability. "Half of them were intelligent, able people and half of them dunderheads. In fact at one time the man commanding the battalion during our retreat to Dunkirk was one of the stupidest people I ever had to work with."[2]

The glorious weather that accompanied Chamberlain's declaration of war continued, and Britain and the troops of the BEF entered into the so-called period of "phoney war" with the 1st Loyals sent to Bourghelles, near the Belgium frontier. Unexpectedly Doll found that his duties were not confined to the medical care of his own battalion. Upon mobilisation the French government had called up two out of every three doctors, and when Doll called to see his French medical colleague he found him bedridden and unable to travel to his patients. So the young British doctor took on the acute visits for his colleague and in addition to improving his rudimentary French he had some memorable encounters.

> I delivered a number of babies, and of course I didn't accept any payment from the French people, but they used to insist on giving me presents— mostly food, which I presented to the mess. Or they would invite me to lunch. I remember the best lunch I've ever had was one Sunday with an apparently dour French family living in a converted railway coach. It turned out that the husband was the local poacher, which accounted for, I should think, at least half the lunch. It was a seven-course meal, each course being prepared on the stove as we sat around. Certainly, if I had to pick out one meal, that was the best of my life.[3]

Doll was a handsome man (and retained an elegance into old age), athletic and clever, and he was attracted by and attractive to women. However, from the summer of 1939 he was not in a serious relationship with anyone in England. In France, while there may have been an absence of love in his life, there was not an absence of sex. In common with many of the BEF, Doll "did on occasion visit a number of brothels".[4] French brothels were government-regulated and free of venereal infection, and he only went to those that "a medical colleague had assured me were free of any infection."[5]

Some years later, while visiting the area with his wife Joan, Doll met some of his wartime friends and the encounter shows that his pursuit of amour had gone beyond the antiseptic confines of the brothel. One of the men asked in French during the course of their visit whether he remembered bringing a child into the world. Doll was not quite sure of the idiomatic meaning of the phrase: "I still go red when I think of it—I remember thinking how Joan would interpret *la petite fille que j'ai mise au monde*. But it was just 'the little one who I had delivered', who I had brought into the world in that sense. So it was all right. But that was, I think, the most embarrassing moment of my life."[6]

At the end of April 1940 Doll's battalion left the defensive position of Bourghelles, which they had been preparing for the previous six months, and went down to Louvencourt near Amiens with the rest of the brigade for a fortnight's intensive training.[7] The exercise had been postponed numerous times over the past months for fear of a German move. Reflecting the same incompetence that had defined Chamberlain's premiership, the relocation of the battalion took them seventy miles out of position on the very eve of Hitler's attack. Now, if the BEF was going to survive the Nazi assault, it was their turn to be heroic.

More than 1,700 German bombers roamed through the clear blue skies of northern Europe on that Friday morning of 10 May.[8] At breakfast the battalion was told about an intense air battle that had gone on in the early hours of the morning. "I soon discovered from talking to civilians, in particular the postman, that the Germans had invaded Holland and Belgium."[9] On the same day Winston Churchill became prime minister, the rapid defeat of France was under way and the survival of the elite elements of the British Army, of which the 1st Loyals were part, was now in question. Over the following three weeks the British were engaged in a bloody rearguard action; it was to be nasty, brutish and short. "Nothing but a miracle can save the BEF now, and the end cannot be very far off," declared Field Marshall Lord Allenbrooke in his diary.[10]

At this point France had not fallen and was still fighting. In the north of France and Belgium, between 250,000 of the 300,000 British troops were encircled in an area some 25 miles long and thirty miles deep around the port of Dunkirk. Finding it difficult to stay ahead of the advancing Germans, on 14 May Richard Doll wrote in his diary, "Today, for the first time, we came under fire."[11] Days of exhaustive fighting and marching and sleepless nights were the rewards for the men of the BEF though occasionally they experienced good fortune. "After about two hours the troop carriers came into sight. As we arrived we were packed into them, irrespective of our company and, at times, of battalion, and as each carrier became full it was sent off. I think it was one of the most delightful experiences of my life—to leave the enemy behind at thirty mph."[12]

The order to begin the evacuation was issued by the admiralty to Admiral Ramsay on the evening of Sunday 26 May, the National Day of Prayer. Two days later and still some ten miles from Dunkirk, a stream of humanity was moving westward on foot, by car or on horseback, their progress interrupted by the lethal attentions of Marshall Goering's Luftwaffe and the Wehrmacht's artillery:

> ... Shells were continually falling along the whole length of the road, usually some 300 to 400 yards off, and aeroplanes were persistently flying over at anything from 1,000 to 1,200 feet. At times when they came low they were greeted by bursts of small arms fire from our troops, but usually they were unmolested. Most of them were returning from bombarding Dunkirk or the beaches, but others must have been reconnoitring our positions.[13]

Certain encounters take on a retrospective historical significance. The evacuation of the army from Dunkirk has become part of British national history, and Churchill was able to exploit a humiliating military disaster as a kind of triumph of British ingenuity and determination, "a miracle of defiance".[14] It was about David and Goliath, snatching glory from defeat, symbolising the true British spirit. What is indisputable is that with Dunkirk the war became a people's war.

Saturday 1 June was a momentous day for Doll. Still responsible for more than a dozen patients in his care, he had to devise a plan to reach the port and evade capture by the Germans who had broken through the final line of defence. "I put it to them that we had two alternatives—either one of us stay with the wounded and wait to become prisoners, or for all of us to get into the transport that I could collect and make a dash for it along whichever road seemed best to me. They voted unanimously for making an attempt to leave, and I chose the direct road back to Dunkirk for our route."[15]

As night fell the port was illuminated by the amber haze of exploding shells. Most of the town's buildings had been destroyed, and for the exhausted troops the scene was disturbing. All had been told to aim for the mole at Malo-les-Bains, a suburb of Dunkirk, but when Doll found the pier it was full of French troops and shells were falling slowly but continuously around it. The obvious danger and the feeling of being so near home increased the nervousness of the troops. Through a combination of self-preservation and the desire to offer a lead, Doll decided to find a different avenue of escape. He could not believe that the British navy would be so foolish as to embark only from the mole, so he began to ask if anyone had seen any boats further along the beach. Soon he found someone who said that about one hour before he had seen British sailors standing in the water begging people to go aboard their ships, some mile or two along the sands in the direction he had come from.

> I tried to explain the situation to the five who were with me and they said that they left it entirely in my hands; so, getting up, I led them along the beach down to the water's edge. After walking for about ten minutes

we saw a dark mass ahead of us and, pushing on rapidly, we found to our joy that it was a crowd of some two to three hundred British soldiers standing in the water while out beyond them were a couple of rowing boats. What was our delight when we discovered that they were actually two companies of Loyals and the odd troops we had collected at Bergues. If ever anybody has been grateful to anyone else, those five men who had come with me were grateful then.[16]

The Dunkirk evacuation involved more than 800 ships, naval and civilian. Of the 338,226 Allied troops who were brought out, 228,500 were British and the rest nearly all French. By dawn on Sunday 2 June the *Maid of Kent* was taking the exhausted Doll and hundreds of other wounded and tired men back to England. It was an historic event and remarkable for its heroism, yet even entering Ramsgate harbour and safety, the retreat to Dunkirk had one last casualty of war for Doll.

I had found a kitten on our arrival at Bergues. Though I had left everything else behind, I had brought it with me and still held it inside my battle dress; poor thing, it was so frightened by the gunfire that it leant quietly against me without making an effort to move. It had stayed with me until we got back to England but when we got home I had to give it to authorities—I couldn't keep the kitten. It was one of the saddest moments of my life.[17]

In June 1940 Britain faced a fascist-dominated Europe. From Salazar's Portugal in the south to the regime of Quisling in Norway, the continent was in a seemingly ubiquitous fascist embrace. For Britain and for Doll it was a time for reflection. His battalion reformed in Rotherham, where he spent the first week writing his diary of the final weeks in France, and recovering his strength for the struggle that lay ahead.

Slowly initially, and then prodigiously, Britain began to mobilise for total war. Ernest Bevin, the Labour minister of labour in the coalition government, was omnipotent in the control and direction of labour, and for the first time, due in part to the influence of the nutritionist and social campaigner John Boyd Orr, food rationing ensured that all British people were eating a healthy diet. The Second World War saw far less division between aspiration and reality. Indeed, the congruence between a public commitment to change and a recognition that pre-war society had been unjust and divisive was the most important legacy of the Second World War for British society.

Ultimately, the British Army could not remain immune from these changes, but the traditional social tectonic plates of the inter-war years were still in place, and when in 1940 Richard Doll contravened them it was part of his life-long refusal to endorse the forces of inequality. Now based in Rotherham, Yorkshire, Doll decided one evening to take a taxi into Sheffield and see what the city was like. "During the journey I had such a fascinating conversation with the driver that we decided we'd continue our talk over dinner. I saw absolutely nothing wrong with this, and we had a most enjoyable time together, but the next day when I told the story in the mess, the response was, 'You can't wear the King's uniform of an officer and have dinner with a taxi driver.'"[18]

Britain was an exceedingly dangerous place after the summer of 1940. Throughout the six years of war, a total of 270,000 servicemen died, but more than 60,000 civilians were killed on the home front. In September 1940 Britain expected a German invasion, and Richard Doll's battalion was deployed near Lyme Regis on the south coast of England. It was another occasion when the medical officer almost became one of those statistics himself.

I was attached to the officers' mess of the battalion that was based on Portland Bill, and one of the officers was a bomb disposal officer whose job was to go round when bombs had been dropped and decide whether there was an unexploded bomb or not in the pit. And he said to me, "I'm just going out—I've been told there are three or four bombs I've got to go and have a look at. Would you like to come with me?" Well, I wasn't that keen, but I didn't see how I could refuse, so I spent the afternoon going around with him some ten miles from Portland Bill looking at craters and trying to decide whether or not there was an unexploded bomb at the bottom of them. During this time we heard a heavy bombardment of Portland, and when we got back I actually found that the room I would have been sleeping in had been destroyed or rather the ceiling had come down and my car, which was just outside, was covered in rubble. I think if I'd not gone out looking for bombs I probably would have been killed so it was a fortunate choice.[19]

At the beginning of 1941 Richard Doll was posted to the Middle East. His friend Archie Cochrane remembered Doll arranging concert parties on the boat to Cairo and organising the singing of "You'll get no promotion on this side of the ocean."* Arriving in Egypt as one of fifty medical reinforcements, he was sent to be the physician at a small hospital in Nicosia, the capital of Cyprus, where urgent cases that could not wait to be moved to Egypt were dealt with by the Colonial Medical Service. Dedicated to the care of his patients, Doll set out to see what the standard of the medical care was on the island. He was horrified to discover that the senior surgeon was believed to be an alcoholic. "In my innocence, I went to see the governor reporting my findings and the hazards associated with it. This was a grave mistake. He sent me a brief savage letter, telling me to mind my own business. Some year or so later the governor developed an acute appendicitis, was operated on by the surgeon, developed a general infection (in the days before penicillin) and died."[20]

---

* Archibald Leman Cochrane joined the Royal Army Medical Corps in 1940, and was posted to a general hospital in Egypt. He was then sent to Crete, where he was soon taken prisoner. There followed the darkest period of his life when, as medical officer for a prisoner of war camp in Salonika, he was confronted by major epidemics, malnutrition and extreme Nazi brutality. During this time he undertook what he described as his "first, worst, and most successful controlled trial" in search of a cure for famine oedema, finding it in small amounts of yeast obtained on the black market.

For the most part, Doll was kept busy dealing with the minor ailments and fevers that caused soldiers to be admitted to hospital. All was well until there was a small outbreak of acute poliomyelitis, an infrequent occurrence among the British troops in the Middle East. Once the disease developed, the patient was immediately evacuated to Egypt.

> On one occasion the hospital was full of soldiers with minor fevers of one sort or another, when one turned out diagnosed with the disease, and the patient was moved to Egypt and the nursing staff set about sterilising the bed—a process that took some 24-48 hours. Another soldier with a fever was, however, sent for urgent admission and as there was no other free bed in the hospital I recommended the matron that he should be admitted to the free bed just left by the soldier with poliomyelitis. "He'll catch polio," said the matron, "if I don't sterilise the bed first." "Nonsense," I said, "he has a high temperature, needs a bed, so put him in it." Two days later, when his temperature came down, he began to show signs of paralysis and turned out to be an obvious case of polio. Any attempt to persuade the matron that he must have had previous exposure to polio before he was admitted was doomed to failure and I didn't even try. This was, of course, in the days before the polio vaccine had been invented and the molecular history of the disease was less well known than it subsequently became.[21]

Mirroring his medical radicalism, Doll's politics pushed against convention. That bastion of the establishment, the officers' mess, was aware of his communist beliefs. Soon after the German invasion of the Soviet Union in the summer of 1941, he volunteered to give a lecture on the Red Army. It is doubtful if the talk was persuasive, but it was certainly memorable to the young doctor. "It wasn't a good lecture, and I declared to never again give a lecture unless I had a thorough knowledge of the subject, and I've never deviated from that rule since 1941."[22] But it was not Richard Doll's politics that affected his tour of duty on Cyprus—it was again to do with contravening the social mores that governed army life.

By his own admission he was not a good linguist yet during his five years on active service he learned French, some Arabic, and his Greek was good enough to enable him "to make an after-dinner speech in it once".[23] The manner in which he became so good at Greek led to his being shunned by the military:

> I had a wonderful Greek teacher while in Nicosia—he would take me to meet his friends in cafés, and through the nexus of his friends I began to learn the language. He was a most remarkable man who spoke French fluently. He may well have been a spy, but the problem for the army was that he wasn't even a non-commissioned officer—it was anathema in the army to go drinking with a non-commissioned officer. And as punishment I went from being a physician in the little hospital in Nicosia to being a medical officer to the Greek Company in Limassol. That was a banishment for breaking the army code, behaving with impropriety.[24]

His attempts to break down the segregation within the military machine brought him to the attention of the secret service. While in Cairo Doll was known to be outspoken and when Sir Walter Monckton, director-general of the Ministry of Information, visited Egypt for political discussions, Doll was invited to meet with him. This marked him out. He certainly shared the view of the Cairo Forces parliament, which had shocked its officers by electing a mock Labour government including communist ministers.[25]

While in Cairo, Doll made an unsuccessful attempt to join a paratroop regiment. There were two reasons why he wanted to join such an overtly attacking unit; the first was the sheer adventure and danger of combat, the second was that after the Soviet Union joined the war on the side of the Allies in 1941 British communists wanted to be real war heroes and genuine zealots. Many were paratroopers, and Doll wanted to join them. Unfortunately, he was turned down on the rather spurious grounds of not having enough teeth. Unless he was expected to bite the Germans, it seemed a harsh explanation for rejecting the belligerent doctor.

Instead, at the end of 1941 Doll took charge of an infectious disease ward in Cairo where he treated the first case of smallpox and the first case of typhus in the British Army in Egypt. He had as many as fifty cases of smallpox while in Cairo and the disease was so foul—Lord Macaulay described it as "the most terrible of all the ministers of death"—that Doll did not take any chances while treating the troops. "I used to vaccinate myself every time I vaccinated anybody else. I should think at least once a week I scratched a little lymph, a little bit of cowpox into my arm because it was a devastating disease, with an eighty per cent fatality."[26] On one occasion in Cairo in 1943 Doll saw a boy with smallpox walking through the streets; by then he was an excellent diagnostician, and although he tried to alert a policeman (he could speak some Arabic) he failed to get anyone to do anything about the infected youngster.

Among the failures, however, there were triumphs, and for his work at the infectious disease unit in the Sixty-Third General Hospital in Cairo, Richard Doll was mentioned in dispatches for his valiant efforts between 1 May and 22 October 1942. Rather than looking upon the honour as recognition for his medical work, Doll believed the explanation was more to do with his style of ward rounds. "We were in the Cairo suburb of Helmiea, and when the general came to inspect the hospital, I think he was impressed that I could introduce him to the patients using their Christian names. That was the way I had been trained, but I had the impression that the general hadn't encountered this before in a military hospital." [27]

Before leaving Egypt, Richard Doll was selected for a truly unusual wartime privilege. As a reward from the officer commanding the hospital, he was allowed to make a thirty-second broadcast that would be relayed via the BBC to his parents in London. He was not going to use the broadcast to merely say, "'Hello Mother, I'm very well.' I wanted to say something of political significance, so I said, 'When you give my books away for paper (people were giving books as part of the war effort) don't give the Left Book Clubs away, as I shall want them after the war.' That was my radio message, and my mother heard it."[28]

Not satisfied with the onerous duties of running the infectious disease unit, Richard Doll called on James Klugman, an MI4 officer in Cairo, to see if there was any way he could help with his work. The two men were friends from London, where they had been involved in political campaigns in support of the Republican government during the Spanish Civil War. Within a few weeks, Doll was offered the opportunity to act as a medical officer on a foray in Crete. A naval unit was to make contact with British agents in Crete and arrange to pick more up on the coast and drop others. A doctor and medical supplies were, however, needed and a group of Greek guerrillas, on whose heads the Germans had put a price, were to be taken off—but only once they had captured a German general, disposing of, if necessary, some German soldiers manning an observation post on the coast. Hence the need for a medical officer as the Greeks might have suffered some casualties.

Doll was instructed to ask his commanding officer for two weeks' leave and permission to draw such medical supplies as required, but not to tell him anything else. Doll received the necessary permission, a rail ticket to Alexandria and instructions to join a particular naval unit. On arriving in Alexandria, he was surprised and somewhat disheartened to find that his naval unit was nothing more than a large launch with a Bren gun mounted in the stern to keep off enemy aircraft and a crew of three young officers and a couple of seamen.

> The launch, moreover, had a top speed of ten knots which I found even more discouraging, seeing that dawn would break shortly after we expected to leave Crete. The officers, however, were in good heart and looking forward to the adventure, so I stowed my gear in the cabin in where I had been given a bunk, and tried to appear as if I was equally confident.
>
> For a couple of days we cruised along the North African coast and put in for a day at Tobruk, which was now entirely deserted. This was awesome; a small harbour almost entirely surrounded by high cliffs, at the top of which we were able to see the perimeter lines that had been periodically defended by Australian and British troops the year before and which they had held against the Italians for ten months before they were relieved by Wavell's advance.
>
> Then the time came to sail to Crete. The launch bobbled about in the Mediterranean in a most unpleasant way. I was not at the time a

good sailor and I retired to my bunk with a bottle of whisky, small nips of which I had discovered in peacetime were a good prophylactic against seasickness. As, however, we approached the Cretan coast the excitement of the moment provided a therapeutic stimulus and I went on deck watching with the officers for the signal to send a boat to pick up the guerrillas. No signal came and we began to wonder what had happened. Finally it appeared, we dispatched a boat, and it returned with a load of Greeks. The general had not been captured, and the German observation post had not been destroyed. We had, however, first, to send a boat back for more Greeks. Eventually some fifty men were packed into the cabin—splendid figures in traditional dress bristling with revolvers and knives—and we set off on our return journey. All thoughts of seasickness had long been forgotten and, as dawn broke, I stood by the wheel with the naval officers looking for any sign of enemy aircraft. None appeared and we returned to Alexandria without incident—at a steady speed of ten knots.[29]

Within a year of the daring operation in Crete, Doll was posted to a hospital ship in the Mediterranean. The SS *Somersetshire* had been badly damaged by German bombers early in 1943. When Doll joined the refitted ship there were six other doctors on board including a surgeon. Now a physician with the rank of major, his job was to administer the anaesthetics for the surgeon's operations. Normally serious surgery was not undertaken at sea, but soon after the ship left port a man developed gas gangrene in his thigh. In those days, before penicillin, the only hope of saving his life was to amputate the leg; for Doll, the operation taught him a lesson about naval tradition.

> I was called on to assist by holding the man's leg as Major Turner cut it off. It was an unpleasant sight and we wanted to get rid of it as quickly as possible, so I took it and threw it overboard. This greatly annoyed the ship's bo'sun, who turned up, and told me in no uncertain terms that he was responsible for burials at sea and that this applied to parts of the body as well as the whole bodies. Shortly afterwards the ship's log ceased to function properly and, hauling it in, the rotating part was

found to be caught up in the bandages that were partly unwound from the leg I had thrown overboard. The bo'sun apparently received a fee for burials, but, in this case, I suppose the outcome must have more than compensated him for its loss.[30]

Doll's hospital ship left the port of Alexandria with secret orders to accompany the landings in Salerno in southern Italy. Once referred to as the "soft underbelly", the invasion of Italy was anything but soft. The ship sailed up the Italian coast at night, past the Lipari Islands which were illuminated by the still active volcano of Stromboli. As the sky began to lighten, his ship was passed on the port side by a flotilla of British warships proceeding north at full speed—a beautiful and powerful sight. When the SS Somersetshire* arrived in the Bay of Salerno it was full of ships, and they anchored some way offshore at a distance from any other vessels. Again, the admiration that Doll had for the bravery and camaraderie of the ordinary soldier was conversely matched by what he saw as the ineptitude of many of the commanding officers. If the BEF had had, according to Doll, its fair share of "dunderheads", the SS *Somersetshire* medical team was commanded by a colonel who was "absolutely hopeless".

> This commanding officer went ashore, taking his batman with him, and we prepared to receive casualties, which gradually began to arrive. What

---

* Dr Otto Fleming, letter to the *Guardian*, August 2005. "During the Italian campaign, 1943, Richard Doll served as a physician on the hospital ship *Somersetshire*, on which I was a nursing orderly. There was strict segregation of officers and other ranks, but he was the only officer who breached this divide. When we were sailing empty on our way to pick up casualties he came down to the mess deck and arranged word games and other activities to foster a spirit of togetherness. He was never condescending but friendly and courteous, without being chummy. This side of his character never left him. When I congratulated him on his 90th birthday he wrote a charming letter which showed him unchanged by success and old age."

was happening on land was impossible to tell and all I can remember was seeing puffs of smoke and hearing the guns. Towards the end of the afternoon, we were nearly full, bombs began to fall, the army officer told us to leave, even though it meant leaving the colonel behind. Fortunately he and his batman arrived just in time, carrying a couple of sacks. They had been picking apples and pointed to where they had found them. "I suppose you realise," the liaison officer said as he left us, "that that was behind enemy lines."[31]

In the spring of 1944 Doll developed renal colic. Upon examining his urine he found it was acid and had pus cells in it, which raised the suspicion that his symptoms might be due to renal tuberculosis. His ship was due to return to England and he was offered the opportunity of staying on board, but he wanted to be treated in the Middle East and elected to get ashore at Naples, where he knew that Paul Wood, a member of the staff at the postgraduate medical school at Hammersmith, was in charge of the medical division. Doll hoped that Wood might diagnose some other condition. Not wanting to endanger Doll's life, Wood left open the possibility of tuberculosis, but thinking it could also be something else, he decided to send him back to England. Within hours an increasingly worried Doll was invalided out of Naples on a boat bound for Algiers. The circuitous route lessened the danger of attack, but if the diagnosis was correct, then it was life threatening.

The journey was uneventful and during it Doll made friends with a lieutenant-colonel who had had a perforated duodenal ulcer and was being sent home for six weeks' convalescence. When the ship reached Algiers the patients were given the discouraging news that a hospital ship had just left for England and the next one would not be sailing for three months. In the days before streptomycin, the possibility that the tuberculosis would have three months to spread caused Doll understandable anxiety. After a few hours in the hospital in Algiers his mood changed for the worse when the lieutenant-colonel entered the ward and said, "Oh, a bit of luck. I've just been offered a place on a plane and I'm going to fly home to England."

While congratulating his friend on his good fortune, he knew it was bad medicine to send someone back to have sick leave while his own operation was a matter of life or death. "I got pretty angry and went to see the registrar, the senior administrative officer of the hospital, and told him that upon my return to England I would go to the War Office and tell them about his method of selecting patients for evacuation."[32] Within two hours another plane had been found that was going back to England and this time Richard Doll was on it. Stopping once to refuel at Gibraltar, he flew back to England lying in the uncomfortable, buffeting hold of a Liberator; it was a very enjoyable journey.

Back in London, Doll accepted the confirmed diagnosis of tuberculosis with stoical optimism. His worst fears—that both kidneys were diseased—were not realised; only the left one had to be removed. In 1944 the operation carried great risks and post-operative care was still fairy rudimentary, but at least he knew the surgeon he wanted to carry out the operation. St Thomas's Hospital, like the other great teaching hospitals, had been evacuated out of London at the beginning of the war. It took ten days for Richard Doll to track down TW "Gaffer" Mimpriss to a hospital in Woking, Surrey. "What attracted me to Gaffer was that as a student I'd seen him operating, and unlike some of the really senior surgeons who showed off and threw things about, he was always unflappable and calm. I thought if I ever need a surgeon in the future that's who I want to have."[33]

The Woking hospital had a surreal feel as Doll was the only patient on the ward, the hospital having been cleared for D-Day. With the attention of the whole nursing staff to help aid his recuperation, he could look up from his bed and see "Hitler's secret weapon", the V-1 rockets or Doodlebugs, flying overhead en route for London.

But the war was coming to an end, and on 8 May, VE Day, the German forces in Europe capitulated and the exhausted British people rejoiced. Among the millions celebrating in the bright London sunshine were Richard Doll and Joan Faulkner. Their fateful meeting on such an historic day marked the beginning of their love affair, and, with the coming of peace, Doll proposed marriage. Professionally, he could once again turn his energies towards the medical needs of the British people. One of the aims of the Socialist Medical Association was "the reduction of human suffering" and over the coming decades Doll's contribution to this ideal would be his lasting accomplishment.

Chapter 4
The Greatest Benefit for Mankind

"Imagination is more important than knowledge."

Albert Einstein

For Britain, the Second World War had been a "people's war" and what followed the cessation of hostilities was a "people's peace".[1] The past would be exorcised and the future transformed. A new generation of idealistic doctors were determined that the medical status quo of the 1930s would not be re-imposed upon society. A fundamental question for socialists who wanted to construct a more caring society was "What is to be done?" The objective was to usher in a new system of medical provision that would overcome disease—care according to need, for everyone, regardless of income.

It was a time of austerity, fogs, witheringly cold weather, reconstruction and great optimism. Optimism in medicine was fully justified by the new mastery of infections through sulphonamides, penicillin and streptomycin. Sanatoria had begun to close. Immunisation was then possible against diphtheria, but not yet against poliomyelitis. Clinical teaching was inspired by the ideal of curing acute illness and eliminating disease forever. The hospital was the dominant centre of all interest, and a career in hospital medicine was the aspiration for all but a minority of the ablest doctors.

For that cadre of left-wing doctors which included Jerry Morris, Archie Cochrane and Richard Doll, characters and lifelong convictions had been formed by the cataclysmic events that brought Hitler to power and plunged the greater part of the world into a devastating six-year war. What distinguished them from so many others of their generation was the depth of their emotional and intellectual reaction to those events, and their indefatigable idealism for the future.

Doll did not feel that the war changed him overtly[2] but he was conscious that unlike many of his medical colleagues, his war had not been boring, and he had survived—just. The qualities of leadership, courage and camaraderie which were present in the 1930s were refined in those years of conflict. There was also the matter of Doll's political persuasion. Tony Dornhorst, a contemporary of Doll's from St Thomas's, remembered the "shadow" who accompanied his friend around London at the end of 1944. "I can't be sure, I think it may have been someone from Westminster School, but when he came back from the war, I believe he was being followed."[3] Doll played down the attention MI5 showed him, but he was conscious that his political work while in Egypt had gained him notoriety back on the home front. This reputation remained as the permafrost of the Cold War started to bite.

But the war had turned Doll's world upside down professionally and personally. In 1939 it was conceivable that he would have become a neurosurgeon; by the summer of 1945, approaching his 33rd birthday, a further six or seven years of training would have been unthinkable. The kaleidoscope of Doll's life was given two countervailing twists at the end of the war. The first was initially unpleasant and ultimately defining—the melee to find a career in a profession dominated by nepotism—while the second, falling in love, set off an emotional trauma that, after a great struggle, provided him with life-long happiness.

Doll needed to find a career in medicine, one that would fulfil his political and scientific ambitions. After Cyprus and the removal of his kidney, he was discharged from the RAMC with a gesture of national generosity. Medical students in the 1930s all recognised the statistical fact that at least one of them would succumb to tuberculosis. Indeed, Doll believed that he contracted the tuberculosis infection while a medical student and that it had been dormant until he reached the Mediterranean. The British Army, however, believed his disease to have been contracted while a serving officer and awarded Doll a thirty per cent invalidity pension, which he drew until his death, aged 92.

His first instinct upon returning to London was to re-establish his links with Gwyn MacFarlane and the work on coagulation that he had found so intellectually fascinating before the war. He had shared that research with another junior doctor, who had a stronger association with the work, and he thought it judicious to ask him if he planned to re-join the coagulation team. When the other doctor replied in the affirmative, Doll decided to look for a position elsewhere. In convalescence he spent six months at Roffey Park, a rehabilitation centre in West Sussex, as a psychiatrist, and decided that it was not the subject for him. He found that it put him in "the position of God"—it was not an experience much to his liking.

Nevertheless, it was not easy to find a job. This was true when it came to the Hammersmith and the legendary Sir John McMichael, director of the Royal postgraduate medical school at the Hammersmith. Doll remembered: "I couldn't get a job at the Hammersmith—because I was a communist, McMichael wouldn't look at me." However, other known communists such as Ian Gilliland were supported by McMichael. Perhaps one explanation, and an emotionally sensitive one, was that McMichael's wife Joan, who was herself a communist, had left him and their two sons for Bill Carritt, who had been the secretary of the League of Nations Youth, an anti-Nazi campaigner in pre-war Germany and a leading communist in the Spanish Civil War. McMichael was pro-Labour and pro the NHS, and, according to his son Professor Andrew McMichael, he supported the anti-smoking movement and Doll's epidemiology. It may just have been that he and Doll did not get on personally.

The Hammersmith was a most unusual institution for the political left. The Home Office had banned communist doctors from teaching undergraduates, but they were allowed to teach at postgraduate schools. The Hammersmith even had its own MI5 man, John Abbott*, who kept an eye out for any overtly proselytising behaviour. One would imagine that since they all knew of Abbott's existence, a Soviet in west London was not established.

When Doll eventually got a job in 1945, he returned to the wards of St Thomas's Hospital as a junior medical assistant to the medical unit. He was conscious—and if he was not, it was soon made known to him—that clinical medicine had advanced during the five years he had been away.

---

* According to Jean Gilliland, her husband Ian once shared a room with John Abbott, while they were attending a medical conference. One evening Abbott got drunk and confessed that he worked for MI5, that he wanted to get out but could not.

Advancement still rested, as it had before the war, on such factors as having been to Cambridge, membership of the Freemasons and obsequiousness to superiors. This was anathema to Doll who managed to rise above these impediments and secured a year's post at St Thomas's, with a special interest in asthma.*

In the years between the wars and the introduction of the National Health Service there was an unedifying scramble for the very few hospital appointments available, and success could only be achieved by being in the good books of senior consultants. Doll did not like this rat-race atmosphere and began to look for opportunities to do research that would emancipate him from the strictures of hospital medicine while at the same time freeing him intellectually to pursue his main interests: mathematics and public health medicine.

Between 1940 and 1945 Britain had moved more rapidly to the left than at any other period of its history. This irresistible shift in the political pendulum was revealed with dramatic effect even before the war with Japan ended. The Churchill coalition broke up with unexpected suddenness in May 1945, a few days after the German surrender. A general election was called for July. Unlike the general patriotic fervour that followed the "coupon election" of 1918, the national mood was more controlled and sober.

No longer in uniform, Doll threw himself into the election campaign, speaking on platforms with other idealistic doctors about improving the nation's health. Philip D'Arcy Hart, the biologist and socialist, remembered seeing Doll during his period of high politicisation: "I saw Richard Doll at meetings in Leicester Square, very handsome, with those blue eyes, and wearing a red beret; he was a communist, and he wanted to change

---

* *Thorax*, volume 1, March 1946, pp. 30-38. Doll set up an experiment to test the hypothesis that the use of helium-oxygen mixtures resulted in a saving of pulmonary effort. Six cases of asthma admitted consecutively to St Thomas's Hospital were treated by respiration of a mixture containing eighty per cent helium and twenty per cent oxygen, and their progress was followed. Doll's verdict on the value of helium-oxygen mixtures in asthma, due to the small number of cases, was "not proven".

society."[4] Doll's politically motivated enthusiasm for health reforms and the Labour manifesto became known to the Labour leadership, and he was asked to stand in the general election for the unwinnable seat of Horsham in Sussex. Doll declined the opportunity. It was a decision he never regretted, believing that he could make a greater contribution to an egalitarian and just society by remaining a physician.

Doll was still a member of the Socialist Medical Association (SMA), led by the inspiring Somerville Hastings. The SMA had promoted from the beginning the creation of an integrated, universally accessible system of preventive and therapeutic medical services. The Labour Party was slow to make health a central issue, but the SMA was of crucial importance in showing how a humane and effective health care system could be achieved. Moreover, the SMA gathered influence in the early planning of the NHS through its membership of the British Medical Association's medical planning commission (created in 1940), despite its often hostile relations with it.[5]

While a member of the SMA in the 1930s, Doll had campaigned for the building of more and bigger houses, and after the destructive bombing by the Luftwaffe the need was even greater. He had become convinced at the end of his clinical training that social conditions, particularly the problems of deprivation, diet and housing, were absolutely crucial to improving the nation's health.

War can lead to medical progress and in Britain it heightened expectations of wider public benefits. The Labour Party's 1945 manifesto was prophetically entitled "Let Us Face the Future", and the way ahead was a new social democracy. All three of the main political parties embraced the Beveridge report on social insurance and allied services—the work of the liberal reformer Sir William Beveridge. Published in 1942—and selling more copies than any previous HMSO publication— it declared war on the five evils that threatened society: ignorance, squalor, idleness, want and disease.

A new consensus pervaded the nation, and for those who defined themselves politically in their fight against fascism, there existed a sense of optimism for the future, a new world in which the equality of sacrifice in the years of war would be matched by an equality of regard in the years of peace.

The result of the general election in July 1945 was a political landslide of seismic proportions. Labour won 393 seats to 210 for the Conservatives. Clement Attlee, once dismissed by Winston Churchill as "a man with a lot to be modest about", had delivered the first majority Labour government. It was a defining moment in the changed atmosphere of the war years, and no doubt a delayed verdict on the bitterness of the 1930s, with its memories of Munich and Spain, Jarrow and the hunger marches. In 1945 it could be argued that the British people put politics before patriotism, and now they faced a cultural transformation. There was much work to be done.

To combat sickness, Beveridge proposed that a new health service be available to everyone according to need, free at the point of service, without payment or insurance contributions and irrespective of economic status. This was a truly socialist policy and one that owed much to the ideas of the SMA and public health activists. A bill was introduced in April 1946; on 6 November it received the royal assent and the appointed day for its inauguration was 5 July 1948.

While fighting politically for a system that would eliminate the human waste created by unemployment, ill health and inequality, Doll was in another battle, this time for his emotional life. By his own admission he had been promiscuous, but with Joan, for the first time, he had found a friend as well as a lover. Yet her inability to leave Hugh Faulkner—principally because of her loyalty to their son—meant that Doll did not commit himself fully and uniquely to Joan until 1947. The relationship became something of a metaphor for Doll's life: it was to be one of great power and influence, but it would come at considerable cost.

If, in 1946, "making a go of it" together was still a distant reality, Joan, in her professional capacity as a member of the Medical Research Council's headquarters' administrative staff, alerted Doll to a research project being carried out by Dr (later Sir) Francis Avery Jones at the Central Middlesex Hospital. An historic meeting followed which marked the beginning of a scientific collaboration that re-directed Doll's career.

Francis Avery Jones was a pioneering clinician and one of those reassuring doctors who just had to speak to patients to make them feel better. He was only two years senior to Doll, but by 1946, under the dynamic medical director Dr Horace Joules, he had established a department of gastroenterology in the Central Middlesex. Throughout the war Avery Jones had been working as a physician and deputy medical director under the direction of the central medical war committee. At the beginning of the war, medical students from the Middlesex Hospital lived in the "Central", where they continued their clinical training, and this was an important step in building up the Central Middlesex as the first district general hospital to play a full role in undergraduate and postgraduate teaching and in research.

Most of the patients admitted with peptic ulcer and its complications, together with the other main diseases affecting the gut, were cared for in Avery Jones's ward. With the help of his Czechoslovakian assistant, it was possible for him to keep good records, particularly relating to gastric and duodenal ulcer and especially on patients who had bled. Links with the Invalid Kitchens of London, the forerunners of Meals on Wheels, encouraged local factories to take a special interest in their dyspeptic workers. In 1946 plans were evolved to extend this work, and an application was made to the Medical Research Council for support for a wide-scale study of occupational factors in the causation of gastric and duodenal ulcer.[6]

Doll stood at a crossroads in 1946. He had got his MRCP before the war, but a career in clinical medicine held no allure; he wanted, if possible, to do some scientific research. In Avery Jones he found an inspiring role model. Quiet and unassuming, Avery Jones worked exceptionally hard and never appeared to be in a hurry or flustered. By his persistent good humour, support of and loyalty to colleagues, he was universally liked. Moreover, being in a county council hospital, he had many more patients referred to him than to any of the specialists in the large teaching hospitals, all of which had to share out the central London patients. He had, for example, one case of perforated peptic ulcer a week, whereas at University College Hospital they might see five a year. He was the doyen of British gastroenterology and founder of its comically and aptly named journal, *Gut*.

So great was the level of expertise it was rumoured that doctors at the Middlesex would say ironically to their students, "What is the best management of a bleeding peptic ulcer?" To which the answer was, "Catch the no. 12 bus to the Central Middlesex."[7] This may have been a heretical thing for a London teaching hospital to advocate but it was none the less true.

The Central Middlesex was not a teaching hospital but it had some of the most outstanding medical staff in London led by the warm, avuncular and humble Dr Horace Joules, who in addition to being a visionary physician was a good friend of Doll's through the Communist Party.* Dr Richard Asher, one of the truly gifted medical writers of the twentieth century (he coined the term Munchausen syndrome), was there, as was Jerry Morris, the epidemiologist, who established his MRC social medicine unit at the hospital in 1948. The Central Middlesex was completely devoid of the medical arrogance of the large teaching hospitals, which had so alienated Doll. He had found the people and institution that would liberate him; he was about to find his metier.

In the years immediately preceding the Second World War, peptic ulcer accounted for approximately one per cent of all deaths in England and Wales: 23,035 deaths were attributed to peptic ulcer out of a total of 2,460,536 in the five years between 1935 and 1939. Indeed, peptic ulcer was the main cause of being invalided out of the forces and being turned down on conscription.

---

* Horace Joules was one of the most persuasive voices in the anti-smoking campaign after the publication of Doll and Hill's work in 1950. Lady Joan Avery Jones, the doctor's second wife, described Joules as "so Red it was unbelievable, he was aggressive—Richard Doll was a more humane communist. Francis and Horace were dedicated to the NHS and the care of their patients."

The application for a wide-scale study of occupational factors in the causation of gastric and duodenal ulcers was supported and sponsored by the industrial health research board of the Medical Research Council with a co-ordinating committee chaired by Professor JA Ryle, and in 1946 Richard Doll was appointed to carry out the work. In the search for environmental factors that might be significant, much emphasis had been laid on the presumed increasing rush and stress of modern life. According to Henry Bockus's standard text book on gastroenterology, "Ulcer is a civilisation disorder and as the complexities of life increase one may anticipate an even greater incidence of peptic ulcer."[8]

After a period of careful and detailed planning, Doll concluded that to compare the incidence of peptic ulcer in different occupations it would be necessary to interview a number of employees directly and to make personal clinical diagnoses. The method of personal interview was, therefore, adopted throughout the investigation. The work was divided into two stages. A preliminary interview was carried out by Marna Buckatzsch, the social worker, who recorded a number of basic particulars about age, sex, occupation and hours of work, together with short clinical notes. The forms were then examined by Doll in consultation with Buckatzsch and put into three categories—"no dyspepsia", "minor dyspepsia" and "major dyspepsia"—according to the clinical questions. All those who were classified as having major dyspepsia were given an appointment to see Doll and a detailed clinical history was then taken.

This method of screening by a preliminary interview with a social worker enabled a large number of people to be seen, but it introduced several possible errors. First, the limitations of human memory made it necessary to set a time limit to the period about which inquiries were made for the presence of symptoms. As a second source of error, the social worker might miss a number of ulcers, and as a third, Doll might show bias in selecting cases to classify as major dyspepsia, since it had been impossible to lay down strict criteria for differentiating between minor and major dyspepsia.

To estimate the size of the errors Doll introduced a "control factor" that helped define the statistical and methodological parameters within which epidemiological investigation subsequently operated. Without the aid of textbooks or direction, Doll invented a novel method of seeking to minimise bias. One in ten of all the cases of "no dyspepsia" and of those of "minor dyspepsia" were chosen at random (done at the end of each day's work by shuffling the record cards of the people seen, and blindly picking out the appropriate proportion) and reclassified "no dyspepsia control" and "minor dyspepsia control". Doll then interviewed these controls to check on the study's validity for deciding whether a person was likely or not to have a peptic ulcer.

Soon after taking up the position with Avery Jones, Doll realised that the work would require some statistical analysis, so together with Joan he attended a short course at the London School of Hygiene and Tropical Medicine on medical statistics taught by Austin Bradford Hill. The three-month course in statistical ideas and methods was for non-medically qualified students, along with the medically qualified. The object was to introduce them to examples of the types of problem they would meet, the methods needed to solve them, the nature of medical statistics and the kind of medical know-how they should seek to be able to use them intelligently. With the medically qualified students the object was to give them a similar knowledge of the simple statistical methods they would find useful in research work but—still more—to make them think numerically and experimentally. Problems in collecting, interpreting and presenting data were dealt with, as were questions of avoiding and detecting bias of sampling. In short, the "arithmetician"—as Hill sometimes referred to himself—wanted his students to think "arithmetic, logic and common sense".[9] Hill already knew Doll through his work with Avery Jones on the aetiology of peptic ulcer as he was a member of the MRC committee set up to supervise the study under Ryle's chairmanship. Doll's attendance on the course at the London School of Hygiene and Tropical Medicine gave Hill the opportunity to get to know the young researcher and judge his character.

The peptic ulcer study proved to be a classic and an important guide to later field workers. Displaying inexhaustible willpower and determination, both of which he had in abundance, Doll set new standards for occupational studies. A total of 6,047 people were interviewed and assessed. The work took Doll to different parts of the country and his persistence knew no limits—on one occasion he climbed to the top of a haystack to interview a recalcitrant farm labourer. It was a measure of his enthusiasm and detailed planning that as few as 1.6 per cent of those he wished to interview failed to come, a lapse that was remarkably small for such a large study. This diligence marked him out to Hill, indicating to the great teacher that Doll was a physician who could think statistically.

Prior to the study's publication in 1951, a draft, written by Doll, was delivered to Hill's unit for statistical scrutiny. Peter Armitage had joined Hill's staff in 1947 and one of his first jobs was to analyse the document. "The report was brought to me by an MRC employee, Dr Joan Faulkner. I had no idea what their relationship was then."[10] Over the next quarter of a century Joan and Richard were to form one of the most influential partnerships in British medical research; while Hill later said of Joan: "A young researcher starting out on a scientific career could not have had a greater public relations agent than Dr Joan Faulkner at the Medical Research Council."[11]

Doll's quiet decisiveness and concern for the human condition did not lead to the discovery of what caused peptic ulcers (not until 1983 did Barry Marshall make the discovery that peptic ulcers were caused by the bacterium helicobacter). But the results of the survey were of great interest: among Londoners between the ages of 15 and 64 the prevalence of peptic ulcer was found to be 5.8 per cent for men and 1.9 per cent for women. This implied that over England and Wales the number of people with a peptic ulcer history was of the order of one and a half million and the number of men who had symptoms each year was over a million. Foremen and others in positions of special responsibility in industry were found to be particularly prone to peptic ulcer, and agricultural workers particularly free from it. Anxiety at work, but not irregularity of meals or shift work, appeared to be aetiologically significant. Striking differences were observed between gastric and duodenal ulcers, notably in their social-class incidence, with the former being more frequent among the labouring classes and rare among the professional, whereas duodenal ulcer was equally prevalent in all social classes.

This led Doll to the following conclusion:

> The survey, if in some respects iconoclastic, points the way clearly toward further fields of study. The deficiency of ulcers in agricultural workers, the social gradient of gastric ulcers and the positive correlation between anxiety and duodenal ulcer are particularly worthy of interest. In the present circumstances, the economic importance of the disease emphasises the need for a co-ordinated effort to solve the problem.[12]

Doll's research with Avery Jones lasted until 1969,* and although he never solved the "problem" of its pathogenesis he did have the satisfaction of revolutionising the treatment of the disease. Their work showed that the standard treatment of putting patients on a diet of "slops"—as milk and fish was known—did not make the slightest difference. In fact, at the Central Middlesex, patients were fed, among other things, roast beef or kippers and onions, and they did just as well as those following the unpalatable and miserable diet that ulcer patients were traditionally prescribed.

Their method of treatment was a vindication of the earlier work carried out by the remarkable Surgeon Captain TL "Peter" Cleave. Among Cleave's unusual ideas was that patients with duodenal ulcer should be given a varied diet including steak, baked potatoes and wholemeal bread at a time when the standard treatment was a very restricted

---

* After Doll joined Hill's department of statistics at the London School of Hygiene and Tropical Medicine in 1947, he continued his clinical attachment at the Central Middlesex, two days a week. Avery Jones gave him responsibility for four beds in his department for the investigation of the methods of treatment of peptic ulcer. Doll, conducting therapeutic trials, established that only bed rest, stopping smoking, liquorice extract and the drug carbenoxolone were at that time effective methods of treatment.

diet of milk, eggs and white fish. Cleave was the senior clinician in the Home Fleet in May 1941 when it was stationed at Scapa Flow waiting for the German "pocket battleship" *Bismarck* to put to sea, and was consulted by the Admiral of the Home Fleet, Sir John Kelly, who had developed abdominal symptoms suggestive of a peptic ulcer. Cleave had him X-rayed and a large duodenal ulcer was diagnosed. The admiral was consequently told that he would have to come ashore and be treated by rest in bed, which was then a normal recommendation. Just then, however, the message came through that the *Bismarck* had been sighted at sea and the admiral refused to go sick, as the fleet was to set sail immediately to find her. Cleave agreed on condition that the admiral followed his diet, a condition the admiral willingly accepted. The *Bismarck* was eventually found and sunk. On returning to Scapa Flow, the admiral was X-rayed again and the ulcer was found to have healed—so much for stress as a cause of duodenal ulcer![13]

Doll was a perfectionist, an archaeologist of ideas; the more closely people worked with him the more respect they had for him. A pioneering scientist, he continued to work on ulcers and carried out the first multi-factorial trial (testing the effect of several treatments simultaneously in a single trial) of the effect of different treatments for gastric ulcer.* Decades after his clinical work finished—and doubtless with some irony—he described his scientific rejection of the therapeutic healing power of "slops" as "the greatest benefit I've achieved for mankind".

Doll's intuitive skills, his rejection of a career in hospital medicine and his good fortune in finding such an inspiring scientific collaborator had brought him to the defining moment of his professional life. Working with Avery Jones was a transition and it was only when Austin Bradford Hill offered him a post in the MRC's statistical unit in 1948 that he elected

---

* Doll R and Pygott F, 'Factors influencing the rate of healing of gastric ulcers: admission to hospital, phenobarbitone and ascorbic acid'. *Lancet*, 1952; volume 1, p. 171.

to make his career in medical statistics and epidemiology—the study of how nature, nurture, age and luck determine the risk of disease.

At that time, epidemiology was not a recognised medical discipline; only a few enlightened policy makers realised the importance it would have in the fight for the nation's health. Collectively Doll and Hill laid the basis for the explosive development of epidemiology by showing how the old science could be refurbished as a tool to discover the causes of non-infectious disease. Neither man knew it yet, but their subsequent collaboration ushered in a new era of research. Moreover, they formed part of an apostolic succession—perhaps the only one in British medical research—that started with Karl Pearson, who established the discipline of mathematical statistics at UCL, then passed to Major Greenwood, the first professor of epidemiology and vital statistics at the London School of Hygiene and Tropical Medicine, to Hill, and subsequently to Doll. The chain would pass into the future, to at least one other heroic figure; but that succession was still very far distant.

Chapter 5
No Hill No Doll

"In the philosophical sense, observation shows and experiment teaches."

Claude Bernard

Hundreds of years from now, when researchers are excavating the history of medical science, the names of Doll and Hill may be there with Harvey, Snow, Pasteur, and Florey. For together they set in motion a fundamental shift in scientific thinking, and ushered in a new epistemology. For the hundred years prior to 1950 the dominant paradigm had been the "germ theory" in which medicine's main preoccupation had been to find some treatment for infectious diseases.[1] After the Second World War, as infectious diseases continued to recede, a new preoccupation with non-infectious diseases such as strokes, heart attacks and cancer began to concentrate the minds of demographers and epidemiologists.

To understand Doll more fully, we must first look to the life and work of his mentor, the inimitable Austin Bradford Hill. "Tony" Hill was a quiet, unassuming, private person[2] whose name is synonymous with the intellectual supremacy of medical statistics. Hill was described in one of his obituary notices as the greatest medical statistician of the twentieth century despite the fact that he held no academic qualification in either medicine or statistics. If, however, greatness is measured by the influence of a person's teaching and scientific example, there can be no doubt that he earned the epithet. During the course of his career he taught an innumerate profession to think quantitatively, persuaded it to adopt the principle of randomisation in its assessment of the efficacy of therapy and laid the academic foundations for the subject of epidemiology in determining the causes of disease.

Hill's contribution to medical science is all the more remarkable when set against the turbulent events of his early life. In the same way that Doll's six years of service in the Second World War had profoundly affected his future, Hill's life was changed by the First World War. Hill took a commission in the Royal Naval Air Service, and in 1917 was posted to the Greek islands in support of the attack on the Dardanelles. While there, he developed pulmonary tuberculosis, which nearly killed him—but which may also have saved him as the life expectancy of pilots was only weeks or months. Back in England in November 1917 with a temperature of nearly 105°F, he was invalided out of the service to die. After nine months in bed at home, he had an artificial pneumothorax (the deliberate collapse of the lung to allow the tuberculosis areas to heal) induced at the Maudsley Sanatorium and slowly began to recover.

During this period of convalescence Hill, by his own admission, read enormously. The canon of classic literature not only provided diverting entertainment but cultivated in him a feel for the English language and a lucidity that made his medical research understandable to all. He was discharged from hospital with a full disability pension indexed-linked for life—the army expected him to die soon or never be gainfully employed again—which he continued to draw until his death in 1991. The tuberculosis infection was so severe that it took Hill—nursed by his mother—two years to recover. In addition to his love of literature he also learned embroidery from his sister, and even took to tapestry while convalescing.

Hill's early ambitions was to follow his father, Sir Leonard Hill, into medicine, but that was now no longer possible; a career and a university course in science would have required attendance at a laboratory for practical work, which his health would not allow. At the suggestion of Major Greenwood, who had been his father's demonstrator in physiology at the London Hospital and had remained a close family friend, he opted for a degree in economics that he could take as an external student at London University. With the support of Greenwood, who had become the medical officer in charge of statistical work at the Ministry of Health and was a close friend of Sir Walter Morley Fletcher, the first secretary of the Medical Research Council, he obtained a grant from the MRC to investigate the reason for the high mortality at fifteen to thirty years of age in country districts, when mortality at other ages was relatively low. While conducting his investigation, he had the opportunity of extending his knowledge of statistics by attending part of the course for a London BSc at University College. The mathematical lectures found him out of his depth, but he was impressed by Karl Pearson's ideas, enthusiasm, and drive—and by the philosophy underlying the mathematics—and he decided on a career in epidemiology with a special interest in occupational medicine.[3]

Hill was intensely interested in medicine, and his life as a medical investigator was a story of ingenuity propelled by curiosity. Because he was not a medical doctor, and could not treat patients, his interests therefore focused on preventive medicine, for which no medical qualification was necessary. He was concerned with what could be done to prevent disease.

In 1933 Hill obtained the readership in epidemiology and vital statistics at the London School of Hygiene and Tropical Medicine, where, five years previously, Greenwood had been appointed as the first professor of medical statistics. Hill's initial contribution to the development of British science began shortly after his appointment, teaching the elements of statistics to medical postgraduates who, in the main, had little affection or aptitude for mathematics. The lectures that he prepared were so effective that he was persuaded to publish them as a series of articles in *The Lancet* and they later appeared in book form as *The Principles of Medical Statistics*, now regarded as a classic text.

At that time the position with regard to the use of statistics in medicine was succinctly described in *The Lancet*'s 1937 editorial that accompanied his first article:

> For most of us figures impinge on an educational blind spot... This is a misfortune, because simple statistical methods concern us far more closely than many of the things we were forced to learn... Many of our problems *are* statistical; and there is no other way of dealing with them. In preventive medicine this is so obvious that it has acquired general recognition. In laboratory work, although it has come more slowly, it is now widely recognised that it is very unsafe to base conclusions on statistically inadequate data. In clinical medicine, it is coming more slowly

still; so slowly that many avoidable errors, and a sad waste of material, still hinder progress.[4]

Hill responded to this situation not by insisting on deferral to a statistical consultant, but by stressing that the workers in medical problems—in clinical as well as preventive medicine, must *themselves* know something of statistical techniques, both for the planning of experiments and the interpretation of figures.[5] Hill persuaded statisticians to immerse themselves in the problems clinicians faced, while at the same time placing on clinicians a responsibility to accept the statistician as a partner "co-equal and co-eternal" in research.

Hill's lectures,* while being both memorable and persuasive, were read from a prepared text over which he took immense trouble. He lectured without the use of visual aids, and so seamless was his delivery, that his audience frequently thought that he was speaking without a text. Hill's daughter, Rosemary Bull, remembered her father's dedication. "When he wrote his lectures he sent us off to the cinema, and then he read his lectures to the dog. He used to say, 'Oh yes, he's becoming very knowledgeable.'"[6] The hallmarks of his teaching lay in finding out the genuine medical importance of a problem, while emphasising the validity of the data being used, combined with simplicity of analysis. Hill did not favour complex statistical techniques; describing statistics as the application of common sense, he liked to be able to explain what was done in his analyses of the data without algebra, in such a way that a non-statistical person could understand it.[7]

That statistical analysis is now an integral part of almost all serious medical research is due to the work of many statisticians throughout the world. The fact that the medical profession in Britain was alerted to its

---

*   Professor Jerry Morris, like Doll, attended the short course "Essentials in Statistics" at the London School of Hygiene and Tropical Medicine. "Bradford Hill was an inspiring teacher—he made me take my own teaching seriously."

need in the 1930s and 1940s was due primarily to its advocacy by Hill.

The statistical journey that brought Hill to eminence can be traced to the closer rapport between medicine and the public one hundred years before. In 1836 registration of deaths, marriages and births had been made compulsory (the first development of its kind anywhere in the world). This was followed in 1850 with the founding of the London Epidemiological Society by a group of leading physicians interested in the observation and control of infection.

Gradually, from the middle decades of the nineteenth century, intellectual and social forces began to be applied to identifying and eradicating infectious diseases. Hill formed a link in the intellectual ascendancy of statistics that could be traced to Francis Galton in the Victorian era, and to Karl Pearson. Statistics began to be regarded as fundamental to establishing order out of empirical observation, and bringing understanding to the patterns of disease, the conditions of life and that most unarguable of all statistics: death. Statistics produced a science that could interpret nature's impact on the health of the nation. Edwin Chadwick, the "father of the sanitary movement", and Henry Mayhew used statistics to argue untiringly that all causes of filth and therefore much disease were, via the sanitary idea, "preventable".

A crucial inspiration to twentieth-century epidemiologists was the concept that statistical inquiry, by determining the underlying causes of ill health such as poor sanitation, could provide the means for the prevention of disease on a massive scale, so "statisticians" potentially had greater effect in improving the health of the nation than "clinicians".[8]

With the background provided by his *Principles of Medical Statistics*, Hill developed the idea of introducing randomisation into trials and in 1946 he persuaded two Medical Research Council committees to adopt the method: first, in preventive medicine, to test the value of a whooping cough vaccine (MRC whooping-cough immunisation committee, 1951) and second, a few months later, in clinical medicine to test the efficacy of streptomycin in the treatment of pulmonary tuberculosis (MRC streptomycin in tuberculosis trials committee, 1948). The results of the latter were published first, and it has undeservedly received the accolade of the first randomised clinical trial.[9]

Randomisation was not a new idea. It had been proposed in a limited way, more than 300 years before by Jan van Helmont, a medicinal chemist, when he challenged the academics of his day to compare the efficacy of their treatment with his statement: "Let us take out of the hospitals, out of the camps, or from elsewhere, 200 or 500 poor People that have Fevers, Pleurisies, etc. Let us divide them into halfes, let us cast lots, that one half of them may fall to my share, and the other to yours... we shall see how many funerals both of us shall have."[10]

The challenge was not, however, taken up. Van Helmont was deprived of the 300 florins he was prepared to bet on the result, and the idea was not developed in a more practical way until the 1920s, when RA Fisher[11] adopted it as a basic principle of experimental design in agriculture. He used it not only to ensure the avoidance of bias in the selection of subjects for treatment, but also to provide an optimal estimate of the likelihood of the differences observed between the treatment groups having arisen by chance, if the treatments were in reality equally effective or ineffective. The two approaches were complementary, with Fisher appealing to statistical theory, and Hill to practical needs.

There can be no escape from the axiom that every new treatment of a disease must be assessed on patients suffering from that disease. Before a drug is ever tested on humans it will have undergone extensive tests in the laboratory, but ultimately only trial in the patient can give the answer to its efficacy or warn of its dangers. Hill was conscious of not wanting to frighten the medical profession with his advocacy of "randomisation" and "random sampling numbers" and the most compelling way of achieving this aim was by citing an uncomfortable truth: "However well, or however ill designed the trial may be, the clinician at the bedside is *always* making it. He is *always* making comparisons. He is *always* using 'controls', even though those controls may consist only of his impression of his past experience with such patients. He cannot escape measurement, whether he like it or not, or whether it be accurate or not."[12]

Of course, at the time, if clinicians had the good fortune to be testing sulphonamides, or penicillin, then obviously they would not remain long in doubt—but treatments like these were rare. Far more often the doctor was concerned with a treatment that may well offer some benefit for the patients, but not the dramatic cure that was beyond doubt. Also the system had led to many false claims for treatments that were useless and sometimes actually harmful, and it hindered, if it did not entirely prevent, the recognition of small advances that could, however, be important if the condition treated was common. It is these situations that the controlled clinical trial was designed to meet.

The main requirement of a method of comparing the therapeutic effects of different treatments is that there must be no systematic bias tending to favour one or other treatment. If treatments are to be compared on different groups of patients it is essential that these groups are similar in all relevant aspects, except in the treatments they receive. The aim of the controlled trial is very simple: it is to ensure that the comparisons that are made are as precise, informative and as convincing as possible.

To achieve that end, Hill substituted the experimental for the observational approach. The simplest—and with acute diseases perhaps the only—approach is the construction and comparison of two quite separate groups of persons. The aim is to make each of these groups a prototype of the general population of sick persons upon whom the investigator seeks to learn the effect of the treatment in question. "To one group is given the treatment, from one group it is withheld."[13] For Hill, that short sentence was the crux of all controlled clinical trials.

The diffusion of ideas and methodologies in medical science is all the more fascinating when ethical questions are raised, and Hill's experimental advance engaged the philosophical presumptions of the Hippocratic oath. It raised the ethical problem: when can a doctor withhold a treatment, possibly of value, from the patient in their charge? Hill joined the Medical Research Council's tuberculosis trial committee in 1946. Its evaluation of streptomycin is seen as a watershed in the development of medical thinking, for it acknowledged that the responsibility for the cure of the sick and the prevention of disease could only be met by investigation and experiment.

Smoking Kills

Following the unparalleled success of penicillin, much research had been going on to detect other therapeutic antibiotics from other fungi that might be effective against bacteria such as the tubercle bacilli, against which penicillin had proved ineffective. In the early 1940s tuberculosis was still the biggest cause of premature death among young adults in Britain and North America.

In 1943 Selman A Waksman of the department of microbiology at Rutgers University in the United States had been systematically testing soil fungi at the New Jersey agricultural experiment station, and one of his assistants, Albert Schatz, had found that streptomycin had significantly diminished the growth of the tuberculosis bacteria. This had proved very effective against the waxy-coated tubercle bacilli, first in the laboratory in 1944, then in tuberculosis in guinea pigs. Preliminary experiments in patients with tuberculosis looked similarly promising. Due to the dire consequences of its diagnosis, news that a panacea was at hand created excitement within the medical community. Yet, apart from an isolated trial of gold therapy in the United States,* the first controlled trial of treatment for pulmonary tuberculosis was started in Britain in 1947.

For Hill, invention was the precursor of necessity. He had already used random sampling numbers in a less emotive field while testing the value of a pertussis vaccine in the whooping cough trial. Moreover, Hill had the intellectual support of Philip D'Arcy Hart and Marc Daniels, the director and deputy director respectively of the MRC's tuberculosis research unit, and both men were eager to conduct an experiment that could be judged by statistical analysis.

The historical context in which the trial took place posed an implicit ethical imperative. The financial austerity in the years immediately after 1945, and the exchequer's reluctance to spend its dollar reserves on ex-

---

* The only effective chemotherapeutic substances were mercury, salvarsan and quinine. Gerhard Domagk (1895-1964) devoted his early life to testing the therapeutic potential of metal-based compounds—gold, tin and arsenic in the United States in 1931.

pensive medicines, meant that a limited amount of the drug was available. In 1946, 110lbs were bought from America, enough to treat up to 200 cases, and, as a consequence, some form of rationing would be required. It was therefore agreed that the restricted supplies should be used to treat patients with miliary tuberculosis and tuberculous meningitis—conditions that in the past had been uniformly fatal. The amount remaining was insufficient to ameliorate the suffering of the many thousands of desperately ill people with other types of the disease.

The first issue that had to be faced was whether it was ethical to withhold the drug from any patient. Hill made this point: "So, I could argue with Sir Geoffrey Marshall—chairman of the MRC committee—from the statistical side, that, as we had not got much streptomycin, it was not a question of being moral to make a trial, it would be immoral not to make a trial."[14] The committee concluded that "it would... have been unethical *not* to have seized the opportunity to design a strictly controlled trial which could speedily and effectively reveal the value of the treatment."[15] The question whether it was ethically justifiable to withhold the drug from any patient was, therefore, answered with an unhesitating "Yes".[16]

The experimental advance that led to the objective evaluation of any given treatment altered the philosophical foundations of modern medicine. For Hill, the definition of all controlled clinical trials was: "To one group is given that treatment, from one group it is withheld." How was this to be achieved so that the arbitrator of such a decision cannot be biased for or against a particular method of treatment or—equally importantly—can not, though in fact impartial, be accused of being biased?

As with any other disease, random allocation of suitable patients to the treatment series is fundamental to the success of a clinical trial in pulmonary tuberculosis. This will ensure, for example, that the patients with the severest forms of the disease were nearly equally divided between the two treatments. Randomisation will not ensure that all the groups are exactly equal in all respects; nothing can do this. It does however ensure that they differ by an extent that is predictable and can be allowed for in the statistical analysis.

To discover the unbiased truth the clinician must be kept in the dark.

The treatment allocation must be inviolable by the doctor. In addition to having an approximately equal number of patients on the two treatments, it is important to keep the clinician in charge of the patient allocation unaware of the next allocation until the patient has been submitted for the trial. If the doctor has prior knowledge, this may influence the decision whether or not to submit the patient, with the resultant danger that as a consequence the two series will not be similar at the start.

The first patients were admitted in January 1947 to the chosen centres—the Brompton and Colindale hospitals in London, and Harefield Hospital, Middlesex. After three months they had still not found enough patients at these sites, and other authorities were approached in Wales, Scotland and Leeds. The trial included 107 patients, 55 of whom were to be given streptomycin for four months, while 52 were given the best treatment previously available—bed rest and, if necessary, the collapse treatment of the lung Hill himself had undergone in 1917.

The allocation of "treatment" to "control" was predetermined by a series of random numbers and placed in a set of sealed envelopes. Literally, the clinician would wait until a patient was presented for inclusion in the trial—and disregarding gut instincts—would then open the first envelope and follow the directive. In this way Hill was able to circumvent the inevitable clinical observations that all well-trained doctors could not resist making: "[I wrote] on a piece of paper T (Treatment) or C (Control) and put it in a sealed envelope. And after [the doctors] decided, Yes, this is the right patient to come in; he'll open the envelope, and he won't know until the envelope is opened which direction in the trial the patient will go."[17]

It was an historic moment, the first time that "blinding" had been used in this way. In fact, as neither group of patients knew which treatment they were receiving, this was the first ever so-called "double-blind" trial. In 1960 Hill wrote that his rather elaborate tecnhique of using sealed envelopes had been developed mereley to ensure that no bias crept in during the allocation. It had no other magical virtues. However, far from making the clinical redundant in the process of care, the randomised clinical trial now gave the best possible answer to the question: is this new treatment effictive?

Two other features also defined the trial as a landmark in medical research. One was the emphasis that was laid on recording events that were to be used to assess the results in such a way that the record would be unbiased by knowledge of the treatment the patient had received. Progress was assessed with monthly X-rays, graded by three specialists who remained ignorant (blind to) the identities of the allocation of patients to streptomycin with bed rest or bed rest alone. Fever, weight and sedimentation rates were also regularly recorded, and bacteriologists who assessed the disease in patients also remained blind to the allocation process.

The overall results left no doubt as to the beneficial effect of streptomycin. Seven per cent of the streptomycin patients and twenty-seven per cent of the controls died before the end of the six months. This was a statistically significant difference. The results were published in the *British Medical Journal* in 1948. The publication documented that this was the first controlled investigation of its kind to be reported and, quite apart from the results, would serve as a model for other such studies.*

Disappointingly, within less than a year—although the group given streptomycin had done better than the controls—it became apparent that there was bacterial resistance to the drug. In this way Hill's insistence that streptomycin be objectively tested was vindicated. However, the problem was solved by combining streptomycin with another recently discovered drug, para-aminosalicylic acid (PAS). PAS was first shown in 1946 to have a profound effect on tubercle bacilli, and in 1948 the MRC undertook a second controlled trial to assess the drug. The same type of case was used as in the first trial, and patients were grouped randomly for different treatments: PAS alone, streptomycin alone, or both drugs together.

The trial demonstrated irrefutably that the combination of PAS and streptomycin prevented the development of streptomycin-resistant strains of tubercle bacilli.** With streptomycin and PAS[18] the survival rate from

---

*   *British Medical Journal,* 1948; volume 2, pp. 769-82.

**   Linda Bryder, 'Tuberculosis and the MRC', in *Historical Perspectives on the Role of the MRC,* edited by Joan Austoker and Linda Bryder (Oxford University Press, 1989), p. 21.

tuberculosis—"the captain of the armies of death"—reached eighty per cent.[19] Hill must have been proud of the achievement; after all the disease had robbed him of the opportunity to follow his father into clinical medicine.

Doll respected Hill. Of course there were other medical scientists he admired and was influenced by—John Ryle, Percy Stocks, Sir Francis Avery Jones and Sir Ernest Kennaway—but he spoke with reverence about very few people apart from Hill. Hill had turned him into a hunter-gatherer of data, initially as his student, then assistant and finally collaborator. Ultimately, with the passage and mysteries of time, it was Doll's name and not Hill's that became synonymous with the hazards of smoking. No one, yet, has taken up the challenge of writing a biography of Hill. Certainly a lack of recognition exists for one of the greatest non-doctors in the history of British medicine. This may be because he left the professional stage prematurely, while Doll never left it; and his legacy should be greater. History has an obligation to Hill, but in Doll's phrase that contribution has been "unfortunately either overlooked or forgotten".[20]

In the world of British science there is no greater national accolade than membership of the Royal Society, the oldest scientific institution in the world. Doll was not the first epidemiologist to become a member of the Royal Society—that tribute had gone to Hill, who was also the only one ever to become president of the society. It was Hill, too, who put Doll's name forward for membership, and in 1966 Doll became a Fellow of the Royal Society (FRS). Perhaps even more than status and position, Hill's greatest contribution to Doll's career was that he passed onto him knowledge and attitudes to science: it was an inheritance that Doll readily acknowledged.

Hill was an outstanding experimental innovator and he applied his considerable intellect to epidemiology in determining the cause of disease. As tuberculosis began to recede as the gravest concern to public health a new lethal epidemic was taking its place. Hill's contribution to its eradication is something we should all be grateful for.

Part Two 1945-1969

The Medical Revolution

Understanding Cancer

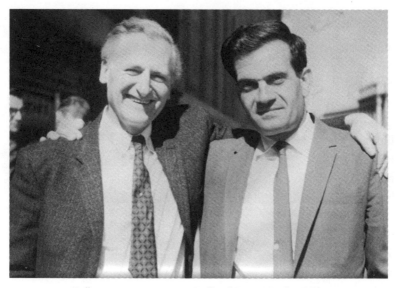
Colleagues against cancer: Doll and Ernst Wynder, 1964

Chapter 6
The Paradigm Shift

"Any work which seeks to elucidate the cause of disease, the mechanism of disease, must begin and end with observations on man, whatever the intermediate steps may be."

George Pickering

Doll believed that in the history of epidemiology John Snow's discovery that fecal contamination of water causes cholera was the most important. A century later Doll's own work, using medical statistics, would contribute another indelible step in understanding the cause of disease.

In the 1930s Percy Stocks, physician and chief medical statistician to the General Register Office, addressed both the doubts and the capacity of his discipline to bring improvements to the nation's health. He wrote, "It is sometimes asked, how statistics can cure disease." For Stocks the solution came by asking another question: "How many researches which have led to real advances in medicine would ever have been started had there not first been some statistics to suggest that here was a problem to be investigated?"[1]

For post-war Britain that moment occurred in 1950 when for the first time the number of deaths from lung cancer—13,000—exceeded those from tuberculosis.[2] This changing pattern of mortality was to lead to a revolutionary advance in understanding the cause of disease and marked one of the major discoveries of medical science in the twentieth century. In the development of knowledge about the origins of a disease, the first and most difficult stage is the search for clues on which a hypothesis can be based. In 1946 Stocks had observed the "startling phenomenon" of a six-fold increase in lung cancer mortality in males in the period between 1930 and 1944.[3]

This statistic drew a historical parallel with the cholera epidemics a century before—in 1849 more than 50,000 died of the disease in England—playing an important role in understanding the cause of disease and the philosophy underpinning public health medicine. For hundreds of years, medicine has struggled with the great mystery of what caused epidemics. Contrasting interpretations had assigned disease causation to miasmas (the spread of fevers via malodorous air) or to contagion theory (infection via bodily contact). The English physician Snow (1813-58) rejected the miasmic theory of infection as cholera affected the small intestine and not the lung. An incomparable master of logical deduction from observations (which did not prevent his epidemiological work from being viewed with scepticism), Snow* brought together statistical research with the experimental design. If Snow had, in the end, undermined a towering monument of theories of miasmatic induction[4] of infectious disease, would an investigation into the new epidemic have an equally profound impact?

Of course, lung cancer—or more strictly cancer of the bronchus— had been known to occur throughout human history but it was thought to be a rare form of cancer until the 1920s when it began to appear more often as the certified cause of death and pathologists began to note more cases on autopsy examination. Indeed, Doll had studied the cases of lung cancers seen at post-mortem at St Thomas's Hospital in the fifty years between 1894 and 1944 and recognised the sharp rise in the decade from 1920. In the 1930s, while still a medical student, he was interested in the association between pipe smoking and cancer of the lip and tongue. On one occasion when he saw cancer of the tongue in a patient he asked a senior surgeon whether he thought pipe smoking or syphilis was the cause (cancer of the tongue being commonly observed in association with syphilitic leukoplakia). Bernard Maybury, the surgeon, told Doll that he

---

*   In 2003 Doll said that in the history of epidemiology "there has never been anything as important as Snow's discovery that fecal contamination of water causes cholera ... I don't think there is anything else comparable with it, and some of the lessons from it have yet to be put into effect." ('Voices. A Conversation with Sir Richard Doll', *Epidemiology*, 2003; volume 14, pp. 375-379.

did not know whether either was responsible for the disease, but he did know "that the wise man avoided the combination of the two."

However, the death rate was rising inexorably and the medical researchers who recorded the nosological (the science of disease classification) evidence came to the conclusion that it was in the main an artefact due to the improved methods of diagnosis that resulted from the successive introduction of chest X-rays, bronchoscopy, open chest surgery and the introduction of effective methods of treatment for pneumonia after the sulphonamide series of drugs began to be introduced in 1936.

In that same year, growing interest in the problem was stimulated by the detailed examination of post-mortem certifications carried out by Ernest and Nina Kennaway. Their work seemed to eliminate the factor of occupation—an association with petroleum products or atmospheric pollution due to gas works or exhaust fumes. Ernest Kennaway thus concluded that: "One obvious factor possibly carcinogenic, to which the lung of man alone is exposed, is tobacco smoke… the consumption of cigarettes, of which smoke is often inhaled, has increased among men and women of all classes. Hence an effect of the kind considered here would be in accord with the absence of social gradient."[5]

Meanwhile pathologists argued about the reality of the increase. Some tried to produce cancer with tobacco tar experimentally in laboratory animals. In 1929 Richard Passey[6] in Leeds failed to produce tumours, while two years later, in Argentina, Angel Roffo[7] produced cancer on the skin of rabbits* with tars from tobacco burned at high temperatures, find-

---

* Angel Honorio Roffo (1882-1947) was an Argentine cancer pioneer who demonstrated the production of tumours by tobacco tar. Other experts were not convinced by Roffo's work, in particular Ernest Kennaway at the MRC. He believed that Roffo had burned his tobacco at too high a temperature to be realistic. Roffo published mainly in German language journals and this may have prevented the wide dissemination of his work. None the less, still today, Argentina's foremost cancer institution is named after him.

ings that were subsequently thought to be inconclusive. The medical establishment was as divided as to the cause of the lung cancer epidemic as it had been a hundred years earlier in explaining the outbreaks of cholera. But since the increase was more pronounced in men than in women, changes in the real disease rates must also have occurred.

The two principal possible causes of the disease put forward were: firstly, atmospheric pollution, whether from homes, factories, car exhaust fumes or from the surface dust of tarred roads; and secondly, the smoking of tobacco. It was clear to all that some characteristics of the former had certainly increased since 1900, and there was no doubting that the smoking of cigarettes had greatly increased. In 1946 (in the edition that contained Doll's article "Helium in the treatment of asthma") the medical journal *Thorax* reviewed what might be responsible for the historically unparalleled increase in carcinoma of the bronchus:

> The causes of the increasing incidence are necessarily difficult to determine but many factors have been held responsible by different observers. Influenza, with its effects on bronchial mucosa of atypical regeneration, metaplasis, and cell-nest formation, has been widely suggested as a predisposing cause. On the other hand, Iceland, where carcinoma is, or rather was, unknown, has suffered from severe epidemics of influenza. Other factors, such as smoking, exhaust gases from motor vehicles, tar particle from roads, have all been held responsible; but the whole matter is difficult of proof, and it is probable that these are factors which prepare the soil rather than sow the seed.[8]

What people were not clear about was principally this: had lung cancer been there all the time, but simply not detected? Or was there something new that encouraged the spread of the disease?

There was an increasing suspicion that smoking was detrimental to the health of British children and that it was responsible for stunting their growth. This factor was invoked at the interdepartmental committee on physical deterioration, appointed in 1903, which investigated the poor health of Boer War recruits. Findings of this report contributed to the pressure for legislation, passed in 1908, forbidding the sale of tobacco to those under the age of 16 and empowering the police to confiscate cigarettes from any child seen smoking in a public place.

After the First World War, tentative moves had been made towards tracing factors responsible for the rise in lung cancer. As early as the 1920s, Edward Mellanby, later director of the Medical Research Council, noted the relationship between the free issue of cigarettes to tobacco workers and lung cancer. Conversely, the much higher incidence of lung cancer in towns than in rural areas tended to throw the weight of emphasis on environmental factors associated with industrialisation and urbanisation, rather than on personal habits.

In Britain lung cancer rose by 1,500 per cent between 1922 and 1947. The annual consumption of tobacco in the UK had increased from 128 million lbs in 1922 to 250 million lbs in 1947, and the percentage of these amounts smoked in the form of cigarettes had risen from 56 per cent in 1924 to more than 80 per cent in 1945. At the same time, car driving and the tarring of roads also increased at unprecedented rates.

British society's total commitment to victory in the Second World War delayed a medical investigation into the nascent epidemic. But with the coming of peace so too came evidence that a sharp scythe had swept through the population of what Winston Churchill referred to as "our island home". In 1947 the Ministry of Health wrote a letter to the MRC petitioning them to find an explanation for the unparalleled increase in the number of deaths attributed to cancer of the lung between the two world wars.

On 6 February 1947 a conference was called at the MRC to discuss the rapid increase in deaths in the United Kingdom attributed to the disease. Among the thirteen attending were Sir Ernest Rock Carling, Percy Stocks, Edward Mellanby, Ernest and Nina Kennaway, Alice Stewart and Austin Bradford Hill, who had succeeded Major Greenwood as director of the MRC's statistical research unit at the London School of Hygiene and Tropical Medicine in 1945. Various hypotheses were advanced at the meeting. Stocks believed that urban atmospheric pollution was the probable carcinogen, while Ernest Kennaway believed that smoking could be a possible causative factor. Other theories put forward were arsenic in cigarette smoke, radioactive dusts and drugs. There was no consensus of opinion.

It was then that Mellanby, the MRC's secretary, said that what was needed was a large-scale study into the aetiology of the epidemic. And it was then, too, that Bradford Hill mentioned that he had a young man in mind for such a job. That young man was Richard Doll.[9]

Hill knew of Doll's interest in cancer, and he had also been impressed with the young physician's capacity to think numerically and experimentally. For Hill it was essential that his collaborator in the investigation should be medically qualified. As Rosemary Bull, his daughter, recalled: "Dad saw himself as an 'unqualified practitioner' and he said he needed a medical doctor otherwise he thought they'd doubt the work and say, 'Oh, it's just statistics.'"[10] Doll was not a mathematician but he had the ability to think like one, coupled with a preternatural determination, as exemplified by his resolve in achieving a response rate of 98.4 per cent in a study of gastric and duodenal ulcer. Somewhat prophetically, Hill wrote: " ... I regard him as a very good worker to whom it is well worth while giving a wider experience in medical statistical work with an eye to the future. As you know, the number of medical persons who take at all kindly to careful statistical work is still small."[11]

The offer of employment could not have come at a better time. Hospital appointments were very difficult to come by for junior doctors—particularly for known communists—even if they ingratiated themselves to their superiors, which Doll was temperamentally opposed to doing. It would be under Hill's tutelage that Doll forged his career in medical research.

High-minded, modern-thinking, well-intentioned men and women were determined to make what Henry Sigerist, the Marxist medical historian, called a "people's war for health". Central to Doll's ideal of a career in medicine was to "understand how the world works and to improve people's enjoyment of life." He envisioned a society in which the benefits of medical science would be distributed to all. He sought to be a valuable member of society and in many ways epitomised Sigerist's concept of the politicised doctor:* "We still need, more than ever, a scientific physician well-trained in laboratory and clinic. But we need more: we need a social physician who, conscious of the social functions of medicine, considers himself in the service of society. There is no point training doctors primarily for city practice among the upper-middle class."[12]

Before Hill and Doll, epidemiology had been concerned almost exclusively with infectious diseases, which tended to look at differences between entire populations—disparities in rainfall, temperature and ecology. With cancer of the lung, the researchers set out to find what were the characteristics and life histories of patients with the disease in comparison with those of patients with other diseases.

Inevitably, at the beginning the relationship between the two men was asymmetrical. Hill was fifteen years older, established as a leading figure in medical science in Britain and unquestionably the senior figure in what became a "momentous collaboration".[13] Politically—and on occasion this created tensions between them—the men were ideologically opposed. Hill, coming from an establishment family, was a Conservative and unsympathetic emotionally or philosophically to the left.

Hill and Doll began planning their search for an explanation in 1947 at a time when Britain had the highest lung cancer rate in the world, and when smoking was generally regarded as innocuous. More than eighty per cent of men smoked, while the economic and social emancipation dating from the First World War led to the habit being taken up by some forty per cent of British women. Smoking was as entrenched among doctors and scientists as it was in the rest of society. Doll smoked a pipe and non-tipped cigarettes, and Hill a pipe. Later Doll wrote: "I was not antagonistic to tobacco when, in 1947, I began to study its effects."[14] Originally Doll

---

* Doll became a member of the Sigerist Society in London in 1947. For Sigerist, the four major tasks of medicine were the promotion of health, the prevention of illness, the restoration of the sick, and rehabilitation. Instead of money grubbing, he urged medical students and physicians to do creative work, to help change the world, to consider themselves "in the service of society".

thought the increase in motor cars and the tarring of roads were likely to be responsible for the epidemic. Hill, typically, was reported to have entered the study "with an open mind".[15]

Indeed, Doll was a man of his time, and it was not until he had started his own epidemiological research into the true extent of the hazard that he stopped smoking cigarettes himself. This was an important event in the history of public health medicine, as indeed was the reason for him taking up one of the nation's favourite social addictions. Doll's father, while a physician in the First World War, had seen at first hand the mass acceptance of cigarette smoking within the British Army. It was an addiction he did not share, and he took a deep dislike to smoking. Seeing it as a waste of money, it so disgusted him that he promised Richard £50 on his 21st birthday if he succeeded in resisting the temptation to smoke. As a dutiful son, Richard willingly accepted his father's puritanically loaded offer. "I was determined to get it."

Unfortunately, the unseen factor in the familial pact was Christopher, his younger brother by almost seven years. Once Christopher knew about the challenge, he never lost an opportunity to tease Doll in front of house guests. He would follow his brother around the sitting room in Montpellier Square, singing in a mocking staccato shrill, "Richard can't smoke cigarettes, otherwise he won't get £50 when he's twenty-one!" Exasperated by the taunting, one evening he launched himself at a proffered packet of cigarettes, saying, "I can't stand this any longer—give me a cigarette." He inhaled deeply, ending the filial torment. Doll was seventeen and he remained a "social smoker" for the next nineteen years—and, like the majority of the British male population who shared the habit, he was oblivious to its dangers.

Hill began their research by drawing up what he described as a "fearsome questionnaire", a ground-breaking case-report form which would establish the life histories of several hundred hospital patients with lung cancer compared to an equal number of hospital patients without the disease. The survey asked people questions such as where they lived; what jobs they had; their social class; whether they ate fat foods or fried foods; whether they had an electric or gas cooker; whether they lived near a gas works. There was no frontal attack on smoking, which formed one section out of nine— eleven questions out of nearly fifty. The questionnaire was deliberately wide-ranging because they wanted to eliminate any bias from the patients' responses. Their observational experiment needed to be carried out on a sufficiently large scale to determine whether patients with cancer of the lung differed materially from other persons in respect of their smoking habits, or in some other way, which might be related to the atmospheric pollution theory.

On 1 January 1948 on a part-time salary of £800 per annum, Richard Doll was formally appointed to direct the investigation along with two (eventually four) "lady almoners", as medical social workers were called then, who would interview the "cases" and the "controls" in the hospitals.

The inquiry, following the classical methods of epidemiology, was to be retrospective. Dr FHK Green was at the time assistant to Harold Himsworth, the long-serving secretary of the MRC. Green wrote to twenty London hospitals, asking them to co-operate by notifying all patients admitted to their wards with cancer of the lung, stomach, colon or rectum. When Doll received the notification, one of the lady almoners visited the hospital to interview the patient using Hill's fearsome questionnaire. In addition to interviewing the notified patients with cancer of one of the four specified sites, the almoners were required to make similar inquiries of a group of "non-cancer control" patients. These patients were not notified. For each lung-carcinoma patient visited at a hospital the almoners were instructed to interview a patient of the same sex, within the same five-year age group, and in the same hospital on or about the same time—"but otherwise chosen at random".[16]

The pioneering researchers were now going beyond the conventional frontiers of epidemiology with the first serious study into cancer and, building on the vital statistics of Percy Stocks, they now sought to explain why the disease occurred. Hill and Doll's aim was to make the field observations mirror an experimental design as nearly as possible. In other words they sought, as in an experiment, to limit the variables.

The patients were closely questioned about their environment, lifestyles and smoking histories. The investigation went beyond what was customary in a medical examination. They were asked: if they had smoked at any period of their lives; the ages at which they had started and stopped; the amount they were in the habit of smoking before the onset of the illness that brought them into hospital; the main changes in their smoking history and the maximum they had ever been in the habit of smoking; the varying proportion smoked in pipes and cigarettes; and whether or not they inhaled. To record and tabulate these details it was necessary to define what was meant by a smoker. Hill and Doll defined a smoker as a person who had smoked as much as one cigarette a day for as long as one year. Each patient in each group was interviewed by a medical social worker, all interviewers using the same questionnaire.

If the thinking behind the study was at the forefront of the subject's techniques, the same could not be said of its technology. Doll recorded the initial statistical findings using a fountain pen. As the flow of information increased so, you might have thought, would the sophistication of the machinery to decipher it. But Doll did not use a calculating machine or the Hollerith electric punch card system for tabulating statistics. As the data came in he recorded what looked interesting, entered it in columns in a record book, and added up the numbers in the columns. "The whole thing was done with a nineteenth-century clerical technique."[17] Being medically qualified, it fell to him to undertake much of the early analysis, and to identify the emergence of a distinctive trend.

In September 1948 Doll wrote an interim report for Green at the MRC based on 156 interviews, recording that: "The results appear to show a definite association between carcinoma of the lung and smoking, an association which is less strong for pipe smokers than for cigarette smokers," although the lack of correlation between inhaling and cancer was "surprising".[18]

With extra funding the one-year study was extended, and Hill and Doll's meticulous statistical techniques started to reveal evidence that neither man had predicted. In October 1949 Doll wrote a detailed report for the MRC in which he asserted that there "was a real association between smoking and cancer of the lung". Lung cancer is fatal, and for those diagnosed with the disease, there was no resolution—death was inevitable and rapid. Where there is no cure, prevention is indisputable. At this point Doll stopped smoking.

For Richard Doll, it was a momentous occasion. At 37 years of age he stood on the threshold of making one of the defining medical discoveries of the twentieth century—the carcinogenic effect of tobacco. Years later he joked about the good fortune that got him selected to assist Hill with the investigation. "He told me that his first thought was to ask Jerry Morris to be his medical assistant, but on reflection thought him 'too left-wing'— if only he'd known!"

Hill was reputed to have found Doll "aggressively ambitious"[19] but what was not in question was his collaborator's commitment to the study. Hill was not like some evolutionary psychologist, prone to dissecting his colleagues' personalities, but he did take some credit for channelling Doll's persistent search for perfection into experimental science. Much later, Hill said:

> He became obsessional. I think at school he'd become obsessional, a religious one. And then he'd become obsessional[ly] left-wing. I never asked him whether he'd joined the party, because it was nothing to do with me. As long as he did his job, I didn't care a damn. And I made him obsessional about research. Once you've got obsessional about re-search, you haven't got time for communism or religion, or anything else at all.[20]

Before the emergence of epidemiology, conditions such as heart attacks, stroke and cancer were collectively known as "degenerative dis-eases," an all-embracing term explaining the existence of cancer as the ineluctable concomitant of ageing. Now, from Hill and Doll, it was evident that not only did cancer have causes, but that the environment and people's lifestyles must play a significant role in the origins of the disease.

In the autumn of 1949 Harold Himsworth weighed the evidence and gave his scientific opinion to Doll. Himsworth,* a patrician figure with elitist leanings, was intrigued by the epidemiological findings. Being a devoted pipe smoker himself, and as a custodian of the nation's health, his interpretation of the findings and the implications for public health were profound. As Doll wrote: "He was convinced by our evidence but he was conscious that our findings would be deeply unpopular. He told us: 'Your study is limited to London, and really you ought to expand it and show that these results are typical of the whole country and not just London before publishing.'"

Following this advice the researchers extended their study to four thoracic centres outside the capital—Newcastle, Cambridge, Leeds and Bristol. By the summer of 1950 the results from these centres were proving identical to the London study. Unfortunately, contemporaneously in the United States another large case-control study into lung cancer was published by Ernst Wynder and Evarts Graham in which they concluded that "excessive and prolonged use of tobacco, especially of cigarettes, seems to be an important factor in the induction of bronchogenic cancer."[21] Initially disappointed at being beaten to publication—they had after all been sitting on the evidence for at least nine months—Doll came to recognise the wisdom of the delay.

To understand Richard Doll more fully, it is necessary to recognise the political and scientific beliefs that guided his work. He always measured the statistical evidence carefully, recognising that the mathematics of statistics is by nature uncertain. He was a political radical while at the same time being a conservative scientist. As early as 1950 a coherent "Doll philosophy" was emerging and one of its central themes had its genesis in

---

*   Himsworth became a legendary figure in post-war British medical research. The only practising clinician to have held the office of MRC secretary, he possessed a remarkable ability to choose outstanding people and to foresee the needs of medical science. He was also—together with Francis Avery Jones and 'Tony' Bradford Hill—a formative influence on Doll's scientific career.

the lung cancer study. It was the principle that if an investigation found something that was unexpected and which was going to be of social significance, then there was an obligation to make sure that the answer was right before publishing the results to the world.

In the middle of the last century there were only about twelve researchers working on the causes of cancer. Doll and Wynder did not know of each other's existence; often in science there are parallel discoveries and that is what happened in 1950. In fact, five papers* were published in 1950 about the dangers of smoking, but the Doll and Hill and Wynder and Graham studies were the most scientifically persuasive because of their size, the precision with which lifelong non-smokers were defined and the argument that led to their conclusion. The American article acted as a catalyst, liberating Hill and Doll from any further deferment, and over the summer they wrote a report based on their London data for Hugh Clegg, editor of the *British Medical Journal*. When Himsworth read it, he was unequivocal in his prediction: "It will be a sensation."[22] On Saturday 30 September 1950, "Smoking and Carcinoma of the Lung, preliminary report", appeared in the *British Medical Journal*, culminating in the now classic observation that "smoking is a factor, and an important factor, in the production of carcinoma of the lung."[23] Nearly forty years later, in an official history of the Medical Research Council, Doll and Hill's ground-

---

* The five papers were: Schrek R, Baker LA, Ballard GP, Dolgoff S, 'Tobacco Smoking as an Etiologic factor in Disease: cancer', *Cancer Research*, 1950; volume 10, pp. 49-58. Levin ML, Goldstein H, Gerhardt PR, 'Cancer and Tobacco Smoking', *Journal of the American Medical Association*, 1950; volume 143, pp. 336-38. Mills CA and Porter MM, 'Tobacco Smoking Habits and Cancer of the Mouth and Respiratory System', *Cancer Research*, 1950; volume 10, pp. 539-542. Wynder EL and Graham EA, 'Tobacco Smoking as a Possible Etiologic Factor in Bronchogenic Carcinoma', *Journal of the American Medical Association*, 1950; volume 143, pp. 329-36. Doll R, Hill AB. 'Smoking and Carcinoma of the Lung, preliminary report', *British Medical Journal*, 1950; volume 2, pp. 739-48.

breaking research was placed in the annals of medical history, as it "provided the basis for what remains to this day the single most reliably established and practicable means of reducing the proportion of deaths from cancer."[24]

To the scientific mind, all knowledge is a matter of probability. Clinical medicine is not a determinist science: diagnosis and prognosis are a matter of probability. Proof in the mathematical sense is unobtainable in dealing with medical problems. Direct experimental verification in humans is possible to conceive but impossible to conduct. This reality led one researcher, in a review of the evidence relating lung cancer to smoking, to conclude: "We are left for 'proof' therefore, with indirect and circumstantial evidence derived largely from considerations of the pathogenesis of the disease in individuals and its observed distribution in human populations: in short, with epidemiological evidence. It is a matter of opinion how many and what facts must be consistent before this hypothesis may justifiably be accepted or rejected."[25]

Theoretically, there are three possible explanations for an observed result in epidemiology. Chance: random error; that the result was due to the play of chance. Bias: systematic error; that, in this case, the result was due to confounding, that it was not smoking that caused the disease, but smoking was associated with something else that did. Causation: that chance and bias are eliminated to such a degree that it could be demonstrated, beyond reasonable doubt, that causation was the only possible explanation.

A fundamental problem in a case-control study is the method by which the controls are chosen. Ideally, they should be on average similar to the cases in all respects except in the medical condition under study. In the 1950 experiment the lung cancer patients and the control group of non-cancer patients were exactly comparable in age and sex, but there were some slight dissimilarities with regard to place of residence and social class. Doll and Hill reported on a group of 709 patients with lung cancer in hospitals compared with a control group of 709 patients who did not have lung cancer and a third group of 637 patients with cancer of colon, rectum or stomach. Of the 649 men with lung cancer, 647 (99.7 per cent) were smokers and two (0.3 per cent) were non-smokers.

When Doll and Hill applied this finding to what statisticians term a "probability test" they felt confident in their estimation because the odds were less than one in a million of getting their results by chance alone. Of the 649 male controls, 622 were smokers, and 27 (4.2 per cent) were non-smokers. Self-evidently, the overwhelming majority of men had been smokers at some period of their lives, but the very small proportion of those with lung cancer who had been non-smokers (0.3 per cent) was "most significantly less than the corresponding proportion in the control group of other patients (4.2 per cent)".[26] For women, while the habit was far less pervasive than among men, smoking was significantly more frequent among those with cancer of the lung. Of the sixty women interviewed with the disease, 31.7 per cent were non-smokers while the corresponding figure for non-cancer controls was 53.3 per cent. In order fully to understand the logic, simplicity and clarity of Doll and Hill's investigation, we must first examine the intellectual foundations of the statistical analysis they applied to smoking and carcinoma of the lung.

RA Fisher, the founder of statistical inference, once famously wrote: "That's not an experiment you have there, that's an experience."[27] Fisher's book, *Statistical Methods for Research Workers*, led Doll to Pearson's X^2 (Chi^2) test for the measurement of a chance result in an experiment. Chances are between 0 per cent and 100 per cent. If something is impossible, it happens 0 per cent of the time, while at the other extreme, if something is sure to happen, then it happens 100 per cent of the time. All events fall between these two limits. Of course, extremely unlikely events do occasionally happen; otherwise no one would buy a national lottery ticket. Therefore, all questions asked about an epidemiological study receive an answer predicated in terms of uncertainty.[28] If the uncertainty is low, the conclusion will be unambiguous and the decision will be safe. If the uncertainty is high, the study must be regarded as inconclusive.

The measurement of uncertainty in statistical analysis is called the theory of probability. This concept of probability provides a measure of uncertainty for various types of phenomena that occur in nature. To understand how Doll and Hill came to the finding that there existed a significant and clear relationship between smoking and carcinoma of the lung we need to understand two other concepts in the canon of statistical knowledge: "significance tests" and "confidence intervals". A significance test is a statistical tool applied to a set of observations to find out if an observed difference is real or just a chance variation.

In Doll and Hill's study the only substantial differences between the case and control groups were in their reported smoking habits. The difference in the proportion of smokers in the case and control groups was clearly significant.* To Doll and Hill the answer was so clear, and their hypothesis testing so rigorous, that when they applied a Chi-square test, the odds against it being a chance finding were in the order of a million to one. As a binomial example—using the chance estimate found in their study—the likelihood of the result being due to chance was about the same as the probability of tossing a coin 20 times in a row and getting "heads" every time.

Confidence intervals define a range of values calculated from sampling observations that are believed, with some probability, to contain the true value of whatever it is we are interested in trying to measure, that is, it is the likely range of the true value. Likely is usually taken as "95 per cent of the time".

In dealing with the accuracy of percentages, statistical surveys are limited, in that, in most cases, it is not possible to interview all the people in a region, country or continent. For example, suppose a public health organisation wanted to estimate the number of smokers in Oxford. They

---

* A P value = the probability of getting a result at least as extreme as this just by chance (i.e. if there is no real effect) not the probability that the result actually did arise by chance. P values measure the strength of evidence, against what statisticians call the "null hypothesis" (or "no effect"); the smaller the P value, the stronger the evidence. P values only deal with chance. In 1950 Doll and Hill found the association between smoking and lung cancer gave a P value of P = .00000064. The likelihood of it being a chance finding was about one in 1.6m.

might estimate it by taking a simple random sample. Naturally, the percentage of smokers in the sample would be used to estimate the percentage of smokers in the city. Because the sample is chosen at random, it is even possible to say how accurate this estimate is likely to be, just from the size and composition of the sample. This is one of the most important ideas in statistical theory. If a public health organisation wants to establish clinics to help smokers break their addiction, they need to know how many of the city's 100,000 citizens are addicted to the habit. So they employ a survey company, which takes a simple random sample of 2,500 people. In the sample 1,328 are smokers so the finding is:

$$\frac{1,328}{2,500} \quad X \quad 100 \text{ per cent } = 53 \text{ per cent}$$

This does not of course mean that the sample would perfectly reflect the smoking habits of Oxford's population; the sample would differ from the whole population: the difference is what statisticians call chance error. Importantly, they can estimate with confidence that, if properly undertaken, the study can be 95 per cent confident that they got the true value to within two percentage points.

In their hypothesis testing, when Doll and Hill measured the relative risk "among male heavy smokers" of getting lung cancer compared to "never smokers" they came up with the figure of 16.3.[29] This means that smokers might be associated with a 16 times greater risk of dying of lung cancer, compared with never smokers. In 100 identical repetitions of this study, the result will be between this range (confidence interval 15-17), 95 times.

To get the right answer in an epidemiological study, an enormous amount of care has to be taken in the planning, execution and publication of the experiment. Doll and Hill's paper is a beautiful example of the concern which should be taken to avoid bias due to unsuspected differences between case and control groups. In 1967 Doll illustrated the susceptibility of epidemiological evidence to distortion when he wrote: "The only safeguard is always to suspect the influence of bias, consider every way it could have entered the study and then test to see if it has."[30] Doll and Hill had found that the patients with pulmonary cancer and the controls were remarkably alike in all the characteristics they recorded, apart from their smoking habits. Scientists do not like uncertainty. To remove the possibility that the disease could have been caused by something other than smoking it was necessary to consider alternative explanations of the results. Could the patients in the study have been unrepresentative? Could the smoking histories of patients have been produced by bias on the part of the interviewers?

Doll and Hill were dispassionate scientists. After comparing the results obtained by the almoners, they were able to discount selection bias by the interviewers as they had interviewed patients with *suspected* diagnosis of one of the three cancers (lung, stomach, rectum); so they had no idea whether the disease would be confirmed. It was not until a month after the patients were discharged from hospital that Doll and Hill came to know the outcome. Incontrovertibly, the smoking habits of those suspected of having lung cancer but who did not have the disease were quite different from the true lung cancer patients and were almost identical with the controls. This eliminated the possibility of bias by the interviewers.

Hill was mindful that all the standard errors and Chi-square tests in the world could not compensate for incomplete, imperfect or biased data. In Doll he recognised "a remarkable capacity for working long hours at the most exacting tasks."[31] This tenacity removed yet another confounding element from the epidemiological study—as it led to a dramatic, reduction in "non-responses". Doll's ability to later persuade an army of doctors to respond to his requests led to an unprecedented follow-up rate of 99.6 per cent: it was an achievement described by Hill as "a monument to his administrative skills".[32]

Smoking was part of the British way of life. As Marna Buckatzsch observed: "In the war everybody smoked because life was so awful. People smoked like chimneys."[33] People had been smoking tobacco for so long it was inconceivable that it could be responsible for so much suffering and death. If almost every man in Britain was smoking, or had smoked, how could it be identified as the cause of the disease? Only a careful statistical weighing of the evidence could see the relationship between cause and effect. For instance, in the lung cancer category, 26 per cent of the male patients fell into the two groups of highest consumption (25 cigarettes a day or more) while in the control group of other male patients only 13.5 per cent were found.

This was clearly significant and indicated a biological gradient; showing a higher mortality in heavy smokers than in light smokers. Also the epidemic seemed to have been triggered by a switch from pipe to cigarette smoking, as fewer than six per cent of lung cancer patients smoked pipes, while more than 94 per cent were cigarette smokers. The one anomaly identified in the study related to inhaling. In fact, the study indicated that the lung cancer patients inhaled slightly less than the other patients.

For cautious men whose pioneering work ushered in the new era of tobacco epidemiology, the belief that the excess of lung cancer in smokers could only point to a causal connection gave them sufficient confidence to make a prediction. "The risk of developing the disease increases in simple proportion with the amount smoked, and that it may be approximately fifty times as great among those who smoke 25 or more cigarettes a day as among non-smokers."[34] After taking all the evidence into account, the difference in the two sexes, the time relationship to the introduction of cigarettes and the increase in the disease, they had come to the inevitable conclusion—"that smoking is an important factor in the cause of carcinoma of the lung."[35]

Doll and Hill had used the statistics provided by Stocks to show that smoking had been responsible for as many deaths per annum as were claimed by the great cholera epidemics of the nineteenth century. Snow's innovatory use of epidemiology was viewed by his contemporaries as an unreliable departure from accepted medical thinking. The removal of the handle from the Broad Street pump on 8 September 1854—so as to prevent access to contaminated water—did little to influence the ideology underpinning Victorian public health medicine.[36] The cholera epidemics in Britain disappeared rather than being blown out of the water on the basis of Snow's theory of fecal contamination. The same prejudices that had confronted Snow were now amassing against Doll and Hill, delaying the knowledge of the dangers of smoking to health, increasing human suffering and hindering the advance of human well-being.

In 1950 Doll and Hill established smoking as a major cause of preventable disease. The knowledge that a fatal cancer could be largely eradicated by epidemiological science was revolutionary and would have a far greater impact on public health than could ever be achieved by curative medicine alone. Unfortunately, with the exception of Himsworth at the MRC and a few notable others, their discovery was widely doubted and generally ignored. For the conclusion as to whether an observed association is causal or not is one of the most difficult things epidemiology has to achieve. Non-infectious epidemiology had no intellectual standing within the medical establishment, and the political class was as addicted to tobacco as the democracy it represented.

During the period of the study Britain had introduced the National Health Service; it was to prove the most important social consequence of the war. Dedicated to the cure and prevention of disease, the NHS was established during the years of financial austerity, under an exchequer whose financial liquidity was dependent on the substantial tax revenue (14 per cent of the total budget) from tobacco. While Stocks continued to provide vital statistics, government policies, determined in a market economy, delayed the acceptance of the dangers of tobacco. Facts do not always speak for themselves: it would take a generation before society recognised the true hazards of smoking and progressively abstained from the habit that led to what had become a very British way of death.

Chapter 7
A Passionate Partnership

"All Thoughts, all Passions, all Delights, Whatever stirs this mortal
Frame, All are but Ministers of Love, And feed his sacred flame."

William Wordsworth

The other change that the war had brought to his life was love. Doll had
met Joan Faulkner at a meeting of communist doctors in the early 1930s,
but her status as the wife of Hugh Faulkner—they had married in 1942
when Joan was still a medical student and their son, Tim, was born in the
same year—subsumed any emotional feelings Doll may have had. They
did not see much of each other during the war, but during Doll's recuperation he called on her. According to Joan, he "rather bowled me over,
because he was rather handsome in those days. He had wonderful thighs
in that marvellous dress uniform, with the trousers made of beautiful
fabric..."

Hugh Faulkner was a figure of influence among London's left-wing
politicos. A doctor whose interests lay not in clinical medicine but in the
organisation of the work of doctors, he had a profound impact on London
medicine. He had also marched against Oswald Mosley's Blackshirts in
Stepney in 1937.[1] His style of oratory was not spellbinding—it had more
of a conversational tone—but this had been one of his great attractions for
Joan and she had an intense admiration for him. Soon, however, admiration was replaced by disillusion. Julian Tudor Hart, a member of the
Communist Party who later became the Dolls' GP, saw Hugh as friendly
and good-natured, but as an impossible spouse for Joan. "I know that
when he came back from the war in Italy he had gonorrhoea. I imagine
that would have been difficult to forgive."[2]

Another contemporary, Nick Rae (later Lord Rae), worked as a
doctor at the historic Caversham general practice in Kentish Town with
Hugh Faulkner, and also saw the defects of his qualities. "I know that
Hugh got jaundice in Italy, and he was certainly enamoured of Italian

women. He said that they threw themselves at him, as if they were saying 'Take me, take me.'"[3] Avis Hutt also knew Joan and Hugh well, both from her work as a nurse treating the injured anti-fascist marchers who had opposed Mosley's Blackshirts and also as a long-term guest in their home during the war years. "Hugh was lovely, a big man, friendly and totally irresponsible. Joan was more cerebral, a cool academic."[4]

The fight for Joan was one of the most "upsetting periods" of Doll's life although he was not to know that on VE Day, 8 May 1945, when Winston Churchill announced through a crescendo of church bells that it was now time, at last, to rejoice. Such was the release from six years of unremitting struggle that there followed a great national outpouring of emotion, an exaltation which, viewed through the periscope of memory, invested VE Day with metaphysical meaning. People were jammed into Piccadilly, soldiers were climbing lamp-posts, and "everyone was wild".[5] Joan and Doll followed the prime minister's advice and allowed themselves "a brief period of rejoicing". The war had transmogrified him from that "callow youth" into a man who was "solid and reliable", and Doll always remembered VE Day—when they sang *The Red Flag* in Piccadilly—as the date of their engagement; and they certainly spent that night together.

Joan Faulkner was an unhappily married woman with a young child, and the portents did not seem favourable but on that May evening a fateful bond was made, and they decided to "make a go of it".[6] Joan, however, was in an invidious position. She loved her son, and the man she had been in thrall to was now exerting all of his emotional persuasion to keep her. Her ambiguity was to last, on and off, for the next four years. To Doll's repeated entreaties of marriage the answer was a resounding "Maybe".

The affair, however, had also brought about an internal crisis within the Communist Party. The Faulkners' home at 21A Belsize Park Gardens was virtually a political satellite of 16 King Street, the party's headquarters, and was redolent of radical activity, passionate debate and bohemian parties. Marna Buckatzsch lived in the area at the time and witnessed the excitement of London's left-wing partygoers, such as the eloquent and fervent Horace Joules and Philip D'Arcy Hart who were part of an opinion-forming circle that would influence post-war medicine. The affair between Doll and Joan was seen by one communist as being so destabilising that he felt compelled to tell Doll over the phone that it was his "political duty" to end it.

Though they were not yet fully committed to each other, Joan was already having an influence on Richard Doll's career. After working at the Royal Free Hospital, Joan joined the Medical Research Council in 1944, eventually becoming the most senior woman on its administrative staff. And, as we have seen, it was Joan's initiative in getting Doll to meet Francis Avery Jones that gained him a foothold in medical research. It was a fortuitous move, not only for Doll's scientific development but also for Joan because it kept Doll in London. In 1946, he turned down an offer from Charles Fletcher, the director of the MRC's pneumoconiosis research unit, to go to Cardiff as an epidemiologist. He rejected the job mainly because of Joan, who was reluctant to leave London and the MRC.

In the summer of 1947, Doll was sharing a flat with some of Joan's friends in Wimpole Mews. He had accumulated no capital, since all of his energies were directed into his work at the Central Middlesex, campaigning for the Communist Party and winning Joan's commitment. Doll already possessed a wealth of knowledge, and in the summer of 1949 he was given a knowledge of wealth when his mother inherited four houses in Streatham in south London. These were sold for £14,000, and this enabled him to borrow £7,000 from his mother and buy a large property near Notting Hill. "Richard came to me one evening and said, 'If I find somewhere for us to live will you leave him?'"[7]

Hugh Faulkner, according to Joan, was "livid" when he heard that she was going to leave him. "He said, 'Richard Doll had a tubercle in the war, and you'll end up a widow!'"[8] On one occasion the two men got into a scuffle. That struggle took on a metaphysical meaning for Doll as he looked upon his fight for Joan as a turning point in his emotional life; and it proved equally significant in his professional career for Joan eventually became a principal at the MRC responsible for epidemiology, social medicine and computers. As well as wanting to make her own mark, Joan was an admirer and supporter of Doll's work and was set on giving him freedom to concentrate totally on science. He had found a friend, lover and scientific companion.

The £7,000 enabled Doll to buy 24 Lansdowne Road* in Notting Hill, west London. The area was popular with the intellectual left and the spacious town house formed part of an elegant square creating a large communal garden: a verdant sanctuary for parents and children. Joan's only stipulation about moving into Lansdowne Road was that it should have a "cosy stove". During the bitter winters of 1946 and 1947 a heater had been indispensable; and she was not going anywhere without one now. She moved in but it would be two years before the two of them could marry.

Together in love, the formation of the NHS in 1948 also saw the couple joined in literature. Inspired by what they had witnessed as junior doctors, *Humanise the Hospitals* was a patients' charter co-written by Joan Faulkner and Richard Doll (their names did not appear on the four-page pamphlet) for the Communist Party of Great Britain.** Though it was their only joint publication, it epitomised a central belief of their thinking that "the patient's comfort is part of his cure."[9]

In time, Richard Doll's name became synonymous with scientific caution. Prone to ideas but not to excitement, he was professionally conservative, only moving his position if the scientific evidence demanded it. Joan Faulkner (she retained Hugh Faulkner's name throughout her professional life) had a reputation for being "frank to the point of cruelty",[10] and Doll believed that under her influence he learned to control the campaigning fervour that was so evident early in his career. Though his reputation within the scientific community was one of exceptional detachment,

---

*   Doll and Joan moved into the five-room flat on the top floor. When Doll bought the house it came with sitting tenants, one of whom was Lady Younghusband, a daughter of the famous explorer Sir Francis Younghusband (1863-1942). She lived in the house for the next 25 years.

**   When Richard Doll read the article in July 2005 while a patient in the John Radcliffe Hospital in Oxford, he said, "Some of our recommendations have still to be implemented."

he believed that Joan had a steadying influence on him. As he put it, "She was more cautious than me."[11]

In the spring of 1948, the British Medical Association was still antagonistic to the ideals of the NHS which was to be launched in July of that year. Rejecting caution for direct action, Doll marked himself out as troublemaker within the medical establishment in a letter to the *Times* on 19 March. It effectively blacklisted him from working at St Thomas's. In the letter, he defended the NHS Act and the compassionate treatment patients received in public authority hospitals like the Central Middlesex compared to the voluntary hospitals such as St Thomas's. Even if he had not wanted it, his closing paragraph ensured his medical career would be in research rather than on the wards of his *alma mater*:

> May I, in closing, make in my turn a dogmatic statement, even though I cannot describe myself as a teacher, and that is that if a human approach to the patient is desired there is much that the voluntary hospitals can learn from the better municipal ones. It was a horrifying experience, after the war, to be brought again face to face with the cavalier manner in which some doctors dispose of a patient's hopes of life in conversation at the end of a bed. There is, I submit, nothing in the Act itself which will "dehumanise" medicine; there is a lot which we all have to learn before medicine becomes thoroughly human.

As late as March 1948 the British Medical Association, led by its president Guy Drain, was unbending in its opposition to the introduction of the NHS. In a BMA-conducted survey, 4,735 of its members were reported to be in favour of the Act and 40,814 against on an 82 per cent poll.[12] It was an unedifying period in the history of British social policy. At the same time, Doll attended a meeting of the BMA in its Marylebone division, where he spoke in favour of the much-needed reforms of Aneurin Bevan, minister of health from 1945 to 1951, only to lose the vote by 220 to four. Faced with such unyielding opposition, it made him wonder just who the other three were!*

At the time Doll was working at the Central Middlesex Hospital for two days a week with Avery Jones as a gastroenterologist. The Central Middlesex was a remarkable institution, with a medical staff that had a defining influence on British public health. Horace Joules, its medical director, was a visionary campaigner, and committed communist. A tall, passionate and imposing man, Joules was Bevan's medical advisor in the planning and formation of the NHS. In 1948, Jerry Morris became director of the new MRC social medicine research unit at the Central Middlesex. This unit was another manifestation of Himsworth's vision for the future—it was here, too, that epidemiological studies were able to transform our understanding of the causes of coronary heart disease. Morris and Richard Titmuss were using non-infectious disease epidemiology in the same way that Doll and Hill were helping to establish the discipline's power to unravel the causes of cancer. In 1957 Morris published his book *Uses of Epidemiology*, which is widely regarded as a medical classic and indispensable to the growth of the subject's acceptance and medical application.

The corridors of Central Middlesex were populated by some of the most able physicians in London: Avery Jones, Joules, Richard Asher, Morris and, of course, Doll. Such proximity did not mean that they shared a similar political orthodoxy—far from it. Doll and Morris admired each other's work, but differed in their political world view. Morris, who came from the south side of Glasgow where "socialism came with your nappies,"[13] had been a houseman at University College Hospital in the 1930s, and was deeply affected by the poverty and malnutrition that he saw within London's working-class communities. For him, the removal

---

*   At a packed meeting of the Royal College of Physicians in London in 2004, Doll told this story while announcing the findings of the fifty-year follow-up of the British doctors' study. While making his way towards the wine, Doll was clasped by the elbow and told enthusiastically, "I was one of the three who voted with you that night."

of these social inequities would come from the traditional socialism of his roots, and for that reason he was antagonistic to the Communist Party and opposed to Doll's advocacy of the communist ideology. The political debates became so feverish that ultimately two of the most politically committed epidemiologists had to make a pact "not to discuss politics".[14] The left was neither united nor homogeneous.

Maurice Backett, who worked with Morris at the Central Middlesex, believed the political forces that were causing the ideological schism were unwelcome. He too, came from a British socialist tradition, and found the exodus from social medicine to a formal communist adherence "frightening".[15] As a scientist, he was also concerned about the dubious biology emanating from the Soviet Union. "Some of us in the Social Medical Society were frightened of the authoritarian bite of the CP at the time."[16] By the time of the Berlin blockade and airlift in June 1948 it was clear that a new enemy had been discovered: rather than the old threat of Germany, it was Russia that was viewed as the potential enemy. The Cold War was well under way, and to be seen, like Doll, to be a communist, or to be overtly associated with communism, was extremely dangerous. While a young doctor, Sam Shuster joined the Communist Party at this tumultuous moment and was conscious of the atmosphere of repression, and admired Doll's courage in adhering to his beliefs. "It's difficult to explain, or even now, quite believe the memory of the fear we lefties had in those times and of the very real fear of the watchers, and what they could do socially and professionally."[17]

In 1949 Richard Doll was named co-respondent in Joan's divorce and engaged Jack Gaster,* a communist lawyer. Fearing the headline "Doctor sues doctor over doctor," Doll gave his name to the court as William

---

* Gaster was one of the most prominent left-wing British lawyers through several decades from the 1930s, and the strictest code of ethics and egalitarianism governed his public and personal life at every stage. (Even in the last year of his life he would not discuss the case.) In 1932 he started a legal firm with the like-minded Richard Turner. His life was one of political involvement. He was, as he liked to say, "never a drawing room socialist". In 1946 he was elected as one of only two

Richard Shaboe Doll. This was, after all, the name entered on his birth certificate, but he was conscious that he used the name of his father, by then bed-ridden with multiple sclerosis. Fortunately, his father did not see the *Evening Standard*'s court report, and the less disheartening than expected headline "Fastest Divorce Ever!"[18] The divorce had been a major trauma. Doll and Joan, now free, decided to marry immediately, and became husband and wife on 4 October 1949 at Kensington register office. There was to be no honeymoon. Fearing more trouble from Hugh Faulkner, they found a temporary safe refuge with a medical friend who had a cottage outside London.

For Joan, falling in love and marrying Doll was a triumph of hope over experience. For Doll, who never doubted for a moment that marrying Joan was the best decision of his life, he would now enter the formative decade of his life. In the evenings at Lansdowne Road, he worked on his scientific papers while Joan listened to music and read. "She said she liked looking at me, I didn't understand why." It appeared they were meant for one another.[19] After the historic publication in the *British Medical Journal* in September 1950, Doll became a full-time member of Hill's statistical research unit. By doing so, he elected to make his career in statistics and epidemiology.

communists on the London County Council for three years, in addition to resuming his legal work.

Chapter 8

The Fight for Acceptance

"General impressions are never to be trusted. Unfortunately when they are of long standing they become fixed rules of life and assume a prescriptive right not to be questioned. Consequently those who are not accustomed to original inquiry entertain a hatred and a horror of statistics. They cannot endure the idea of submitting their sacred impressions to cold-blooded verification."

Francis Galton

Harold Himsworth's prophecy that the publication of Doll and Hill's findings would "cause a sensation" did not materialise. However, George Godber, an indomitable figure and a supporter of the epidemiological research who became deputy chief medical officer at the Ministry of Health, remembered that Doll and Hill's work "provoked a hostile situation".[1] The hostility came from all sides: from within the medical establishment, the political class and the tobacco industry, which took care to persuade the media that no one should pay any attention to Doll and Hill's conclusions.[2] As for the general public, the response was one of indifference. Smoking was such a common habit that people could not accept that it could be doing them any harm.

Moral and medical opposition to tobacco had existed in Britain since the anonymous publication in 1604 of *A Counterblast to Tobacco* by King James I. This broadside on what was viewed as a disgusting habit had little impact. Over the following two centuries resistance came from quasi-religious and anti-tobacco societies and, in the twentieth century, from the National Association of Non-Smokers, founded in 1926. But they made little headway. The invention of the Bonsack cigarette-rolling machine in 1880 had revolutionised smoking habits. Capable of producing more than 70,000 cigarettes a day, it ushered in the era of cheap mass production, and established the tobacco industry on an industrial scale. Galvanised by the shared upheavals and collective unity of two world wars, Britain in

1950 was addicted socially and pharmacologically to cigarettes. Indeed, it was common practice for doctors to offer their patients a cigarette to dispel any anxiety before an examination. Puritanical opposition had dissipated. Ironically, the concept that cigarette smoking could cause cancer was such a simple one that it militated against its acceptance.

The newly constituted NHS obliged the minister of health to provide "a comprehensive health service designed to secure improvement in the physical and mental health of the people of England and Wales and the prevention, diagnosis and treatment of illness."[3] The discovery that the most common fatal cancer could possibly be eliminated by a change in people's lifestyles thus presented a unique opportunity for public health medicine.

A great deal of medical research merely modifies and expands existing fundamental propositions, but occasionally real experimental advances are made in medical knowledge. Doll and Hill's main purpose was to identify cause and effect relationships between diseases and environmental factors. By asking people how many cigarettes they smoked each day it was seemingly possible to measure the relationship between smoking and lung cancer (although the crucial mechanism by which a normal cell became malignant was then still a mystery).

On Friday 5 October 1950, Doll announced the results of the study to a joint meeting of the Royal Society of Medicine and the British Medical Association in London.[4] Hill was in attendance but it was Doll who addressed the meeting. This was symptomatic of their professional relationship, with Hill often preferring his protégé to be the advocate of their collective discoveries to the lay press. In fact, Hill was consciously wary of the media and thought it an impediment to his research. "I don't want anything to do with the media: I just want to do my work."[5] (On one occasion, while waiting to appear on BBC television's *Panorama* programme, Hill had to be physically prevented from leaving the studio by Richard Dimbleby when told that their interview about polio vaccination was to be edited.) Conversely, Doll was also, in the vernacular of today, "media savvy"—confident, precise and able to explain complex scientific ideas simply. Some suspected that his sister-in-law, the film producer

Josephine Douglas,[6] had advised him on how to work with the media, and how to project a reassuring televisual presence. Yet, if Hill was a persuasive thinker, and Doll an articulate communicator, how do we explain the paradox that existed in 1950: a growing financial and intellectual investment in research, yet public indifference to practical prevention?

Positioned between the scientists and the Ministry of Health were two influential advisory bodies: the Central Health Service Council (CHSC) and its standing advisory committee on cancer and radiotherapy (SACCR). As early as January 1951, Horace Joules, a member of both advisory groups (formally a heavy smoker, he gave up after reading Doll and Hill's article), agitated for a publicity campaign about the dangers of smoking. At the same time, the media baron Lord Beaverbrook instructed his journalists not to write articles about cancer—seeing it as an unpalatable subject[7] for the sensibilities of his readership. The perceived horror of cancer led to it being virtually unmentionable; while doctors had few methods to combat the disease and only rudimentary advice to give about avoiding it. Joules saw that now, finally, preventive action could be mobilised for little cost and to great effect.

Unfortunately, his eagerness for action was opposed by the formidable figure of Sir Ernest Rock Carling, the distinguished surgeon and later chairman of the International Committee on Radiological Protection. Carling was a confirmed heavy smoker who was sceptical about Doll and Hill's mono-causal explanation for the rise in lung cancer incidence, and said that "it would be premature to base conclusions on it."[8] In deference to his pre-eminent status as chair of the SACCR, it was decided that no cancer awareness publicity should be initiated by the Ministry of Health. Officials were worried that education would lead to a public panic and a majority within the committee were afraid that society was susceptible to unfounded cancer phobia[9] and that further research was needed.

Sir John Charles, the chief medical officer, was pusillanimous when asked by the crusading Joules to take direct action against the epidemic. Godber, who succeeded Charles in 1960, recalled his predecessor's lengthy reports, which on one occasion contained the sentence "the mysterious and inexorable advance in lung cancer". Subsequently, whenever

Horace Joules met the saturnine Charles he used to glower and mutter "mysterious and inexorable".[10] Some thought that Charles's resistance to Doll and Hill's work was because "he didn't want to offend the [tobacco] industry and the public".[11]

Doll and Hill were not campaigners, at least not for their own scientific findings. Both scientists believed that the research worker's job was to obtain the results, to report them and to comment on them if asked but to leave it to other people to act on them. Doll incorporated this idea into his scientific philosophy, which precluded him from becoming emotionally attached to evidence, while at the same time providing a safeguard against accusations that his epidemiological conclusions were politically motivated. He wanted to use statistics[12] for the common good, but to achieve this he rejected the campaign trail and intentionally embraced the ideal of the dispassionate scientific rationalist. "I regarded my job as being to find out what the facts were. If you once get involved in deciding what attitude to take on the basis of the facts there's a danger your inquiry becomes biased."[13] This conscious detachment was not shared by all epidemiologists. Jerry Morris, for example, was a proselytising public health propagandist who championed the need to inculcate people with uncomfortable information that they might wish to ignore. For him, scientific discoveries came with responsibilities; he was an unashamed "analyst, advocate and activist".[14]

One reason why the medical profession was so cautious in its response to the Doll and Hill findings was that scientists do not like uncertainties. If there had been a survey of doctors and scientists in the early 1950s, the majority of them would have doubted the association between smoking and lung cancer. Many would have accepted that an association had been shown, but not that it implied *cause* and *effect*. After all, Doll and Hill had shown that hospital patients who were non-smokers also got lung cancer. Their finding contradicted the intellectual foundations of causation in diagnostic medicine, namely Koch's postulates.* Formalised in

---

*   Robert Koch (1843-1910) consolidated bacteriology into a scientific discipline; his genius with the microscope established the germ concept of disease. Koch

1882, these stated that to prove an organism was the cause of any disease certain necessary conditions had to be satisfied: that the organism could be discoverable in every instance of the disease; that the germ could be produced in a pure culture; that the disease could be reproduced in experimental animals through a pure culture removed by numerous generations from the organisms initially isolated; and that the organism could be retrieved from the inoculated animal and re-cultured.

Koch's eternal place in medicinal history was assured in 1882 when he discovered the bacillus causing tuberculosis, *Mycobacterium tuberculosis*. This established the aetiology of the disease: no bacillus *ergo* no causality with the disease. The discovery of bacteria such as diphtheria, typhoid, and the tubercle, had been the foundation for the great advances in infectious disease medicine since the last decades of the nineteenth century. The concept behind these postulates was the idea that a disease had to have an identifiable causative agent. Self-evidently, Doll and Hill's research was doubted by those medical researchers who gave primacy to Koch's postulates in determining causation. Certainly, Doll and Hill did not think that cigarette smoking was the cause of lung cancer; but they did believe that it was *a* cause of *the* disease. Doctors had not yet come to understand that chronic diseases could have multiple causes.

Meanwhile, within the CHSC Horace Joules continued his unyielding agitation for preventive action against the increasing death toll from the disease. He described lung cancer as "the most important clinical condition in British medicine at present... Young men ought to be told of the risks which they ran in becoming heavy smokers."[15]

In the summer of 1951 Doll and Hill faced an impasse. Apart from Himsworth and Joules, few other opinion formers believed their conclusions. Another approach would clearly need to be used if the weaknesses inherent in retrospective studies (all being hospital patients) were to be

---

isolated and identified *Vibrio cholera* in Alexandria in 1883 showing that the bacillus lived in the human intestine and was spread mainly by polluted water—thereby vindicating the work of John Snow.

overcome. At this time an idea began to incubate in Hill's mind. In place of the retrospective survey, Hill envisaged a "forward-looking"[16] approach, an experiment to determine the frequency with which the disease appeared in the future among groups of people whose smoking habits were already known. With a well-designed experiment it would be possible to eliminate, or at least allow for, some of the weaknesses inherent in the "retrospective" observational approach.

Doll immediately saw how this innovatory idea would satisfy Galton's aphorism (quoted at the beginning of this chapter) while fulfilling the requirements of the scientific approach to medical inquiry. Doll thought that he should regard his accustomed beliefs with scepticism and should develop fresh beliefs only on the basis of observation and experiment. As he wrote: "Our responsibility—having concluded in our 1950 study that smoking was a cause of lung cancer—was to see if we could disprove it and the obvious way to try to disprove it was to say, 'Well, does it predict, does knowledge of smoking habits predict whether someone will get lung cancer or not?'"[17]

In 1948 Bradford Hill had been asked by Charles Hill,* the secretary of the British Medical Association, to design a study—a type of productivity survey—to help determine salary levels for British hospital doctors and consultants when the NHS was established. In 1951, while recovering from a bout of flu, he had time to think, and his mind turned towards finding a cohort of people for his "prospective" experiment: he settled on the medical profession. British doctors appealed to Bradford Hill for three reasons. Firstly, they were a homogenous group trained in observation and likely to give accurate information about their smoking habits. Secondly, being doctors, they had to keep their names on the medical register and as a consequence would be easy to follow up. Finally, as most doctors would have good medical care, the medical causes of any deaths among them should be reasonably accurately certified.[18]

---

* Charles Hill was created a life peer in 1963, taking the title Lord Hill of Luton. Known as the "Radio Doctor" for his broadcasts on the BBC from the Ministry of Food in 1942.

Doll found Hill's idea inspiring and, like a good experimentalist, he thought it wise to test it on a random sample of doctors. In fact it was not truly random: they took the first name at the top of each left-hand page of the medical directory until they had 200 names, and then wrote them an invitation to participate. Incredibly, and to his own disbelief, Himsworth's name was one of those selected. The results of the pilot study were encouraging, with a 75 per cent response rate. Doll and Hill felt confident that a prospective study of smoking habits within a clearly defined population would provide evidence of the probable cause of lung cancer.

Hill then phoned Himsworth and asked for £2,000 to fund the study. In October 1951, with the assistance of the BMA, Doll and Hill sent a letter together with a short questionnaire to the 59,600 doctors in Britain. This British study evolved into the first major prospective study of smoking and death anywhere in the world.[19] At the time doctors smoked more than the general population because they could afford to continue the habit after the age of retirement, while manual workers tended to smoke less in old age—if they reached it. In November 1951 Hill wrote an open letter to British doctors in the *British Medical Journal*: entitled "Do You Smoke?"

> Last week I sent a letter personally to every man and woman on the Medical Register of the UK asking them to help me. I asked them to fill in a very simple form about their smoking habits.
>
> This, I think, is a new method of approach. May I therefore repeat my appeal through your column? If every doctor, whatever his field of work, will spare only a moment or two this research can be founded on a firm basis and in time give, I believe, firm and important answers.[20]

In addition to giving their name, address and age, they were asked to fill in a simple "questionary". This old-fashioned name for a questionnaire was the only thing about the study that was not ahead of its time. The doctors were asked to classify themselves into one of three groups, based on: whether they were, at the time, smoking; whether they had smoked but had given up; or whether they had never smoked regularly (that is, had never smoked as much as one cigarette a day, or its equivalent in pipe tobacco, for as long as one year). All present smokers and ex-smokers were asked additional questions. The former were asked the ages at which they had started smoking and the amount of tobacco that they were smoking and the method by which it was consumed, at the time of replying to the questionnaire. The ex-smokers were asked similar questions but relating to the time at which they had last given up smoking.[21]

The response was so great that the Post Office opened a sorting office at the London School of Hygiene and Tropical Medicine, and it took almost a year to finish opening the replies. Hill drew on the help of his daughter, Rosemary. "We were sorting the data into smokers and non-smokers, he said, 'That's the first move.'"[22] Doll also used child labour for the benefits of science when he employed Jean Gilliland to bring order to the doctors' questionnaires: "The replies had to be sorted alphabetically, and Richard Doll paid my seven-year-old daughter, Ann, to help too."[23]

A total of 41,024 physicians replied, and 40,564 questionnaires were accurately completed. Doll and Hill eliminated the men under 35 and the 6,185 women—since lung cancer was uncommon in both these groups—so their prospective study was carried out on the remaining 24,389 male doctors over the age of 35. As cancer incidence varies greatly with age, the researchers decided to use death rates standardised for age when comparing the mortality among the doctors in the different smoking categories.*

---

* Mortality in a population is usually measured by an annual death rate, for example, the number of people dying during a certain calendar year divided by the estimated population size midway through the year. Often this ratio is multiplied by a convenient base, commonly 1,000, to avoid small decimal fractions; it is then called the annual death rate per 1,000 population. If the death rate is calculated for a population covering a wide age range it is called a *crude death rate*. Mortality depends predominantly on age. The essential idea in standardisation is to introduce a *standard population* with a fixed age structure.

Epidemiology is both an art and a science, but it differs from other branches of medicine in that it is more cold-blooded—patients are not cared for and compassionately returned to full health. It is perhaps because of the unpalatable nature of their findings that Doll and Hill were not lionised for their contribution to public health. Instead they were often criticised for being "spoilsports", described as "grey-haired"[24] and subjected to ill-informed and tendentious criticism in the press. Hill would send these articles to his elder brother, a lawyer, marked "Query libellous"? But invariably the answer was "No, vulgar abuse".[25] Even some of the physicians in the study accused Hill of being "callous", and at a cocktail party another doctor said, "You're the chap who wants us to stop smoking." Hill, deploying his characteristic detachment, replied, "Not at all. I'm interested if you go on smoking to see how you die. I'm interested if you stop because I want to see how you die. So you choose for yourself, stop or go on. It's a matter of indifference to me, I shall score up your death anyway, and it will be very useful to me."[26]

Doll and Hill's work had already led to a great deal of scientific controversy. In 1952, for example, Hammond and Horn[27] began a much larger study for the American Cancer Society, specifically (so Hammond told Doll) to disprove the relationship between smoking and lung cancer that had been observed in the case-control studies. Hammond started the American Cancer Society's study to show that Doll and Hill were wrong, while Doll and Hill started their cohort study not to show that they were right or wrong: but to see if they were right or wrong.

More evidence that smoking was a cause of lung cancer came from Doll and Hill in 1952. After interviewing nearly 5,000 patients they were able to show the relative mortality rates for different levels of smoking as estimated from the case-control study of 1,357 deaths from lung cancer in men. Himsworth's directive to extend the study had provided corroborative support of their earlier paper. Also, with the larger numbers, they were able to demonstrate more clearly that the incidence of the disease became more common as the consumption of tobacco increased. They were still unable to implicate atmospheric pollution as a cause of lung cancer* (though conceivably it could act in conjunction with smoking).[28]

This second case-control paper is particularly interesting to historians of science because, for the first time, a citation is given to the epidemiological study on smoking and lung cancer by Eberhard Schairer and Eric Schöniger in Nazi Germany in 1943. In their 1950 paper Doll and Hill did not acknowledge Schairer and Schöniger's work but they had cited the case-control study carried out in Germany by Franz H Müller, who in 1939 presented the world's first controlled epidemiological study of the tobacco-lung cancer relationship.[29]

When the National Socialists were elected to power in 1933, Germany had been the most scientifically advanced country in the world. Hitler was a zealous reformed smoker (Franco and Mussolini were also non-smokers while Churchill, Stalin and Roosevelt were heavy smokers). The Nazification of German science was paralleled by a national campaign against the dangers of tobacco addiction and it was portrayed as antipathetic to the Nazis' central tenet of racial dominance: Strength through Joy. Doctors had been active participants in the Nazi project and joined Hitler's National Socialist Party in greater numbers than any other profession (45 per cent were party members, compared with 20 per cent of

---

* On 21 December 1971 in the *Oxford Mail*, Doll was reported as saying that it is not always essential to argue on health grounds alone, but if you do then certainly the facts must be right. "Take diesel fumes. They're extremely unpleasant and, they ought to be curtailed for this reason alone. But to argue that they cause disease is extremely dangerous, without the facts. Hill and I couldn't relate them at all to lung cancer and years of study have shown that it's extremely difficult to show they have any effect. My own personal view is that you should be prepared to oppose pollution on aesthetic grounds, not always to bring in health when the evidence may not be very clear. The trouble is people often get worked up about the less harmful things while they tend to ignore the ones that are actually harmful."

teachers). Doll had fought against all that the Nazi Party represented, yet when it came to examining scientific discoveries he invoked the ideals that Charles Darwin believed a scientist should exhibit—to have no wishes, no affections: a heart of stone.

The chaos that followed the outbreak of the Second World War had a distorting effect on science, on its discoveries and its obligations to history. For example, in 1948 Willem Wassink in Holland communicated a case-control study, larger than that of Müller, which also deserves a place in the accumulated knowledge of the dangers of tobacco.[30]

The contribution of Schairer and Schöniger is significant for two reasons. Firstly, it is important for what Doll called their "percipient" discussion on the meaning of their findings, and secondly, for the accusation that Doll and Hill were neglectful for not acknowledging the work in their 1950 paper and, more seriously, that Doll had acted perfidiously—consciously not referencing this earlier epidemiological investigation.

Schairer and Schöniger's work was financed by Karl Astel's Institute for Tobacco Hazards Research founded in 1941 at Jena University with a 100,000-Reichsmark grant from Hitler's chancellery. However, the issue of *Zeitschrift für Krebsforschung* in which Schairer and Schöniger's paper appeared did not arrive in Britain during the war and was not catalogued in the cumulative medical index. At the same time, post-war West German society tended to disregard scientific research sponsored by the Nazi regime, as to respect it contravened the accepted wisdom that National Socialism was redolent of depravity and a bestial disregard of humanity. What is undeniable, however, is that the combined studies of Müller and of Schairer and Schöniger (both were small, with a combined total of 179 lung cancers) helped initiate anti-tobacco legislation including the banning of smoking in many public places by the Nazi Party.

Doll and Hill's report, published in the *British Medical Journal* in 1952, cited all the American, German and British studies as being mutually supporting. Equally indisputable was Doll's recognition of their work in a paper in 1963 when he wrote, "The first studies [retrospective inquiries] were carried out in Germany more than 20 years ago (Müller, 1939;

Schairer and Schöniger 1943).*

Much later, in 1994, Schairer and Schöniger's study was liberated from relative historical oblivion by Davey Smith, Ströbele and Egger[31] whose thought-provoking article led Doll to re-examine the contribution made by German scientists:

> Judged by the modern standards of epidemiology, Schairer and Schöniger's work fails on several grounds: (1) the small number of cases of lung cancer (93 men and 16 women), (2) the use of surrogate informants for the patients who had died from cancer and living inform- ants for information about themselves for the controls, (3) the low response rate to the questionnaires about the cancer patients (53 per cent for those with lung cancer, 40-60 per cent for those with cancers of the tongue, oesophagus, stomach, colon, and prostate, and an even lower rate [39 per cent] for the controls) and (4) the use of controls in only one narrow age group (53-54 years) selected to correspond with the average age of the lung cancer patients (53.9).

Schairer was a professor of pathology and Schöniger was his doctoral student and the deficiencies of their study led themselves to observe "the association between tobacco consumption and lung cancer is therefore statistically, and causally only likely" and that "larger investigations are required." These larger investigations were carried out by Doll and Hill, and their discovery of new unimpeachable methods of control for bias and measurement of statistical error pointed with greater clarity towards proof of causation.

Schairer and Schöniger were not the only scientists to have sought a correlation between smoking and premature death whose work was dis- carded or forgotten. In 1938, Raymond Pearl,** an American statistician

---

*   'Investigation into Cigarette Smoking and Atmospheric Pollution in the Aetiology of Lung Cancer', *Methods of Information in Medicine*, 1963; Vol. 2, No 1, pp. 13- 19.

**   In a letter to the *Financial Times* in June 2004 Samuel Grober wrote: "Without in any way detracting from Sir Richard's (Sir Richard Doll "Tobacco's Nemesis" 26

at the Metropolitan Life Assurance Company, recognised the deleterious effects of smoking from studies of family history records taken from the Johns Hopkins School of Hygiene and Public Health. "The smoking of tobacco was statistically associated with an impairment of life duration and the amount of degree of this impairment increased as the habitual amount of smoking increased."[32]

In his scholarly work, *The Nazi War on Cancer*, Robert N Proctor, an American historian of science, examined the work of German scientists into tobacco addiction and the reasons why they had been neglected by historiography. "Müller's pre-war paper is occasionally cited, but Schairer and Schöniger's is little known. A 1953 German bibliography on the smoking-cancer link does not even mention Schairer and Schöniger's paper; nor does an otherwise admirable 1990 historical review of lung cancer-tobacco epidemiology."[33] Proctor went on: "Sir Richard Doll, the man most often credited with documenting the link, told me in February of 1997 that he had never seen the Schöniger and Schairer piece. (I sent him a copy.) Science can be a forgetful enterprise."[34] Proctor is a great admirer of Doll, but certainly does not credit him as the discoverer of the cigarette-lung cancer link. "Doll's work was of a deepening and synthesis, and discovery of new methods of control for bias and measurement of statistical error. One could almost say that Doll proved the case to smokers."[35]

Doll did not like sloppy ideas. He could read German, and it was unthinkable that he would reference a scientific paper if he had not read it. Moreover, non-infectious disease epidemiology was in its infancy,

---

June 2004) accomplishments, it is pertinent here to mention the work of Dr Raymond Pearl at Johns Hopkins University in Baltimore in the late 1920s and 1930s. His research clearly showed the correlation between smoking and cancer and his work was published in the contemporary journals. I know this because I was a graduate student in the botany department at the University of Maryland agricultural experiment station in 1938 to 1942. Dr Mark Woods, our professor of plant pathology, who specialised in diseases of tobacco, repeatedly told his smoking students of Dr Pearl's work and tried to get them to quit smoking."

there were few serious papers to read, and even fewer practitioners in the field. Perhaps one explanation for Doll's statement to Proctor was that he meant he had not seen the German paper while preparing the 1950 case-control study with Hill. Doll and Hill were not the first medical researchers to establish a link between tobacco and lung cancer, but what they did was to nail the subject down using solid science and new theories of causation.

A qualitative difference exists between the strength of the scientific evidence about cigarette smoking and lung cancer that was available in the 1940s and the 1950s. Proctor did not think Doll's neglect of German tobacco research was a matter of perfidy. "I think it's more a matter of forgetfulness, combined with a pinch of self-aggrandisement (as one often finds in great men). Doll may well have read Schairer and Schöniger's paper at some point and then simply forgotten that he'd read it... I know, though, that he was not terribly happy about my having unearthed this earlier German work."[36]

Doll believed that "science will always win in the end" but that science does not take place in an historical void; scientists can become heretics, heroes, or casualties of history. He addressed these themes in 2001 when summing up the Nazi-sponsored investigation into tobacco smoking and death. "Schairer and Schöniger's article marks an important phase in the development of knowledge about the harmful effects of tobacco and has, until now, failed to receive the recognition that it deserves. It would be wrong, however, to suggest that it proved, beyond reasonable doubt, that smoking was an important cause of the disease, a conclusion that the authors themselves never claimed."[37]

Questions in Parliament from Somerville Hastings, by then a veteran Labour MP and founding president of the Socialist Medical Association from 1930-51, together with mounting epidemiological evidence and equivocal media reporting of the possible relationship between smoking and death had the effect of bringing the Imperial Tobacco Company into the debate.[38] The company was highly respected and generated over 14 per cent of the government's tax revenues, so its vital place in the nation's financial well-being was conspicuous to the treasury. This political leverage enabled the company to gain access to Doll and Hill at the London School of Hygiene and Tropical Medicine in November 1952.

Doll and Hill were prepared for the encounter. The Imperial Tobacco delegation included its secretary EJ Partridge, DA Clarke, an economist, and Geoffrey Todd, their statistician. Dr FHK Green, the assistant secretary of the MRC, took the minutes. Even at this early stage, the tobacco industry was suspicious of Doll* and would have preferred him to be absent from the meeting as he "seemed to have made up his mind on the subject".[39] The meeting, as Doll recalled, was friendly (indeed, for many years the relationship between Doll and the British tobacco industry was polite) and centred around three statistical points raised by Todd.

> Firstly, that smoking histories were too unreliable to use, secondly, that the correlation between cigarette consumption and lung cancer in different countries was too small, only 0.5, and thirdly, that lung cancer was obviously due to atmospheric pollution. Bradford Hill responded that if smoking histories were unreliable this must have made the association appear weaker than it actually is, the correlation coefficient** was unusually high and should be regarded as strengthening our conclusions, and that if lung cancer was due to atmospheric pollution, go and show it because we could not! That rather set them back.[40]

---

*   Dr Neville Goodman, the senior medical officer in the Ministry of Health responsible for cancer, wrote to Green with information that the company wanted "to repeat on a larger scale the Doll-Hill inquiry, in which they claimed many flaws".

**   The correlation coefficient has played an important part in the history of statistical methods. It is used to measure the relationship between two variables. To understand this point it is easiest to think in the extremes—it can range from -1 to 1. The correlation is the degree to which things (variables) change together (their co-relation). This can be measured and it is called the correlation coeffi-

None the less, Todd carried out a study based on his initial statistical objection, which Imperial Tobacco wanted submitted to the SACCR as a counterbalance to Doll and Hill. Such action was to be expected. What was less predictable were the objections raised by the pathologist Richard Passey. He voiced his scepticism of a too easy acceptance of the thesis that the great majority of lung cancers were due to excessive cigarette smoking. Instead, he postulated that lung cancer manifested itself at a particular time of life, not after a latent period determined by carcinogenic dose and length of time of exposure.[41] In February 1953 he conveyed his misgivings in the *British Medical Journal*: "When doctors disagree it is bad for the patient. It may be that a proportion of lung cancers in man are induced by tobacco smoking: at the moment we do not know, but let us be sure of our evidence before we scare our public. As a profession we have that responsibility."[42]

This criticism of Doll and Hill led Sir John Charles to seek outside arbitration in the form of a panel of experts led by Sir George Maddex, the government actuary. After weighing the evidence the statistical panel vindicated Doll and Hill and recommended as proven "that there is a real association between smoking and cancer of the lung".[43] On 23 November, years of campaigning by Joules were grudgingly recognised when the SACCR recommended:

> The evidence was sufficient to justify advising the minister that the association was real and that the panel's suggestion that the association was causal was acceptable. Young persons should be warned of the risk attendant on smoking and it should be made clear that the risk apparently increased in proportion to the amount of tobacco smoked. The risk from cigarette smoking was apparently greater than from other forms of smoking.

---

cient. The important thing to remember is that the values are associated. The 0.5 figure established by Doll and Hill is a relatively strong correlation for this type (smoking and its relationship to lung cancer) of ecological association.

Yet far from being rewarded for dedication to public health, Joules lost his place on the SACCR, although he retained membership of the Central Health Service Council; he was perceived as a member of the "awkward squad", a political troublemaker.

The tobacco industry, moreover, kept up its scepticism. In December 1953 Sir Alexander Maxwell, representing the tobacco industry, gave Himsworth a memorandum reaffirming the industry's doubts about Doll and Hill's work and making an offer of £250,000 to the MRC "for specific research into the real cause of cancer of the lung".[44]

The politicians were reticent for another reason. Iain Macleod, the Conservative minister of health, was acknowledged as a man of insight and ability.[45] However, in 1954 while the government knew something of the harm smoking did, it needed the tax revenue so much that it did not want prevention to succeed. For Doll it was another notable example of the way government policies were determined in a market economy. Before making a public announcement on the dangers of smoking, Macleod wrote to John Boyd-Carpenter, the financial secretary:

> I need not say anything about the financial implication of any ill-considered statement in this field for we all know that the Welfare State and much else is based on tobacco smoking. I would, however, like to make a point here about the political implications of delay. Moreover, the prime mover in all this is a man [it can only have been Horace Joules] of extremely advanced left-wing opinions and would not hesitate to embarrass the government if nothing appears soon... My only anxiety is to make whatever statement should be made as quietly as is possible but I feel that we must move soon if events are not to overtake us.[46]

On 11 February 1954 Macleod called a press conference at which he announced that the tobacco companies had offered £250,000 to the MRC for further research into the subject. He also spoke about the ambiguous nature of the debate while paying tribute to the pioneering work of Doll and Hill and other workers "who have given us what information we have".

What was most striking about Macleod's statement on the strong reasons for refraining from smoking was that he chain-smoked four cigarettes while making it.

Later that year, Doll and Hill published their preliminary findings on the adverse health consequences of cigarette smoking on British doctors.[47] The findings with regard to lung cancer had confirmed those predicted from the retrospective case-control studies. On relatively small numbers—789 deaths had occurred among male British doctors, and of those 36 were from lung cancer—the researchers felt sufficiently confident to write of the increases in mortality from non-smokers to "light" smokers, from "light" smokers to "medium" smokers, and finally from "medium" smokers to "heavy" smokers. The study was also notable for the discovery of a previously unforeseen cause of death. "The resulting rates reveal a significant and steadily rising mortality from deaths due to cancer of the lung as the amount of tobacco smoked increases. There is also a rise in the mortality from deaths attributed to coronary thrombosis as the amount smoked increases." It had not escaped their notice that the specific association postulated made it incumbent upon them to conclude: "We thought it necessary, in view of the nature of the results, to lay these preliminary observations before the survivors of the 40,000 men and women who made them possible."

Importantly, a short time later, the results in the United States from the once sceptical Hammond, based on almost 5,000 deaths in 190,000 American men had shown a correlation between smoking and lung cancer and smoking and coronary disease.[48]

On Thursday 24 June, Doll and Hill gave their conclusions to hundreds of guests at a Royal Society *conversazione* in Burlington House, Piccadilly. The *Daily Mail* reported that Doll had succeeded in persuading his wife Joan to stop her forty cigarettes a day habit. "My husband bribed me to give up smoking. He gave me £10, and with the money which I had already saved I went out and bought a dress."[49]

One of the major contributions of the study to public health medicine—and one that Doll and Hill did not predict—was that once doctors understood that smoking was not just killing their patients, they realised it was also killing them. As a result they became the first social group in Britain to give up in large numbers. Knowledge that quitting could have such a dramatic effect on death rates would, in time, advance public health medicine as profoundly as the introduction of inoculation or the therapeutic application of penicillin.

Chapter 9

Man's Relationship with His Environment

"The objective of science is to gain power to control nature in the interests of humanity."[1]

Richard Doll

There was never an occasion when Doll regretted the sacrifice that the Second World War had imposed on his life. The six years of conflict had, after all, been exciting if sometimes dangerous and to him, as a committed anti-fascist, of political necessity; however, they were irreclaimable. No British generation had been asked to forfeit so much productive time for the cause of national survival. As a result, Doll was on a determined course. Free of obfuscation and under Hill's leadership he applied himself with inimitable single-mindedness to the cause of saving people from avoidable diseases and premature death. Fortunately for medical research—particularly at the beginning of his career—he had few interests outside science. Joan helped fill this cultural lacuna, and with the years came a greater artistic hinterland and a growing love for literature and the intellectual freedom it afforded him.*

In the five years from 1951 to 1955, while following up the deaths of British doctors, Doll published (alone or as a co-author) 26 papers—nine

---

* On 8 July 2003 Doll gave a graduation address to medical students at Aberdeen University. While listing the great advances in medical research over the previous hundred years he used literature as an aid to navigating the future. "But if the world changes, and changes in some respects dramatically, as I suspect it will, one thing will not change, or rather will continue to change only very slowly and on an evolutionary scale, and that is the psychology of the people who inhabit it. Those of you who will deal directly with patients will still be dealing with irrational fears and jealousies, with greed and aggression, with stoicism and self-sacrifice, and, as

dealing with gastroenterology, thirteen with cancer and four with miscellaneous subjects. In 1954 he collaborated with Peter Armitage in a study of the age distribution of human cancers and a multi-stage theory of carcinogenesis to explain it. This watershed study—in the era before molecular biology—set in train a path of mathematical reasoning to explain the progression of the disease at a biological level.

Politics and science moved in parallel for Doll. On 25 May 1951 Guy Burgess and Donald Maclean fled the United Kingdom after they had been exposed for passing valuable intelligence to the Soviet Union. The men defected three days before a planned interrogation by MI5 after being tipped off by US-based fellow Cambridge spy Kim Philby. Also in that year, Doll co-founded—with, among others, Joan, Lionel Penrose, Horace Joules and Ian Gilliland—the Medical Association for the Prevention of War (MAPW). Doll became its first president and was on the editorial advisory panel of its journal *Medicine and War*. (This scientific alliance pre-dated the Russell-Einstein Manifesto,** which was established in July 1955 while the Cold War was at its most intense.)

The formation of such a moral-force scientific pressure group carried great risks of censure for its members. Jean Gilliland recognised the danger

---

I still believe, with a majority who are simply seeking experienced advice and are grateful for it. Our professional education does not, however, prepare us to recognise and respond appropriately to all these facets of human nature—at least it does not in England. What does is good literature: Tolstoy's *Anna Karenina* and *War and Peace*, George Eliot's *Middlemarch*, Vikram Seth's wonderful account of Hindu and Muslim life in *A Suitable Boy*, and Bernhard Schlink's account of German adjustment to the post-Hitler world in *The Reader*. How much more fit we are to deal with the ineluctable facts of real life, when we have read such novels."

** On 9 July 1955, Bertrand Russell read what became known as the Russell-Einstein manifesto at a press conference in London. Signing the manifesto was one of the final acts of Albert Einstein's life. In a letter to Einstein on 5 April 1955, Russell wrote: "I have been turning over in my mind, and discussing with various people, the best steps for giving effect to the feeling against war among the great majority

her husband faced from the political status quo: "It was a big deal. Did they have to think twice? I think they did, but they were so full of conviction, that they looked upon it as something they had to do."[2]

The MAPW announced its existence on 20 January 1951 in a letter to *The Lancet*: "We appeal to all our fellow doctors who think there may yet be an alternative to merely providing treatment for casualties; we ask them to join us, in the spirit of our chosen profession of healing, in doing all in their power to halt preparation for war and to bring about a new and determined approach to the peaceful settlement of disputes and to world disarmament."

On 17 February 1951, the group, again in a letter in *The Lancet*, voiced their opposition to warmongering paranoia:

> It is not, in our opinion, true that the sole danger of war rests with the Russian aggressiveness. Clearly it would not be possible to reach agreement here on what constitute real threats from the east; but the nature of propaganda makes it inherently likely that some, at least, of the published threats are exaggerated. Moreover, we believe, that some recent actions of the western powers may not unreasonably be interpreted by others as being aggressive (whatever have been the intentions behind them). To specify, there is the advance beyond the 38th parallel in Korea, the occupation of Formosa, the decision to build a new German army, and the release of Krupp and other Nazi supporters.

The period reflected the kind of paranoia portrayed in Stanley Kubrick's film, *Dr Strangelove*. Certainly Doll and his medical colleagues believed the rumours that America favoured a "first-strike" on the Soviet Union before it became too strong and had its own weapons of mass

---

of men of science. I think the first step should be a statement by men of highest eminence, communists and anti-communists, western and eastern, about the disasters to be expected in a war."

destruction. The response in US military circles was one of "rude shock"[3] at the Soviet Union's success in exploding its first atom bomb in 1949— four years before western intelligence predicted—and this led many Americans to make up their minds that war with Russia was inevitable and America should make the first move. British intelligence warned Prime Minister Winston Churchill in the early 1950s that the US was ready to wage a "preventive" atomic war on the Soviet Union. The director of naval intelligence, Vice-Admiral Eric Longley-Cook, warned Whitehall that the Americans' fascination with the ideas of preventive war was fuelled by McCarthyism and spread beyond the US defence department into the minds of the American people.[4] Churchill's initial scepticism was dispelled after detecting for himself an increasingly warlike mood in Washington during a visit to President Harry Truman in 1952 when he failed to secure a veto on the US nuclear strikes from British bases.

It was against this political background that Doll's work developed. From his student days Doll had been interested in the social environment as a cause of disease. There were a number of important occupational diseases that were then prevalent, with lead poisoning being the most characteristic one. Dating from the epidemiological work of the English surgeon Percival Pott (1714-88) linking scrotal cancer to the soot to which child chimney-sweeps were exposed, work-related diseases had attracted medical investigation, if little government regulation

When Doll began to work with Hill investigating the reasons for the dramatic increase in the mortality attributed to lung cancer, his attention was drawn to the analysis of the national mortality data that the Kennaways had carried out in 1947, which showed the disproportionate frequency with which occupations in the coal gas industry were referred to when lung cancer was recorded as the cause of death. In view of the fact that the manufacture of coal gas caused many workers to be exposed to fumes from partially combusted coal, which was likely to contain powerful carcinogens, their findings were highly suggestive, but they were not considered proof of a hazard. This, Doll thought, would be obtained if he could define a cohort of gas workers, divide them according to the extent of their exposure and follow them up to see how their mortality from lung cancer compared with the national average.

He therefore approached an old friend, Dr REW Fisher, medical officer to the South East Metropolitan Gas Company, and Fisher drew up a list of company pensioners classified to their last occupation—a classification which, if far from perfect, clearly separated those who worked in the ovens known as retort houses, where exposure might occur, from those who worked outside in people's houses. Follow-up soon showed that the retort house workers had about double the "normal" mortality for the disease. Doll and Fisher wrote a paper describing the findings, but by this time the gas industry had been nationalised and permission for Fisher to publish his findings was refused.

Fortunately Doll was an independent worker, employed by the MRC, and he published the findings without reference to Fisher's crucial help.[5] This cohort study's aim was to compare the mortality experience of subgroups, such as high exposure with low exposure, in order to establish whether exposure to the agent might be contributing to mortality. As well as alerting the industry and its workforce to the carcinogenic hazard (due to the large amounts of benzpyrene in the air) the study was also memorable for incorporating an advance in statistical analysis.* The survey was continued and expanded, successfully defining the limits of the hazard, and showed there also included a risk of scrotal cancer (which had been suspected).

Coal gas, at the time of the study, contained a material proportion of carbon monoxide (a common way of committing suicide was to turn on

---

* This is one of the first examples of the person-years method. In this approach the number of deaths in the group, or in the subgroups, is expressed in terms of the number of deaths expected if the individuals had experienced the same death rates as the population of which the group is part. In this case it was the existence of the disease in the workers (25 deaths against 13.8) compared to that of male inhabitants, of the same age distribution, of metropolitan London.

the gas and lie down with one's head in the gas oven). In the late 1950s the annual number of suicides began to increase, accounted for wholly by an increased number due to gas poisoning. Dr Frank Tym, medical officer to one of the four regional gas boards collaborating in the study, believed that the proportion of carbon monoxide in the gas provided by the board was progressively increasing and had reached the dangerous level of 13 per cent. Doll persuaded the Medical Research Council to draw attention to the increasing number of suicides and seek information about the carbon monoxide content of gas. To his surprise the MRC was told by the Ministry of Supply that the carbon monoxide levels were unknown and that there was no information to suggest an increasing trend. Some years later, with the expansion of North Sea gas, the carbon monoxide content began to be reduced and so did incidences of gas poisoning—until eventually there was none. (Interestingly, there was no contemporaneous increase in suicide from other methods and it looked as if many potential suicides, no longer able to put their head in the gas oven, decided not to kill themselves at all.*)

Not all great medical advances change the course of clinical knowledge. Occasionally, however, there are certain discoveries of such originality that they expand the previously assumed limits of medicine. In 1954 Doll helped establish the principles of cancer progression and epidemiology in mathematical form, decades before modern molecular biology advanced our understanding of genetics and evolution. In collaboration with Peter

---

* The marked decline of suicide rates in England and Wales following detoxification of the domestic gas supply during the 1960s and 1970s was profound. Between 1963 and 1975 the national rate declined by three per cent precisely in step with the decline in gas toxicity. The absence of displacement to other methods was a truly striking societal phenomenon.

Armitage—another member of Hill's MRC statistical research unit—they proposed a sequential stage of cancer induction that could be measured, and possibly predicted.

The evidence of human cancer incidence seemed to show that most of the common cancers increased very rapidly with age. This increase begins at about the age of twenty and continues at least until the age of 75 and probably beyond. Armitage and Doll set out to establish a theoretical law of cancer risk in individuals that would explain the epidemiologically observed patterns of the disease in large populations. They built a mathematical theory that sought a quantitative explanation for the stages of progression, the rates of change between stages and the consequences of the rate for incidence in populations.

Doll had been impressed by the work of CO Nordling[6] who, using statistics for cancer in men from Britain, France, Norway and the US, proposed a probability model of intriguing symmetry: that over the age range 25-74 years, the death rate increased proportionately with the sixth power of age. He also believed that the observed relationship would be explained if a cancer cell was the end result of seven successive mutations.* Moreover, the nineteenth-century hypothesis, that biological ageing increases the susceptibility of certain tissues to the induction of cancer, had been supplanted by a new theoretical concept. In his monograph on the pathology of cancer, RA Willis wrote, "We now know that cancer is a disease of the elderly, not because senile tissues predispose to cancer, as was once supposed, but because of the unusually long latent period elapsing between the application of carcinogenic stimuli and the development

---

*   In 1951 Fisher and Hollomon advanced the theory that the observed relationship between age and mortality could result if about six or seven cells were transformed independently. However, Armitage and Doll showed that if transformation happens by one step in each of several independent cells, then tumour incidence should increase with about the sixth power of carcinogenic dose. Instead incidence rises approximately linearly with dose, thereby making Fisher and Hollomon's hypothesis untenable.

of tumours. Occupational and experimental tumours show that these periods often occupy large fractions of the life spans of the affected animals."[7] Doll and Armitage believed that in some tissues the carcinogenic process required such a long time to be completed that the disease could appear only rarely at young ages.

Efforts to derive theoretical laws from changes in the death rates with age were not new, but it was not until the middle of the twentieth century that attempts were made to build a mathematical model for mortality from cancer. Armitage and Doll were not only collaborators, they were also friends. Working in rooms on the same corridor at the London School of Hygiene and Tropical Medicine, they developed an intellectual liquefaction. Through scientific intuition, innovative reasoning and analysis of the statistical data, they established a biological theory of the process of "multiple mutations" that even today, in the era of high throughput genomics, is widely accepted. Armitage intuitively understood the medical and biological rationale behind Doll's imaginative thinking:

> Richard's idea was that several specific changes had to take place, in a specific order. He had been impressed by animal experiments, particularly by Berenblum and Shubik, showing that some carcinogenic agents are effective mainly at the start of an induction period, whereas others have full effect when applied near the end. He also wanted to ensure that an external agent would affect the chance of only one change at a time, so as to preserve a proportionate dose-response relationship.[8]

Doll, with Hill, had shown this association between smoking and lung cancer: it was one of the reasons why people began to believe in the science of epidemiology.

Although a few of the rare genetic conditions may strongly predispose to cancer, and some more common genetic conditions may less strongly predispose to it, there is no such thing as genetic immunity from cancer. Cancer arises from a combination of three elements: nature, nurture and luck. In large populations nature and luck appear to average out and only nurture remains as a subject for quantifiable inquiry.

One of the elements responsible for the great leap forward in understanding causal relationships in the pathogenesis of cancer was the growing availability of reliable vital statistics. Even for a thinker of such virtuosity as Nordling, one of his observations reveals the evolutionary nature of the discipline:

> Among the multitude of still unexplained statistical data concerning cancer, mention might be made of the great difference in cancer frequency between whites in the north-eastern United States and among those living in the southern part of the country, as well as between Negroes in these two parts. The fact that environment rather than race appears to be responsible for these differences is encouraging, since it indicates the possibility of greatly reducing the incidence of cancer.[9]

Nordling was correct in positing the importance of the environment, or rather the personal behaviour of the people living in the north-eastern part of the country. The excess of cancer, in all probability, was due to the higher levels of cigarette consumption.[10]

Nordling's innovative probability model stated that the observed relationship between age and mortality would be explained if a cancer cell were the end result of seven successive changes and if the occurrence of each mutation remained *constant* throughout life. What Doll and Armitage set out to do was to examine the relationship between mortality and age for cancer of different sites for each sex, and to see whether Nordling's hypothesis could account for the data when it is recognised that the strength of the carcinogenic factors may be variable. In building their mathematical analysis they did not assume that the changes leading to the development of cancer were necessarily mutational. In their groundbreaking 1954 paper they wrote, "All that needs be postulated is that the changes of state should be specific and discrete and that each stage should be stable. It will be assumed that the changes must proceed in a unique order."

Everyone is exposed to carcinogens and our DNA is constantly being bombarded by internal and external pathogens, which, in early life, one assumes, are being successfully repelled by tumour suppressants. With the progress of time, this defence mechanism becomes confused or weakened and as a consequence is less resilient. One of the effects of ageing is to increase the chance of cell division. This implies that, for the development of tumorous cells, it is necessary for a certain number of cellular divisions to have taken place, between each of which there has been a certain period of time.

The concept of carcinogenesis as a multi-stage process also makes it easier to understand the mechanism of the latent period, which occurs after exposure to a carcinogenic agent before the appearance of a tumour. Armitage and Doll found one of "nature's experiments" compelling in a mathematical sense and in terms of how the disease might evolve. In 1947 Kennaway had demonstrated that circumcision postponed until the fourteenth year of life failed to give the complete protection against cancer of the penis that it provided when carried out on the eighth day, as in the Jewish faith; in other words, some change must take place within the first 14 years of life which eventually leads to the development of the disease after a latent period which may be as long as seventy years.

At the outset Doll and Armitage would have thought it unlikely that a single theory of carcinogenesis would explain data from such different sources as animal experiments and human mortality and morbidity records, each subject to many difficulties of recording and interpretation. Recognising it to be fortuitous, they nevertheless welcomed the discovery that their primitive model fitted such a wide variety of data. Armitage acknowledged that their model was simple and naïve.

> It assumed a succession of six or seven specific changes in a cell line, each change occurring at a specific but constant rate. It predicted the power law observed for many sites, at least as a good approximation, and we suggested that the departure found for other sites could be explained either by fluctuating external carcinogenic agents or hormonal effects. We did not regard our model as anything but a crude

representation of what might be happening. However, it enabled us to explore the possible effect of external agents applied at different times.[11]

Doll's own work on industrial lung cancer confirmed this temporal phenomenon. After following men who were employed for at least five years in the retort houses of various gasworks he found cancer incidence to have been higher in men who were first exposed at age 30 years or over than among those who were first exposed at age 25 years.[12]

On the hypothesis that cancer is a multi-stage process, the incidence of the disease will depend on the periods when the carcinogenic factors are most active and on the stages in the process of carcinogenesis affected. This insight led Doll and Armitage to consider a varying rate of production of the *first* of a chain of *six* changes:

> An increased rate of production for a short time during early life will provide a larger number of altered cells to be acted upon by other factors in the future, and will therefore appreciably affect the incidence at, say, age 60. The same increased rate of production of the first change applied for the same short period during middle age will, on the other hand, have little effect on the incidence at age 60, since there will be but little time left for the altered cells to be acted upon.[13]

Such an observation had a profound effect on Doll and subsequently on public health medicine. By 1954 Doll and Hill were convinced of the dangers of tobacco and felt morally obliged to alert the British doctors of the hazards of continuing to smoke. Biologically, there was no *a priori* reason to suspect that once a smoker—who may have been smoking for twenty years—had quit that the elevated danger of getting lung cancer would recede. Initially, Hill did not believe that stopping would do any good[14] and when it became clear that those doctors who stopped smoking materially reduced their chance of getting the disease Armitage and Doll's multi-stage theory of carcinogenesis was confirmed. For, in a multi-stage process, if the first stage were involved, the rate after stopping smoking would continue to rise in the same way as for continuing smokers. If, on the other hand, the last stage was affected, one would expect the rate to drop immediately to the rate for non-smokers and to follow the rise for non-smokers. In fact, what Doll later discovered was that no delay occurs before the effects of stopping can be seen, as tobacco smoke affects both early and late stages in the process of cancer induction. The incidence of the disease will, therefore, stabilise almost immediately when smoking is stopped instead of increasingly progressively with age.[15]

In the case of human biology if we have more than one of something, we often have two. At the time of writing the paper on the multi-stage theory of carcinogenesis Doll had only one kidney. Perhaps his altered anatomical state will serve as a good example of how the theory could be applied to a real life and death situation. As Doll only had one working kidney, an accident or infection to that kidney would kill him. Suppose that the chance of knocking out that kidney is the same tomorrow as it is the next day, and the day after, and so on. If, among those other people with only one kidney, we measure the fraction of surviving individuals who die because of failure of that one kidney on each day, that fraction will be constant over time. Each day brings the same unchanging risk per day for those who have survived. The rate of risk per day is constant, neither accelerating not decelerating with time.

Now, consider those who have two working kidneys. To die of kidney failure, they must suffer two events: first loss of one of their kidneys, followed by the loss of the second. In this case, the probability of failure per day increases with the passing of time. This acceleration of the death rate with time happens as follows. We must first wait for the loss of the first kidney. The probability of losing the first kidney increases with time. Then, after the loss of the first, we must wait for the loss of the second. The loss of the second happens at the same rate each day. So the death rate is the probability that the first kidney is diseased, which increases with time, and the rate at which the second kidney fails, which happens at the same rate each day.

The key is that one must multiply two different kinds of number to get the death rate. The first is the probability that all steps except the last one have happened. That probability is the amount of time that has passed raised to the number of steps to get to the point that only one more step remains. The second is the rate per day (or year) that the final step happens.*

For those with quantitative intuition this formula may be instructive:

Cumulative probability = constant x $(time)6$

X = cumulative probability of getting lung cancer by 35

$X = (1/2x1/2x\ 1/2x1/2x1/2x1/2)\ P$

NB annual probability proportional to $2x\ (1/2)6 = (1/2)5$

[--]
Infant   35   70

Cumulative probability of getting lung cancer by 70 =P

Six different things have to happen in one cell (maybe with some restrictions on the order they can happen in, maybe not).

Six "stages" = lifelong cumulative probability x (age) 6
Which means annual probability x (age)5

Epidemiology is about prediction, and in 1954 Armitage and Doll proposed a probability model of cancer induction based on the experiments that were taking place in nature. They did not know what was happening at the cellular level, and in fact we still do not know much more today. We know that in a great majority of cancers** a number of changes

---

*   This example is entirely the brainchild of Steven A. Frank. I have merely superimposed Doll's actual physical state onto the multi-stage theory. Doll lived for more than 61 years with one kidney.
** About ninety per cent of all cancers worldwide are epithelial cancers.

have to take place in a cell and a number of these changes have to take place in the DNA of the cell before a malignant change will be initiated which will turn into cancer. However, the precise mechanism is not yet known.

About ten per cent of lung cancers occur in non-smokers, but in statistical terms it is a rare disease in this population. Doll recognised both the play of chance and the role of nature, nurture and luck in the mechanism of cancer induction.

> The fact that only, say, 20 per cent of heavy cigarette smokers would develop lung cancer by 75 years of age in the absence of other causes of death does not mean the 80 per cent are genetically immune to the disease any more than the fact that usually only one cancer occurs in a given tissue implies that all the stem cells in the tissue that have not given rise to a malignant clone are also genetically immune. What it does mean is that whether an exposed subject does or does not develop a cancer is largely a matter of luck; bad luck if the several necessary changes all occur in the same cell when there are thousands of such cells at risk, good luck if they don't.[16]

The American biologist Steven A Frank spent three years researching the future consequences of the Armitage and Doll theory. In his book *Dynamics of Cancer Incidence, Inheritance, and Evolution*,[17] which builds on the intellectual achievements of the multi-stage model, Frank posits that quantitative perspective may become increasingly important in cancer studies. The mathematical modelling structure proposed by Armitage and Doll will still be insightful in connecting genetic changes to biological pathways as, if things remain the same—which they undoubtedly will not—a third of us will develop cancer and a quarter of us may die of it.

As president of the Medical Association for the Prevention of War, Doll's interest in radiation had been further heightened in 1952 when

Britain became the world's third atomic power. Before the Second World War there was little reliable knowledge about radiation. There were X-rays, and small amounts of radium were in existence, but its use was limited to doctors and scientists. Radium was an extremely rare material whose production could be measured in grams; but after the war it was manufactured in kilograms and tons. No one knew what hazards this revolution in its use might bring, and it was not until some years after the war that it became possible to study the effects of radiation accurately.

In Britain, the International X-ray and Radium Protection Committee had been in existence before 1939, and then went into abeyance during the war. The new nuclear world was seen by Ernest Rock Carling and WV Mayneord, professor of physics at the Institute of Cancer Research at the Royal Marsden Hospital, as one of unimaginable changes. What was needed was a new committee. Out of their determination to understand and measure the new hazards of radiation came, in 1950, the International Committee on Radiological Protection (ICRP).

Doll, too, wanted to understand the science that led to the devastation of Hiroshima and Nagasaki, and more importantly to gauge the repercussions of America's H-bomb on the health of the world's population. Accordingly, early in 1954, he enrolled on a course on radiological hazards at Sir John Cass Institute in London.

In the autumn of 1952 preparations had begun at Bikini atoll for the American thermonuclear weapons tests, which were to begin in March 1954. The *Bravo* bomb weighed 23,500lbs, and was mounted seventeen feet above sea level. On 1 March at 6.45 am, the countdown began on the planned explosion of the five- to six-megaton yield H-bomb. Within one minute a fireball rose to 45,000 feet sucking up debris into a tenebrous cloud that reached to the edge of the atmosphere. Due to a miscalculation the explosion was far greater than predicted—nearer fifteen megatons (colossally more powerful than the bomb dropped on Hiroshima). It was the biggest test explosion the Americans ever carried out. In addition to military personnel and local inhabitants being exposed to radiation fall-out, the entire crew of the unfortunately named *Lucky*

Dragon, a Japanese fishing boat 85 miles from the hypocentre of the explosion, were also contaminated.

The fear that science, in a destructive application, could now endanger cities, peoples and the entire developed world set off a political chain reaction. The Japanese demanded a formal inquiry, and the fear that the new generation of H-bombs could obliterate the largest city on earth alarmed the American people.*

Concern over the H-bomb was also voiced by powerful forces outside the United States: Prime Minister Nehru of India, the philosopher Albert Schweitzer and Pope Pius XII, who in his 1954 Easter message called for efforts to ban nuclear war. But nowhere was the debate more vigorous and long lasting than in Britain. Radioactivity was literally "blowing in the wind" and people began to realise how little was known about it. Operation Gandhi, the Committee of 100, and the Campaign for Nuclear Disarmament coalesced into a powerful moral and physical movement determined to neutralise the nuclear threat. *Bravo*'s destructive horror created a worldwide movement that was to have a powerful effect on the nuclear weapons programmes of the superpowers and Britain, and ultimately led to the partial Test Ban Treaty of 1963.

In 1954 scientists did not know what effect the fallout would have on the world's population. At the time, those concerned were only thinking in terms of congenital abnormalities resulting from small doses of radiation, and the idea that small doses might cause cancer was not suspected. It may well have been politically expedient, but when research began to appear about the risks of leukaemia in the survivors of the atom bomb explosions in Japan, suggesting the possibility of a proportional relationship, Doll felt a scientific compulsion to study the effects of thermonuclear explosions.

---

* Lewis Strauss, president of the US Atomic Energy Commission, was asked on 31 March by a journalist if an H-bomb could be made large enough to destroy New York. He answered, "The metropolitan area, yes." The answer had an electrifying effect.

Using early data for leukaemia detected among the survivors of the Hiroshima and Nagasaki nuclear bombs, together with the evidence of the disease found among American radiologists, Doll projected an intriguing hypothesis. He wrote, "Animal experiments suggest that the incidence of leukaemia is directly proportional to the dose given and that, in this regard, it is immaterial whether the dose is given all at once or is spread out over a long period."[18]

Ionising radiations are carcinogens to which human exposure is ever present. In estimating the total dose received from cosmic rays, radioactive substances occurring naturally in the earth's crust and atmosphere and from radioactive substances in the body, Doll put a figure on the probability of developing leukaemia from naturally occurring radiation. Advocating the theory "if carcinogenesis is analogous to the production of genetic mutations"[19] he was able to plot the arc of the difference between the number of leukaemia cases that would occur naturally and the number attributable to nuclear explosions. Proposing that there was no threshold dose below which no effect is produced, in May 1955 Doll made a remarkable scientific prediction:

> The integrated life dose which the inhabitants of the USA have, on average, been subjected to as a result of test explosions over the four years preceding March 1955, has been estimated by the US Atomic Energy Commission to be of the order of 0.1r to the whole body. The total number of cases of leukaemia directly attributable to the explosions is, therefore, estimated to be of the order of
>
> $$\frac{0.1}{400} \times \frac{2.5}{100} \times 150,000,000$$
>
> i.e. about 900. In Britain, with one-third of the American population subjected to one third of the dose, the number liable to occur is estimated to be of the order of 100.[20]

Doll then sent his paper to Himsworth at the MRC and asked if it was worthy of publication, as even the title contained the word "tentative". Himsworth advised against, seeing it as so speculative that it might damage Doll's reputation as a scientist. Although Himsworth was not at all left-wing, he was supportive of Doll politically as well as professionally, and his advice was usually followed. The paper reflected the development of Doll's scientific thinking together with his interpretation of the role of epidemiology. It moved the science beyond the merely descriptive to answer questions of cause and effect in disease. Doll decided not to publish and put all thoughts about it into suspended animation.

Some forty years later, he received a phone call from a journalist asking, "Do you still think the Bravo explosion caused one hundred cases of leukaemia in Britain?" The journalist had discovered Doll's original memo to Himsworth in the files of Sir John Cockcroft (then director of the Atomic Energy Authority) when they were opened under the thirty-year rule. Doll was alarmed to be told that the paper was going to be used as evidence in a court case portraying him as an incompetent epidemiologist. Not having kept a copy, it was only when he re-read his long-forgotten three-page investigation he realised that far from being unusually speculative, his figure was not far from modern probability estimates. Rather than being embarrassed, he thought his 1955 paper "bloody good" and finally published it in 1996, in the *Journal of Radiological Protection*.

For Richard Doll work was an all-consuming passion. Peter Armitage thought him a workaholic, and "uneasy if he isn't working".[21] Within the London School of Hygiene and Tropical Medicine, Doll was seen as a semi-detached member of the staff, a sedulous researcher who kept teaching to a minimum. Armitage recognised that the last thing that Doll wanted to do was write a text book to go over standard stuff. Nor was the school a social nexus for Doll as his circle of friends came more from the world of politics and clinical medicine.

By the early 1950s Doll's reputation was spreading beyond the frontiers of British medical science. What made him so original was his status both as a doctor and a statistician. He was also so intellectually clever that it could, according to Malcolm Pike, one of his later collaborators, "make him a very scary person to be around".[22] In this respect he was an enigma.

He was seen by his contemporary John Pemberton as "sensitive, courteous and kind" yet when Marie Kidd, a research worker on the British doctors study, walked with him around the wards of the Central Middlesex Hospital, "he emanated intimidation in an unconscious way."[23] Of course, the 1950s was an era of much greater deference, and social segregation still persisted, at least in some respects, as if the war had never happened. It was an era when doctors were revered, respected and rare. Doll was a communist, but he had been brought up in Knightsbridge, he had been to Westminster School and St Thomas's, he was a high-status person and he knew how to behave in such a role. As a consultant walking through the gastroenterology ward, he would be treated in a deferential manner, whether he demanded it or not. Malcolm Godfrey, who began working with Joan at the MRC in 1960, acknowledged that Doll mellowed with time, but in the early days, "He could be acerbic. He was very precise and exact, you had to be careful."[24]

Doll certainly had a courageous mind and in the innately politically conservative world of London medicine his stance alienated him from the establishment. What was not in question was his productivity; and it was not surprising that the variety and ingenuity of his epidemiological studies then came to the notice of one of the most prestigious academic institutions in the United States. In February 1954 Doll took a phone call from Harvard University offering him the position as head of their school of public health medicine. Joan's cautionary influence had not yet precluded him from putting his political beliefs before professional advancement. Doll's immediate response was bold and morally in keeping with his commitment to peace and opposition of bigotry. "Not as long as McCarthy is there." The Communist Party was an illegal organisation in America. Between 1950 and 1954 Senator Joseph McCarthy carried out a pitiless campaign into alleged communist infiltration in US public life.

At the time Doll was offered the appointment at Harvard, McCarthy was at the apogee of his powers. Opposition to McCarthy's vociferous witch hunt existed within certain liberal-minded groups and institutions in America but Doll's declaration was not sufficient to deter Harvard from trying to get their man. Soon after the call from Boston, Doll was visited in London by the American John Enders (who shared the Nobel Prize in 1954 for his work on the polio virus) asking him to reconsider the offer. But while Hill remained director of the statistical research unit, Doll could not imagine working anywhere else. And his reply to the offer remained as forthright: "Not as long as you've got Joseph McCarthy."

The 1950s was the defining decade of Doll's professional life. In choosing epidemiology he brought insight and imagination to a subject that was on the threshold of an age of discovery. Together with his work on tobacco, he also pioneered epidemiological studies into the hazards of radiation, the prevention and cure of cancer and innovative methods of detecting occupational dangers of the disease. All of these subjects— although he did not know it—would occupy Doll with varying degrees of intensity for the next fifty years. One historic investigation in the asbestos industry transcended the decades and visibly displayed the political fault lines that divide science and society. By identifying what is now recognised as the world's most important industrial carcinogen, his work also serves as an example of epidemiology's capabilities— and its limitations— in discovering human exposure to a fatal cancer risk.

Chapter 10

The Rise and Fall of Asbestos

"If I know myself, I work from a sort of instinct to try to make out truth."

Charles Darwin

In April 1953, Richard Doll received a letter from John Knox, medical officer for the asbestos company Turner & Newall Ltd (T&N), an event which marked the beginning of one of the most compelling stories in the relationship between medical research and industry.

Doll's subsequent 1955 paper[1] was a pioneering work that provided early conclusive evidence that asbestos fibres cause cancer. Over the course of the following thirty years Doll's standing was to undergo a transformation: initially seen as a critic of the industry, he would later be portrayed as its defender.

The background to the story started with the death of Nellie Kershaw, a former T&N worker from Rochdale, in March 1924, an event that has been recognised as a landmark in medical history. The subsequent inquest was the first on an asbestos worker. The coroner ordered a post-mortem, and microscopic examination of the lungs confirmed that she had died through breathing asbestos. When the pathologist, Dr William Cooke, wrote up the case in 1927, he coined the term by which the disease has since been known—"pulmonary asbestosis".

Following Cooke's published report[2] on the Kershaw case, the pace of medical writing on asbestosis suddenly increased. In 1928 and 1929, a dozen separate medical publications carried discussions and reports about the disease. By now, the factory inspectors were monitoring the situation closely. Most of the Rochdale inquests of the time were attended by Dr Edward Merewether, a medical inspector of factories who was to become a leading authority on asbestos disease. In 1928 the government had commissioned Merewether and Charles Price, an engineering inspector, to prepare a study of workers' health in the asbestos textile industry.

The findings of their report[3] were unambiguous. Choosing workers with as "pure" an exposure to asbestos as possible, Merewether and Price selected 363 asbestos workers from an estimated UK workforce of 2,200. The sample was deliberately weighted with employees who had long employment histories and many workers from Turner Brothers Asbestos (later Turner & Newall) were included. Around one quarter (95) of the sample had asbestosis, and 21 more had early signs of the disease. The incidence of the disease increased with duration of employment: excluding those employed for less than five years, the incidence of asbestosis was about 35 per cent. After twenty years four out of five workers still in the industry had asbestosis. The prevalence of the disease prompted calls for action by the government, and in 1930 talks were held with the industry's leading manufacturers. Legislation followed within a year, with three linked measures:

a. The asbestos industry regulations (1931) were introduced to control the dust levels.
b. A medical arrangements scheme was set up to screen new employees and monitor them annually by means of a government medical board, which could certify and suspend the sick. Autopsies were to be performed on suspected cases and asbestosis was to be confirmed by a special death certificate.
c. The asbestos industry was to be brought within the Workmen's Compensation Act by an asbestosis scheme. Workers disabled by asbestosis were to be compensated by the industry—and the dependants of those who died were to be awarded by a lump sum death benefit.

This was a remarkable piece of industrial legislation because, due to the investigations of Merewether and Price, Britain was the first country officially to recognise asbestosis. In addition, the 1931 regulations were to prove exceptional for their longevity. Even with the increase in asbestos-related deaths after the Second World War, the safety standards remained unchanged until 1968.

Most of the known occupational hazards of cancer have been discovered as a result of clinical acumen, backed up in the course of time by epidemiological investigation of varying degrees of sophistication and eventually confirmed. This was certainly the case with lung cancer in asbestos workers. Richard Doll was always aware that "if there is one general rule in the assessment of epidemiological evidence, it is that no conclusion of any sort can be reached until the totality of the evidence is taken into account."[4]

At the same time as carrying out his retrospective study on smoking, Doll was also investigating other suspected causes of lung cancer. In 1934 the London pathologist Dr Stephen Gloyne[5] had reported cases of carcinoma of the lung among his asbestosis autopsies. He reported to Merewether the possibility of an association between the two diseases. Intrigued by a further study by Gloyne,[6] Doll had a meeting with him, and wrote to Merewether in May 1948[7] informing him of the MRC study with Bradford Hill on smoking. He stated that he did not consider the evidence linking asbestos and lung cancer to be very convincing but would "like to look into it a bit further".

This was the catalyst for Merewether and Gloyne to introduce Doll to Dr Hubert Wyers, works medical officer for Cape Asbestos, the main competitor of T&N. In 1946 Wyers had completed a doctoral thesis on the association of lung cancer with asbestosis; he suggested that improved safety measures might be warranted even without greater scientific proof. Doll was keen for the association "to be logically proved", as he wrote to Wyers in June 1948. He continued:

> What is wanted is a definitive population which can be observed to see what proportion die of cancer of the lung in a given period—a proportion which can be compared with expectation, based on general mortality figures. A possible way of doing this might be to define your population as being "certified cases of asbestosis" and then to follow them to death. Best of all would be to limit the population to cases certified arising out of the periodic medical exam at specific factories, but I imagine that would reduce the numbers too much. I don't know whether you've had anything like that number certified at the Cape company since 1931.

A meeting at Cape Asbestos was finally arranged for 24 March 1949. Wyers wrote, "I had prepared all the figures with the exception of the series of certification dates and to my surprise I find that the company's records are exceedingly scrappy."

Frustratingly, just at the very moment when it appeared that the first cohort study into lung cancer in asbestos workers was about to begin, Cape Asbestos withdrew its consent. It is unclear exactly why the company undermined Wyers' collaborative efforts, but what is clear is that when Doll formally approached the company "they just said 'no'."[8] There was an understandable level of corporate paranoia in the British asbestos industry, and the introduction of the 1931 regulations brought a sense that it was under more intensive observation than other sectors of the industrial economy.

This was certainly the accepted logic at T&N. Their factory in Rochdale had been established in 1855 to weave cotton, and it was not until 1879 that experiments were started with asbestos. By the 1920s its dominance made it synonymous with the country's asbestos industry. By the early 1950s it accounted for about sixty per cent of Britain's asbestos industry, and its factory in Rochdale was the largest asbestos textile factory in the world. As it turned out the hygiene standards at Rochdale were widely regarded as "best practice" in what was undoubtedly a dangerous industry. Certainly if the T&N board were going to venture where Cape Asbestos had feared to go by putting their factory under an epidemiological microscope, they expected to be vindicated with a record to show that there was no association between asbestosis and lung cancer.

From the early 1940s the firm had been linked with the work of the Saranac Laboratory in upstate New York. The research facility there had been funded as part of the famous Trudeau Sanatorium for tuberculosis at Saranac Lake. Its director, Dr Leroy Gardner, had begun a new line of research—the effects of asbestos inhalation—with the support of leading American firms. Among Gardner's sponsors was T&N's American subsidiary, Keasbey & Mattison. Reports of Gardner's research, which were confidential and not for publication, were also sent to Rochdale.

In 1952 John Knox attended the seventh Saranac symposium at Saranac Lake where the subject of pneumoconiosis— including asbestosis and its link with pulmonary cancer—was discussed. This prompted Knox to have another look at the problem when he returned to Rochdale. He re-examined the hundred or so post-mortem reports of the workers, noting all the lung cancer cases. The count now seemed higher, but, as Knox realised, the matter could only be deciphered by a professional statistical study. After gaining the approval of the board, Knox wrote to Doll at the London School of Hygiene and Tropical Medicine. His letter, dated 12 April 1953, is a key document in the discovery of occupational cancers:

> Dear Dr Doll
> As medical adviser to a large asbestos works in Rochdale I have been reviewing my accumulated reports on autopsies conducted on workers here who were alleged to have died of asbestosis. This series goes back to 1930 when asbestosis was put on the industrial map and numbers 115 cases to date. In the present instance I am anxious to contribute to the carcinoma lung question in association with asbestosis and would like your opinion on my material. Your published work demonstrates your own interest in the etiological factors in connection with carcinoma lung and I think I have some material of interest. My statistical ability is nil and I have the approval of my firm Messrs Turner Bros Asbestos Co to approach a medical statistical authority to discuss this question.

After being rebuffed by Cape Asbestos, Doll eagerly accepted the offer to collaborate with an industry noted for its suspicion of interventions from the outside world. On 14 April Doll confirmed his participation in the study:

> Dear Dr Knox
> I was delighted to get your letter as I have for long been interested in the association between lung cancer and asbestosis and have been very dissatisfied with the existing evidence...

Even with the asbestos industry regulations—passed in 1931 and effective from March 1933—dust was an accepted fact of life for workers in the factory. In 1954 Doll's investigation faced two major problems. First was the latency period of at least twenty years (more than 26 years was the average period for the cases of lung cancer and asbestosis later reported in the paper) before the development of malignancy—even in 1954 it was still too early to draw firm conclusions about the future risks the workers would be exposed to. Second—and this was the issue, more than any other, upon which Doll's reputation as the industry's critic or defender rested—was that asbestos is not a uniform mineral. Between 1933 and 1974 chrysotile (white) asbestos was used throughout the period in the factory, but its amphibole varieties, crocidolite (blue) in particular, and amosite (brown), were also used in asbestos textile manufacture.[9] It was the amphibole varieties that were truly lethal.*

From being little more than a curiosity at the beginning of the twentieth century, asbestos came to have a thousand or so uses by the 1950s, when more than 150,000 tons were imported and processed in Britain each year. That asbestos made a tremendous contribution to human welfare through its insulation power and indestructibility by fire and friction is incontrovertible, but what was equally incontrovertible was that its manufacture provided a risk of severe disability and death. Doll and Knox were to set about measuring just how great that risk was. Perhaps more than with any other occupational hazard, the dangers of asbestos production made one of the central themes of epidemiological inquiry even more sensitive: that of balancing benefits and risks.

---

* In 1946 Cape's physician, Dr Hubert Wyers, highlighted that workers regarded chrysotile as the least dangerous, while "blue asbestos is regarded… to be more dangerous". As regards amosite, "its reputation as regards health [is] utterly pernicious; it is seldom now used." See Wyers, 'That Legislative Measures Have Proved Generally Effective in the Control of Asbestosis' (Glasgow University MD, 1946), p. 48.

On 7 May 1954 John Knox had lunch with Doll in London. It was the start of a celebrated collaboration that was to become long-lasting and controversial. For an epidemiologist determined to measure scientifically the risks to health in a specific industry, T&N presented an ideal opportunity. Unlike Cape Asbestos, the employment records for the Rochdale factory were anything but "exceedingly scrappy"—the combination of the company's scrupulously kept records and the fact that the overwhelming majority of the workers lived in the town made it a relatively straightforward task to measure the local mortality statistics against those experienced in the general population. (This punctiliousness and the detailed records of all aspects of company history were later utilised by American lawyers under "discovery" procedure during litigation in 1995.)

The two men devised a study in which the lung cancer incidence from T&N's "scheduled workers"* was compared with the death rate from the disease in the general population between 1935 and 1953. On 16 December 1954 Knox wrote to Doll confirming that the company was carrying out his statistical instructions; the final paragraph stated: "I'm very pleased indeed that the work is to be done. It should be a most important guide to us as regards the efficiency of the preventive measures."

The investigation was limited to a small group of men who had been employed for at least twenty years. The date of birth, date of completing twenty years' work in the scheduled areas and, where applicable, date of ceasing employment and date and cause of death were obtained for each man from the records of the firm's personnel officer. The first published application of this person-years analysis had been carried out by Doll in 1952[10] and represented a methodological advance in epidemiology.

Within a matter of months Doll had concluded his analysis. All the subjects in whom both lung cancer and asbestosis were found had started employment in the industry before 1923 and had worked in the factory at

---

* These were men working in so-called "scheduled areas"—areas which were scheduled under the asbestos industry regulations of 1931 as being dusty.

least nine years before the regulations for the control of dust had become effective. The results were striking.

> One hundred and thirteen men who had worked for at least 20 years in places where they were liable to be exposed to asbestos dust were followed up and the mortality among them was compared with that which would have been expected on the basis of the mortality experience of the whole male population. Thirty-nine deaths occurred in the group whereas 15.4 were expected. The excess was entirely due to excess deaths from lung cancer (11 against 0.8 expected) and from other respiratory and cardiovascular diseases (22 against 7.6 expected). All the cases of lung cancer were confirmed histologically and were all associated with the presence of asbestosis.
>
> From the data it can be concluded that lung cancer was a specific industrial hazard of certain asbestos workers and that the average risk among men employed for 20 or more years has been of the order of ten times that experienced by the general population.[11]

The report continued, "The great reduction in the amount of dust produced in asbestos works during the period has been accompanied by a reduction in the incidence of lung cancer among the workmen so that the risk before 1933 is likely to have been considerably greater—perhaps 20 times the general risk."

Having identified the hazard that workers experienced in the past, Doll was then cautious about predicting how this knowledge could determine future danger. "Whether the specific industrial risk of lung cancer has yet been completely eliminated cannot be determined with certainty; the number of men at risk, who have been exposed to the new conditions only and who have been employed for a sufficient length of time, is at present too small for confidence to be placed in their experience."

In the 1950s the asbestos industry was at its most expansive and profitable, and as the T&N board read the Doll and Knox report they became increasingly concerned about the paper's main discovery—a lung cancer risk which was ten times the norm for those exposed to asbestos for twenty years or more. The anxiety first showed itself in the board's refusal to allow

Knox's name to be associated with the paper, despite his indispensable role in its creation. This was the beginning of a struggle between the forces of scientific freedom and corporate suppression. The board's decision was relayed to Doll in a letter from Knox on 4 January 1955: "I gather that my name on the paper might not be acceptable as it would naturally suggest Rochdale as the place of origin."

Doll's findings could not have come at a worse time for T&N. No asbestos firm had ever admitted publicly that there was a cancer risk; indeed, the industry had always projected itself as a protector of life, not a bringer of death. In desperation the company then sought to preserve the status quo by using censorship and intimidation—and refused permission to publish the article.

Knox was given the job of erasing the evidence; his letter of 25 May was apologetic:

Dear Dr Doll

I have now had the decision of my chairman on the paper and after submission of the matter to the parent board (Turner & Newall Ltd) it has been decided not to allow publication at the moment. The subject of carcinoma of the lung in however obscure a connotation is thought likely to attract undesirable publicity. My feelings, of course, are of deep disappointment and I hope that later on a reconsideration of this decision will be made ... I do appreciate very much the effort you have put into this work and am most conscious of all the labour involved. For you it is, perhaps, a very small piece in a very large jigsaw but if it helps at all towards the completion of the picture the time spent will not have been lost.

In the same way that tobacco companies were to dismiss as "unscientific" any evidence linking lung cancer with their products, Turner & Newall described the report's findings as "inaccurate". In fact, by 1955 Doll's findings relating to the occupational hazards of nickel-refining, asbestos and coal gas had all been objected to by the respective industries. Denial, suppression or coercion were the natural first reactions of industries under attack. Richard Doll was a young determined epidemiologist, and one who had encountered corporate intransigence, intrigue and intimidation before: capitulation was unthinkable. On 8 June he replied to his collaborator:

Dear Dr Knox

I was shocked to hear of the decision of your board not to approve publication of our proposed paper. In the circumstances it will obviously not be possible for your name to appear on it. For my own part I feel that any further findings with regard to the cause of cancer must be made available to all research workers in the subject (and not limited to those few with whom we may personally be in contact). There is no knowing, but what may appear at first to have only a limited application in the industrial field may eventually prove to provide an important link in the chain of reasoning by which knowledge of the general causation of the disease may be determined.

I would not, of course, have undertaken the work in the first place, had I imagined that there would be an attempt to limit the dissemination of scientific data.

I think perhaps the best thing for me to do is to go ahead and submit the article to the *British Journal of Industrial Medicine* under my own name—regretfully removing all reference to yours.

I wonder whether perhaps your board have had the opportunity of considering those aspects of the problem, which I have put forward, and whether they would consider reconsidering their decision?

Free of any pre-conditions—throughout his salaried career Doll worked for no fee—and with the institutional support of the London School of Hygiene and Tropical Medicine, Doll stood firm against T&N's overtures of censorship. This did not, however, stop the company from making them. When, in the summer of 1954, RG Soothill, T&N's chairman, invited Doll to Rochdale for dinner, the chairman's appeal for silence was motivated by a greater moral imperative than the mere protection of company profits: that of national preservation. "It was just suggested to me," wrote Doll later, "that it would be contrary to the interests of the country to publish it. It was suggested that it would discourage workers from coming to work in the factory, that there would be a fall off in the production of asbestos, and this would delay the development of aircraft and hinder British defence against the Soviets."[12] Unknown to Soothill, at the time of the meeting Doll was a member of the Communist Party.

A remarkable feature of Doll's work, and one not confined to the asbestos study, was that his science transcended his political beliefs. This ideological immune system, like many of the central pillars of his work, can be traced to the influence that Austin Bradford Hill had on his scientific methodology. "He taught me early on that if you were going to contribute to a subject it was very important to separate the presentation of evidence from the discussion of what should be done on the basis of that evidence."[13]

Looking back at these dramatic events through the "discovery" records and court transcripts of the Chase Manhattan trial of 1995,* a remarkable secret history of Machiavellian intrigue unfolds. It took forty years for the truth to emerge and, when it did, it revealed the lengths to which the board was prepared to go to suppress Doll's research paper.

From intimidation T&N had then moved towards litigation. In the summer of 1954 the board drafted a barrister's letter to pressure Doll into withdrawing the paper. It stated that a published article "would be wholly premature and undesirable from all points of view".[14] The letter was never sent, however, and Richard Doll remained resolute in the face of the coercion. He sent the article to Richard Schilling, editor of the *British Journal of Industrial Medicine*, still hoping that T&N would eventually allow its publication, but determined to carry on regardless. Schilling, professor of

---

* In 1995 Chase Manhattan Bank lost its $185 million action against T&N for the removal of asbestos from Chase Plaza, its Manhattan building, built in 1959. Under "discovery" procedure, Chase was granted access to T&N records at their place of storage in Manchester, where a vast amount of material was microfilmed. In 1991 Chase lawyers, led by vice-president and senior council Michael O'Connor, won a major discovery ruling that gave the bank sweeping access to all documents in the T&N repository.

occupational medicine, and Richard Doll had studied medicine together at St Thomas's; both shared a love of cricket, with Doll being a wicket keeper and Schilling a fast bowler. They knew each other well, and were good friends.

Some forty years later, in the Chase Manhattan Bank lawsuit, Schilling recalled under oath being paid a personal visit by a member of the T&N board: "Well, I remember very, very clearly a man with dark hair, who was a director of Turner & Newall's, coming to me when I was working in the physiology lab department of the University of Manchester, asking me to suppress the publication of this article."[15]

Doll and Schilling made a stand for academic freedom when they declined to withdraw the lung cancer article in 1955. They were also conscious of the earlier failure to set up a collaborative study with Cape Asbestos, and the fact that no meaningful epidemiological study could be undertaken without the consent and co-operation of industry. Even after the volte-face they had experienced at the hands of the T&N board, Doll's letter to Schilling on 3 September 1954 expressed a shared realisation:

Dear Richard

I have given some further thought to the problem of publication and I think I would like you to hold the paper over till the April issue so as to give the firm an opportunity to show whether they are genuinely anxious to have further research undertaken. If they are, it should be possible to make an estimate (within a month or two) of the survival rate of workers taken on in the last 25 years. Should the survival rate be shown to be the same as that for other inhabitants of Rochdale, we could make an addendum to the paper of a half a dozen lines pointing this out and promising more detailed results later. If, on the other hand, the survival rate is not yet normal (and I doubt if it is), the sooner the firm are made to realise it the better.

Then at the end of the typed letter Doll added in his spidery handwriting a sentence that has been apportioned almost religious importance by some observers: "Unless I offer them quid pro quo, we may never find out."

While researching his exhaustive book *Magic Mineral to Killer Dust: Turner & Newall and the Asbestos Hazard*, the industrial historian Geoffrey Tweedale interviewed Richard Doll and said to him, "After they tried to put the boot in, why did you continue to work with them? I certainly wouldn't."[16]

As an experienced epidemiologist working in the febrile atmosphere of occupational health, Doll was no stranger to the demolition tactics employed by industries against his work. "It was a natural reaction, and continues to be, for big business to do that. I had trouble with the nickel industry, with the gas industry, and that was even after it had been nationalised!"[17] By mid-1954 Richard Doll had proved irrefutably that workers in the Rochdale factory had been exposed to great danger, but what was not known was the existing risk to workers' health, and more importantly, what the scale of the hazard would be in the future. For this to be determined, Doll needed to build on the knowledge of his first cohort study and apply it to a more recent group of asbestos workers and measure their pattern of disease against that experienced within the general population. To achieve this Doll needed to persuade a reluctant T&N—who were desperate to prevent bad publicity—that such a study would be beneficial to all. The final sentence of his paper, controversially to some,[18] was written in the past tense: "The risk has become progressively less as the duration of employment under the old dusty conditions has decreased."[19]

Although the paper was eventually published in 1955 without naming the company, the location of the factory or the identity of the co-author, Knox undoubtedly had an influence on the final wording before it went to press. On 11 August Knox wrote from his home:

> I conveyed your message to the chairman last evening, and had a further long chat about the whole business. I think my position is quite clear now. It is admitted that I am not now a protagonist and that my personal position should no longer be considered as a pawn in the game ... I was most grateful to you for your patience and consideration on my work last week. It was an educating experience to have your personal view of this new paragraph on the diminished risk point. I think this

should be considered as an important piece of new evidence for a review of the present position on publication.

No routine dust measurements were made before 1951[20] so dust levels between 1933 and 1950 could only have been guessed at, and all that could be said of earlier conditions was that they were substantially worse than in 1933. Science is neither optimistic nor pessimistic, yet these opposing emotional states feature in the controversial history of asbestos—Knox took an optimistic view, while Doll kept an open mind as to whether all risk had been eliminated.

Yet just as the board's initial paranoia was beginning to recede and the more positive elements of the cohort study were being emphasised, news of the research was leaked to the national media in a most unconventional way. The T&N board was "aghast" that the *Times*, on 18 February 1955, published parts of the annual general report of the London School of Hygiene and Tropical Medicine:

> Dr WRS Doll, of the Medical Research Council, has made a study of lung cancer in conjunction with Dr JF Knox, the industrial medical officer of an asbestos works… In the investigation the causes of death were determined of all men employed for 20 or more years in parts of the works exposed to asbestos dust. The number of lung cancer deaths which had occurred among them (all in association with asbestosis) was about ten times the number expected.

Surprisingly, and much to the relief of the company, Doll's definitive study failed to make a bigger impact in the wider world. This quiescence, together with some of the more positive findings, had the effect of persuading the board that further collaborative work should be undertaken. It is possible to understand why the company was relieved that a national outcry did not occur but why did the workers not make a more belligerent stand? Geoffrey Tweedale offers a balanced historical explanation.

The feeble response was due to the fragmented nature of both the unions and the factories. Some of the factories made textiles, some made ropes, others insulating material, and as a consequence there was not a unified voice. In addition, and this was not to change until the 1970s with the emergence of mesothelioma, asbestos was seen as a traditional British industry that carried a risk to the workers. In Rochdale there was another disease—byssinosis (an industrial disease of the lungs caused by the inhalation of cotton dust)—which affected workers in the cotton mills and probably killed more workers in Rochdale than asbestosis.[21]

After Doll published his study the company agreed to continue to provide him with employment records for independent analysis, which were eventually used to demonstrate a significant continuing hazard. Doll's scientific detachment established his reputation of impartiality. His strategic aims were to ensure that the epidemiological evidence would be described accurately, and to ensure that true hazards were discovered sooner rather than later and that mistaken claims of hazard or safety would be minimised.

Beyond the controversy, one element of the story was incontestable: the originality of Doll's study. For almost a decade he had been working in the forefront of a burgeoning new science. It is true that in Austin Bradford Hill he had a colleague who had established the central principles of epidemiology, but by the 1950s Doll was now expanding the subject's frontiers, and, according to Sir Donald Acheson, the benchmark 1955 asbestos paper was

> a classic in its own right, which would have gained Richard Doll a place in the history of epidemiology had it been his only publication... Almost as an aside Sir Richard's paper also gives one of the first and unquestionably one of the simplest descriptions of the man-years method of calculating expected numbers. Subsequently this technique rapidly became established as the standard way to measure risk in cohort studies. Previously risk was usually estimated by a "snapshot" of

the situation at the beginning of the period of exposure, thus wasting much of the available information.[22]

Acheson, who was the chief medical officer throughout much of the 1980s, also made a contribution to the asbestos debate[23] and was conscious of the need for epidemiologists to be circumspect in their dealings with the industry. "You had to be scrupulous about the way in which you behaved in relation with everything to do with an inquiry into an industrial process. Because they were looking for anything they could do to reduce your credibility. You had to be cleaner than clean."[24]

Doll's scientific skill lifted him above the political maelstrom, and he then set about persuading the Turner & Newall board to allow another study. "Eventually they realised that it would be a good thing to follow up their workers to see if the hazard had gone, and there was reason to think the hazard might have gone; and I got their permission."[25]

Doll was not a propagandist, and he refused to use his discoveries in medical science as campaign platforms. Often his *modus operandi* was to study an industry or manufacturing process, identify any hazard, eliminate that danger, and where possible for the trade to continue within socially acceptable standards. In the case of the asbestos industry this was to become an increasingly unattainable aim. There was no denying the will of the company and Doll to continue their collaboration but the initial trust had been shaken. When Doll asked for records of workers employed for ten years after 1 January 1933, Knox's letter reflected the emotional shift:

... Before we go any further with the study I have been asked to require from you whether the results are likely to secure any publicity through your annual report or other publication. I personally understood from you that you regarded this particular matter as only of domestic interest to us in judging the effect of our protective devices, but if I have been mistaken in this regard perhaps you would let me know. The recent publicity in the press has upset the board here and the directors would like to know where they stand with regard to the projected study before going any further with it.

Responding to Knox on 6 July 1955, Doll set the historical record straight. "On April 5 1955, I wrote at your request to confirm that if I assisted in the analysis and interpretation of your new data, neither the data nor the results would be given any publicity without the company's approval. This assurance still stands and I do not think that I ought to have been asked to repeat it."

When the moral and historical audit is drawn up, Doll's behaviour should be viewed as "cleaner than clean"—yet this determination to be beyond reproach personally, and independent scientifically, led to a celebrated disagreement with a member of his own team in the 1970s—a time when the industry was under unprecedented attack.

The human intellect is moved more by affirmatives than negatives, and after the initial shockwaves created by Doll, the board viewed further collaboration with optimism. Indeed, the results of the cohort study when they were published in 1965[26] seemed to exonerate the company—the analysis did not show the horrendous hazard that had been there a decade before, and even declared "it is possible that the specific occupational hazards to life have been completely eliminated." The statistician David Hill, son of Bradford Hill, worked on the analysis, and gives vivid testimony to the improved conditions. "What I recall from my time on the asbestos study was talking to some of the workers who had been in the Rochdale factory since the 1920s—and after the 1931 regulations, which cleaned up the factory, the men said what they first noticed was that there was a clock at the other end of the room."[27]

The management had succeeded in cleaning up the factory dramatically, and they genuinely believed that there was no excess of lung cancer in people who started working there after 1933. The use of epidemiological methods to discover an occupational hazard is, however, far from ideal. Not only do they require that some cancers should be caused before the hazard can be detected, but the long induction that is common with cancer means that irreversible changes will certainly have been produced in some members of the apparently healthy exposed group, and that they will continue to cause an increased risk of cancer for many years to come after the agent is discovered and removed.

As the industry, and its profits, grew in the 1950s and 1960s, so did public concern over the dangers inherent in the material's ubiquitous presence. In parallel with the known hazards of asbestosis and lung cancer, a new and devastating disease began to appear both inside and outside places of manufacture. The new catastrophe facing an unsuspecting society was mesothelioma, which affected the outer lining of the lung and pleura and was nearly always fatal.

The disease was first diagnosed in 1959, and a special meeting was called at the MRC by one of its most senior medical officers, Doll's wife, Dr Joan Faulkner. The meeting was attended by, among others, researchers Earl King and John Beattie (funded by the Asbestos Research Council), John Gilson (the director of the pneumoconiosis research unit) and John Knox. Discussions ranged informally over the whole problem of asbestos and the threat of mesothelioma.[28]

A decisive breakthrough came in 1965 with the publication of an article in the *British Journal of Industrial Medicine* by researchers Dr Muriel Newhouse and Hilda Thompson.[29] Their findings were definite. Not only occupational exposure was dangerous. Casual and brief exposure through living near an asbestos factory, inhaling fibres from a relative's clothes or working in a factory insulated with the material—all these could trigger mesothelioma.

But why was it that in Richard Doll's 1968 study of the Rochdale workers no increased risk of cancer was found?[30] This can be explained by the Knox-Doll methodology, which had a crucial characteristic: it looked at cancer only among scheduled asbestos textile workers and only at one factory where exposure had been mostly to chrysotile (white asbestos). By the 1960s dust control in Rochdale meant that the conditions for workers represented the cleanest in the industry. Yet even this could not offset the feeling that the status quo was irreversibly shifting, social and medical forces were coalescing and their combined weight would lead to the decimation of the industry.

The ideological change, together with the accumulation of medical knowledge, had altered the way the industry was viewed in the eyes of the public by the 1960s. Richard Doll recognised why his definitive work in

1955 had not attracted more attention, and how diagnosis was influenced by social and political mores:

> I think it was because it was thought that it was in relation to asbestosis—which was a condition that you got with heavy exposure—and people didn't think that small amounts of asbestos that they would come across in normal life were hazardous. And that attitude hung around for quite a while, in fact, I was quite susceptible to it for a long time. The evidence for lung cancer was under conditions in which you got asbestosis. But asbestosis, when one talked about it in the 1950s, was not the condition so called in the 1970s; it was then invariably a disabling disease. Whereas in the 1970s, the definition had been changed to "any detection of abnormality in the presence of asbestos fibres". Which was very different indeed.[31]

Between 1968 and 1971 Doll chaired a Department of Health and Social Security inquiry into asbestos that accepted there was a cancer risk to the public and that "no amount of exposure is completely free from risk." It made several recommendations: asbestos products should be labelled, waste tipping should be controlled and local authorities should implement safety checks.[32] Yet as Doll himself later recognised, there was initial opposition to the advice offered:

> We wrote a report recommending six things about asbestos, in particular the banning of crocidolite (blue asbestos) and not one of them was put into effect, yet all of them were accepted some ten years later as a result of other pressures. But the Department of Health circulated our recommendations—it was accepted by the main committee on cancer, that wasn't what held things up—to other government departments because it affected them in various ways, and it was those departments that had an objection to every single recommendation, and as a consequence not one of them was adopted by the department.[33]

Indeed, as late as 1967 a *Lancet* leading article had argued that "there is a danger that workers' representatives may overrate the dangers of dealing with asbestos." The leader went on to say "situations arise where the use of asbestos can save more lives than it can possibly endanger."[34]

Within British epidemiology Doll was known for his intellectual ability, his left-wing views, his freedom from bias when confronting medical evidence and—whatever the sacrifice—his instinct to find out the truth. But as Julian Tudor Hart observed, political activism based upon the findings of scientific investigation was not permitted: "Should scientists and epidemiologists campaign and be advocates of their discoveries? Having produced the evidence he didn't feel that he [Doll] should be the advocate of that evidence. He thought it would be undermining."[35]

This judicious reserve when working in a moral and ethical minefield was in vivid contrast to another dominant researcher in the field of occupational health medicine—Dr Irvine Selikoff (1915-92), director of the environmental sciences laboratory at Mount Sinai Hospital in New York. Selikoff was an irrepressible force, a man dedicated to publicising the dangers to the workers in the industry, and to the American public. For more than two decades the combined social forces of organised labour, a politicised environmental movement and an aggressively litigious society crystallised around the remarkable Selikoff.

In October 1964 the New York Academy of Sciences organised a major international conference on the biological effects of asbestos. What would normally have been no more than an obscure gathering of academics attracted unexpected publicity. The conference helped launch the asbestos campaign for the charismatic Selikoff in a dramatic way. Selikoff's approach was different to that of his medical contemporaries outside America. Unlike Doll, who had to rely on T&N for data, Selikoff worked outside the industry. He obtained the personnel and medical records of trade unions in New York and New Jersey whose members worked every day with asbestos insulation. His results were truly staggering and showed how dangerous the industry was to the health of the workers. He investigated 1,522 workers. Of 392 examined after twenty or more years' exposure, 339 had asbestosis. Selikoff's findings, presented at the New York conference—alongside several papers on mesothelioma by other researchers—marked a turning point in public perceptions of the asbestos hazard. Between the 1960s and the 1980s he was to become the leading American expert on asbestos and health and the industry's most memorable and persuasive antagonist.

After spending more than twenty years working in epidemiology, Doll had become one of the most respected medical scientists in Britain and the foremost authority on the causes and prevention of cancer. He had brought medicine and mathematics together in such a compelling way that in 1969 he was offered the post of Regius Professor of Medicine at Oxford University.

When Doll took up his chair in Oxford he recruited some talented scientists to add to the cream of his MRC unit from London. A new generation of disciples, who learned under his tutelage the science of epidemiology, began to take up and develop further those areas of inquiry he had pioneered. Peter Smith, for example, joined his studies on radiation; Richard Peto became the collaborator on the British doctors smoking study; and Julian Peto, Richard Peto's younger brother, began working on the asbestos study.

Julian Peto was a skilled statistician and it was his job to build on the achievements of the 1955 and subsequent studies of the Rochdale workers. As had happened twenty years earlier, an epidemiological investigation sent a tremor through the British asbestos industry.

The introduction, more than half a century ago, of properly randomised trials in which the treatment allocation was rigorously concealed was a watershed in the evaluation of the effects of medical treatments.[36] No other epidemiologist had done more than Doll to advance the role of the randomised controlled trial in medicine—at the heart of his work was a determination to minimise bias. So as to diminish the likelihood of planting any seeds of a preconceived view of the asbestos industry in Peto's mind, Doll told him nothing of the attempt to censor his work. "I discovered that incidentally in the course of time. He just said, 'There's the cohort, let's update it.' He left me pretty much alone, he wasn't breathing down my neck, and we just did it. I started working with Leo Kinlen, and sort of took it over."[37]

After gaining a first in mathematics at Balliol College Oxford, Julian Peto had studied statistics at Imperial College London under David Cox. When he arrived in Oxford,

> I found myself in the same position Richard Doll had been in twenty years earlier. In 1968 he had published a paper showing that there was no excess of lung cancer in people who started working in Rochdale after 1933. But when I updated that study, which we published in 1977, the excess cancer risk in those workers became visible. Up to that time the factory genuinely believed that they had solved the problem, and Doll just had an open mind; at the end of the 1968 paper he wrote *it is too soon to say*—so he was not too surprised when the excess emerged. Our findings were not as horrendous for the company as his 1955 discovery, they were not that wicked. We found a doubling of the risk of lung cancer for long-term workers—[which] was horrendous by the standards of the 1970s.[38]

Before the publication of their collaborative study[39] in 1977, Peto gave a paper while attending a conference in America on the possible future dangers for asbestos workers based on the existing safety levels. "The results of the 1966 follow-up show that no detectable excess of lung cancer or respiratory disease had emerged after up to 33 years' follow-up, but by 1974 substantial excesses were evident. This is a nice illustration of the difficulty of detecting new industrial hazards."[40]

On 30 January 1977 the *Sunday Times* ran a special report on Peto's claims that the official safety level was in fact far more hazardous than previously realised. The journalist Oliver Gillie came to the profession from genetics, which he had taught at London University. Peto knew him well, and had even babysat his children. To some, and most importantly to Doll, the article gave the impression that Peto had colluded with the newspaper and given away privileged information based on dose-response records provided by T&N. This was seen as a transgression of trust and one that was incompatible with ethical scientific practice.

He very nearly sacked me, because he thought I was campaigning over the work I was doing. And he regarded that as completely unacceptable. I wouldn't give Oliver Gillie the paper, because I told him to leak things would be suicide, but he got the paper from the American publishers and splashed it all over the *Sunday Times*. "Official safety limit for asbestos may put one in fourteen at risk"—and the reason Richard was so furious was that he thought that I had leaked it to the press, and that I was campaigning, which I wasn't at all. I rang Oliver and said, "For Christ's sake, you could have let me see the article." I kept all the correspondence and I sent it to Richard Doll, and when he realised what had happened it was all right. But it was a dodgy period.[41]

Following the turbulence created by Gillie's article, more humiliation came Julian Peto's way in the pages of the *Oxford Mail* [42] under the headline: "Don denies asbestos allegations." Doll, who was the don in question, said that the report used invalid assumptions to test ideas. "I think some of the assumptions are certainly invalid. I don't think we have any justification for doubting the safety levels. But there is no such thing as absolute safety with a material which can cause lung cancer."

Doll's 1968 study made at the Rochdale factory had appeared to show that workers there were no more vulnerable to disease than other people. The asbestos industry made much use of this study in its publicity material. In 1969, in a leaflet called *Asbestos—Public not at Risk*, it reported that "the incidence of lung cancer among a population of asbestos workers is now no greater than in the general population." It conceded that there had been a recent increase in the asbestos-caused cancer mesothelioma, but then concluded that "if control measures over 36 years have been as successful as this," the recent increase in mesothelioma was likely to be "the crest of a wave ... which will decline in the next decade."

In fact when Doll and his team followed up the Rochdale workers in 1974, they found a marked increase in deaths from lung cancer and chest disease. Out of 678 men, 33 died of lung cancer (including mesothelioma) when only 18 were expected to by comparison with workers in other industries, and 31 died of chest disease when the expected figure was, again, 18.

The official standard for dust levels of an average level of two asbestos fibres per cubic centimetre of factory air (which meant that in a working shift of eight hours 16 million fibres may have been inhaled into the lungs) in Britain's asbestos factories was set in 1968 by the British Occupational Hygiene Society. It was intended to usher in a new age of safety and protection for workers in an industry with an appalling health record. The 1968 level, reaffirmed in January 1977 by the Health and Safety Commission, was intended to reduce the risk of asbestosis so that less than one person in a hundred working a lifetime in the industry became diseased.

In addition, according to Peto's calculations, the chances of the Rochdale workers getting lung cancer—which killed eight per cent of men over the age of 65—would increase by 25 per cent. The problem was one of judgment: should calculations be based on optimistic or pessimistic assumptions?

The two-fibre limit of 1968 was set after a study of 290 workers at Rochdale by the British Occupational Hygiene Society. In 1966 only eight of them had asbestosis. But when the workers were re-examined in 1970 (by the company's doctor), 26 men had asbestosis and X-rays showed that almost half of the 290 had signs of lung changes.

Julian Peto was conscious that conclusions must not be wrong as people's lives and livelihoods were on the line:

> Roughly speaking, the lung cancer rate was doubled—this was over a fifty-year period—and in those days there were people who went in at 15 and worked until they were 65. This suggested that there could be a doubled lung cancer risk at what was supposed to be a safe level. It got a lot of publicity, and Richard immediately battened down the hatches in a most extraordinary way, although it didn't last very long. I was annoyed at the time because he told me not to talk to the press and then he made a statement to the local Oxford paper, and I can still remember the quote that I was "playing with mathematical models" and that we had no reason to doubt the safety standards. The funny thing is, when we published in 1985—although we'd updated the study the results were the same—the estimate we gave was essentially identical to the one he'd disowned in 1977.[43]

Once this unacceptable hazard of the level of fibre inhalation was proven, even greater regulation had to be imposed. The government's advisory committee on asbestos (ACA) was headed by the chairman of the Health and Safety Commission, Sir Bill Simpson. In the summer of 1977 fevered public meetings were held bringing together those voices of community and industry that were irredeemably divided. The ACA published the submissions in the same year, and Simpson and his colleagues then considered the evidence.

The committee's conclusions, published in two weighty volumes in 1979, contained the proposal that for dust in the workplace the control limit for exposure to chrysotile should become one asbestos fibre per cubic centimetre by the end of 1980, with 0.5 of a fibre the target for amosite. The tighter threshold reflected the influence of Peto whose presentations to the committee were strongly critical of the British Occupational Hygiene Society's two-fibre limit.*

One of the most intriguing parts of the asbestos story is the personality of the two main scientists involved, the one in the US and the other in the Britain. In his work, Richard Doll was dispassionate, affable and inscrutable, while Irvine Selikoff was passionately politically motivated, scintillating and with the power and the desire to campaign. Julian Peto knew both men and saw how they diverged scientifically.

---

* "From these data estimates have been made of the quantitative relationship between ambient exposure and the mortality from lung cancer and mesothelioma. These results together with other published data, suggest that the lung cancer rate among chrysotile textile workers is approximately doubled following a cumulative exposure of 100 fibre/ml year, irrespective of age at first exposure." Peto J, Doll R, Hermon C, Binns W, Clayton R. and Goff T, 'Relationship of mortality to measures of environmental asbestos pollution in an asbestos textile factory'. *Annals of Occupational Hygiene*, 1985; 29: pp. 305-55.

What you've got to remember is that the workers in Britain weren't that interested, they had a fairly balanced view. The risk wasn't in the same league as it had been in the 1950s. The other thing they realised early on was that it was going to destroy the industry and was going to take their jobs away. So the workers in the factories were either indifferent or slightly dubious about the whole thing. They weren't campaigning about the lung cancer risk as a health issue; never did. Whereas in America Irvine Selikoff had set up a study of the American Insulation Workers' Union—a trade union that did all the asbestos insulation—and they had horrendous death rates, with four- and five-fold excesses of cancer. The people who went into the union at age 20 had a virtually 20 per cent lifetime risk of mesothelioma—it was extraordinary—and I analysed some of the data. Also, Selikoff was an amazing individual—he just launched a campaign against asbestos in America which really took off. But when people campaigned with their data, as Selikoff did, Richard Doll pointed out areas of scientific weakness, and he was right to do that.[44]

Mis-certification of lung cancer had often occurred in the past before it was realised how common the disease had become. Mis-certification of mesothelioma must have been even more common, for pleural mesothelioma was not even generally realised as a specific type of cancer until the late 1950s,[45] while peritoneal mesothelioma was not generally recognised until after the conference on the biological effects of asbestos held in New York in 1965.

In 1979 Selikoff and his colleagues[46] sought clinical and pathological evidence of the cause of death, as well as the certified cause of death, of all members of the asbestos workers' union in North America who were enrolled in their study on 1 January 1967 and who died within the following ten years. Useful additional information was obtained for 71 per cent of the 2,771 deaths, and this enabled the causes to be categorised in two ways: by the underlying cause on the death certificate and by the "best evidence" that the investigators had obtained.

In 1982 Doll and Julian Peto were asked by the Health and Safety Commission to undertake a further review of the adverse effects of asbestos on health. Their definitive study[47] contained a celebrated piece of deductive investigation, and questioned Selikoff's scientific methodology:

> It is not clear how intensively the clinical and pathological inquiries were pursued. On the basis of British experience of the reliability of death certificate diagnoses, it seems surprising that equally intensive inquiry of all deaths should have caused 37 per cent (93/252) of those attributed to types of cancer that were not eventually regarded as asbestos-related to be transferred into the asbestos-related category (cancers of the oesophagus, stomach, colon-rectum larynx, oropharynx or kidney), while none of the 670 cancer deaths that were originally in that category should have been transferred out. Even if all mesotheliomas are omitted, the contrast is still great: namely 39 out of 198 (20 per cent) against none out of the 554.

If Selikoff could be looked upon as someone with biased judgments and with a quasi-religious certainty of being right, he nevertheless did more good than harm, as Julian Peto recognised. "Selikoff correctly identified a lot of mesothelioma that had been missed. But, as Richard pointed out, everything got transferred from non-asbestos related to asbestos-related causes, but nothing was transferred back the other way. So it couldn't possibly have been an objective review. So there were straightforward scientific weaknesses like that."[48]

In Britain the hazards of asbestos were well-known before they were implanted in the public mind in the 1960s and 1970s by newspaper headlines warning of "the dust of death" and the "asbestos time-bomb". The documentary *Alice—A Fight for Life* made by Yorkshire Television and broadcast in 1982, however, had a dramatic effect on public opinion and T&N's future. *Alice* was a harrowing two-hour film following the battle against disease of a 47-year-old woman with mesothelioma who had worked for a short time in Cape's infamous factory in Hebden Bridge. The documentary was used as a crusading vehicle against the asbestos industry, seeking to bring the dangers of mesothelioma and other asbestos-related diseases to the public conscience.

Doll was aware of the dangers of mesothelioma and this had been reflected in his efforts to find how much crocidolite was used in the Rochdale factory. On 16 October 1962 Knox had written Doll this detailed reply:

> ... On the question of the type of asbestos used in the factory. I have followed, of course, with interest the findings of the South African workers on the question of mesothelioma and have not found any evidence that the disease is being missed here. There is only one case of endothelioma in our recorded group of lung cancer and this is the type of tumour which is now being called mesothelioma.
>
> I have made inquiries from the production director, and in our textile unit here the amount of crocidolite used has always been very small. Over the years you mentioned from 1920 onwards it has not averaged one per cent of the total amount of asbestos used in the factory...
>
> In 1920 the amount of chrysotile used was about 10,000 annually and now it would be about 20,000 tons annually. In view of these factors you may not require the specific amounts of blue asbestos used here in any greater detail, but if you still think there is anything substantial to be gained, the actual amounts could be extracted.

The film *Alice* captured the zeitgeist. Its impact hit T&N's share price and sent shock waves into the heart of the Rochdale community. In 1955 the company had tried to prevent Doll's voice reaching the people; in 1982 they looked to him to placate the increasingly hostile world. Then approaching his 70th birthday, Sir Richard Doll—he had been awarded his knighthood in 1971—was by now a giant in medical research; there was no greater authoritative medical researcher to adjudicate on a contentious scientific problem. In the summer of 1982 Doll and Joan went to Rochdale, and after watching the television film he spoke to the audience of managers and trade unionists.

> It so upset the workers, because it made them feel they were all being killed off. I went up at the request of the industry to talk to the workers and try and get it in proportion what the effects were. I cannot remem-

ber much about the film now, but one thing I do remember very clearly was they filmed people as they walked from the bottom of the hill to the top, where the factory was. As they had walked up they were short of breath, they did this to give the impression that all the workers were short of breath because of the factory, which was quite untrue; they were not, the vast majority were not suffering any complaints at all.[49]

In the 1980s a rising tide of litigation began to engulf T&N—an experience shared by all the asbestos companies. By 1982 the insurers of US asbestos firms had already incurred costs totalling $1 billion. In that eventful year three defendant manufacturers—the most notable of which was the industrial giant Johns-Manville—took refuge in a federal bankruptcy law known as Chapter 11. But Chapter 11 was not an option for T&N in Britain so it had little choice other than to continue paying compensation. Medical advances which introduced greater certainty in diagnosis; the activities of trade unions; the availability of legal aid—all these factors made the legal outlook more threatening for the company, and in the 1980s the number of writs served on T&N began to mushroom.

Responding to increasing public and political pressure, the government tightened safety regulations further. A review requested by the Health and Safety Commission on the control limit for asbestos was issued in July 1983.[50] Donald Acheson, who became chief medical officer the following year, was a co-author of the report and twenty years later he was able to give some historical context to the rise and fall of asbestos:

Martin Gardner and I showed that mesothelioma did not occur with chrysotile. It occurred with amosite and crocidolite—and as far as I know that is still the case... That does not mean to say that it is safe, because you do have the interaction with tobacco, but I would guess that if you were a non-smoker and worked only with chrysotile, you probably would not get any problems.

But perhaps it is as much because these words are almost impossible for anyone other than someone who has worked with the damn things, like I have, to be able to explain let alone spell those elements. The health agencies say, "For God's sake, what is all this about?" And this is what the EU is doing now—they say, "Let's do away with asbestos completely. Finish."[51]

At the same time, John Gummer, the Conservative under-secretary of state for health and safety, asserted that there was no safe level, and that "a single fibre could do real damage which may not be seen for 20 years or more."[52] Mesothelioma, besides its devastating impact on individuals, sounded the death knell for the British asbestos industry. With no safe threshold (a level below which there was no danger) even relatively trivial amounts of dust could be lethal.

In 1971 the medical services division of HM Factory Inspectorate had established a prospective mortality study of men in a limited number of workplaces which were covered by the 1969 Asbestos Licensing Regulations; this was subsequently extended to cover most fixed workplaces, and in 1986 to all individuals having statutory medical examinations under the regulations. In this cohort, from 1971 to 1991 there were 183 mesothelioma deaths. Over the same period 10,985 mesothelioma deaths occurred nationally. The vast majority of workers at risk from asbestos were not employed in occupations where this risk was recognised. Quite simply, the fact that most new cases of the disease were found outside the asbestos plants meant that the Doll and Peto factory-based study was not picking up the true hazards that society faced. Looking back, Peto saw vividly the parameters of epidemiology's capacity and its limitations in discovering human exposure to a fatal cancer risk:

It was extraordinary—we were focusing on whether the factory regulations were accurate and making them more stringent, and I simply wasn't involved in the wider pattern of exposure. And when the results of the twenty-year study came out there were less than 200 mesotheliomas in the cohort group, while over the same period there were over 10,000 mesotheliomas in Britain. So what they'd regarded, and what we'd regarded, as the major problem if you like, was two per cent of the problem. And that's how bad it was—the asbestos factories had cleaned up; in the case of Turner Brothers they had cleaned up in the 1920s pretty dramatically, the Rochdale factory was cleaner in the 1930s than a lot of builders' yards were in 1975. I published my dose/response paper in 1977 and by 1980 asbestos use had ceased. But, we were all surprised and horrified when ten years, fifteen years later, just how huge the mesothelioma epidemic was going to be.[53]

Most of the asbestos imported into the UK between 1960 and 1980 is probably still in place in buildings; and carpenters, electricians and other workers involved in building renovation, maintenance and demolition may still suffer unsuspected exposure. These workers often operate individually or in small and unmonitored groups, and it may be impossible to obtain reliable information on the extent of their exposure. For Doll, there was a logical explanation as to why the measured analysis of factory pollution was relevant. "The thing about studying industry is that you could get some dose/response relationship, whereas you had no idea at all what the exposure was in builders' yards, or what dangers carpenters who were boring holes in the walls of people's houses faced; you just had no idea what the situation was like there."[54]

Although the UK's death rate from asbestos disease in per capita terms is four times that of the United States, asbestos victims in the US are four times more likely to sue for damages. The contingency fee system (which allows lawyers to take on a case without a fee for a share of the damages) and punitive awards in millions of dollars helped produce the biggest wave of litigation in history. In 1991 the insurance industry had paid out $2 billion in American asbestos cases, with Lloyd's syndicates paying half that total.

Ten years later, the *Wall Street Journal* reported in its columns: "Like the ubiquitous material itself—once prized for its fire-retardant and insulating qualities—asbestos lawsuits are proving to be ineradicable. Asbestos has spawned more lawsuits than any other product in the history of personal-injury litigation. The US Supreme Court has called asbestos litigation an 'elephantine mass' that defies the normal values of judicial litigation."[55]

Mesothelioma is nearly always fatal, and it is a disease with a particularly devastating course. The cancers characteristically take many years to develop. Few if any occur less than 15 years after first exposure and because the amphibole fibres persist more or less permanently in the lung, the risk of developing mesothelioma increases progressively with time since first exposure. This is in sharp contrast to lung cancer, the incidence of which peaks ten to twenty years after exposure and falls off. Therefore, the disturbing reality was that the peak incidence of the disease resulting from the use of amosite in building materials and for insulation in the 1960s would not be observed until the second decade of the twenty-first century—when mesothelioma may be responsible for a half of one per cent of all deaths in men. Most of such deaths will have been caused by the uncontrolled exposure of building and maintenance workers before the end of the 1970s.

In 1994 Julian Peto and his colleagues defined the true extent of the disease's future death toll. "The prediction that British mesothelioma rates will continue to rise for many years is fairly secure. Whether the eventual total will be of the order of 3,000 deaths per year, as the simple cohort analysis suggests, depends on several factors... Irrespective of future trends and past errors of diagnosis, total asbestos-related cancer deaths in the UK must be substantially greater than the number of recorded mesothelioma deaths."[56] The report's concluding paragraph stated: "The campaign to remove all asbestos from schools and other public buildings on the grounds that occupants might be at high risk was founded on fear rather than evidence."[57]

After forty years researching the carcinogenic effects of asbestos use in Britain, how did Doll feel the general public viewed his work?

> Initially I think they thought I was a critic of asbestos, but, subsequently, they came to regard me as a defender of it because I believed things have gone too far, with claims that exposures to tiny amounts are impor-

tant. I believe you can get mesotheliomas from small amounts, but the fact that you've had a week's exposure to asbestos while working in a garage and then you develop lung cancer doesn't mean that your lung cancer was due to asbestos—which is what the public tended to believe. They were encouraged by doctors like Selikoff, who were involved with the environmental movement; they tried to argue that every cancer that could be caused by asbestos was caused by asbestos, if the person had had any exposure. I used to deny this very strongly.[58]

Four decades after writing his first research paper on asbestos, Doll was still acknowledging—at least in a limited way— its social benefit:

> ... to continue to use white asbestos, for a few limited purposes such as the production of asbestos cement. For asbestos cement products can be manufactured without giving rise to any material occupational hazards, and they can provide major health benefits, as when asbestos cement pipes are used for large-scale distribution of uninfected water. The difficulty in achieving a balanced approach is partly that the material has been given such a bad name that rational discussion about it has become almost impossible and partly that the scientific evidence is, in some respects, still unclear.[59]

Doll and Julian Peto's epidemiological research into asbestos came at personal and professional cost. Buffeted by the countervailing interests of the industry and the environmental movement, both scientists have occupied a unique position in one of the twentieth century's seismic industrial medical stories: the rise and fall of the use of asbestos. Julian Peto owes his career in medical research to Doll, and is more qualified than any other observer to pass judgment on the role of his former boss in that story.

> He was both a critic and a defender of the industry. He thought that what he was going to do was what he had done for the other industries he had studied—which was to detect intolerable risks, for safe regulations to be imposed, and for the industry to carry on. That is what he thought he was doing. He said very early on that blue asbestos should

be banned, because that was in a different league. The thing is he was right in a sense. Well, he was wrong in that if there had been more hysteria about asbestos earlier on a lot of deaths would have been prevented. Because people were wondering what the risks were, this led to a situation where nothing was done until the late 1970s. But in a purely scientific sense it may well be true that most uses of white asbestos are relatively innocuous and the world is not doing itself a favour by getting rid of it.[60]

In Britain the continued use of asbestos is not now a major issue because other reliable substitutes have been found; none the less the new century has seen more criticism of the work of epidemiologists by the industry's defenders. Julian Peto has been accused of hysterical exaggeration of the risks of chrysotile even though the 1985 paper he co-authored with Doll assumed that the crocidolite used in the factory at the same time caused half of all the mesotheliomas. When Peto told Doll about the personal attacks on him being made in the *Sunday Telegraph*,[61] Doll drawing on his half-century in the firing-line of medical research told him: "Ignore it."

Chapter 11

The Anatomy of a Scientific Dispute

"The value of a scientific hypothesis lies less in the number of the observations that it can explain than in the number that it can successfully predict."[1]

Richard Doll

The most important discovery in the history of cancer epidemiology is the carcinogenic effect of tobacco. Epidemiological science changed the ways in which causes of disease would be investigated and understood, but this would only be after Doll and Hill had successfully repelled a withering attack from Sir Ronald Aylmer Fisher, a genius of statistical science.

One of Doll's intuitive skills was the ability to discern patterns. By 1953 he could see how the epidemic was unfolding. The temporal and geographical observations Doll made with Hill led him to a prophetic statistical prediction.

Of all male deaths in 1950, four per cent were attributed to lung cancer; at ages 45-54 the proportion was 10 per cent. There is no reason to suppose that these figures have yet reached their maxima. On the contrary, the trend in mortality rates suggests that lung cancer will reach an even more prominent position. It is difficult to estimate the actual number of deaths that will occur. Trends do not always continue smoothly... The maximum mortality from lung cancer, unlike that from every other major form of cancer in men, is not in the oldest age group ... If it can be assumed that the death rates under the age of 45 have now become stable, and that the trend in the age distribution continues until the distribution is similar to that of, say, cancer of the stomach, a rough estimate can be made of the number of deaths which will eventually be attributed to lung cancer. On such assumptions— admittedly highly speculative but, I think, not wholly unreasonable— the number of deaths, for a population of the same age and sex composition as at present, will eventually reach 20,000. In fact, the future population will almost certainly contain a higher proportion of old persons, so that the number recorded in 20 years' time (1973) may be as great as 25,000.[2]

Doll was wrong: it was 26,000.

In 1956 more solid results came from the study of British doctors. By this time Doll and Hill had some fifty months of observations. The outstanding finding in the cohort study was that the quantitative relationship with smoking was almost exactly the same as they had found in the case-control study. This showed that not only qualitative but also quantitative estimates of risk could come from a case-control study. As they got more data, so the dose-response relationship became firmly established and they found it to be practically identical with that deduced from the case-control study. In 1956 a total of 1,854 deaths of British doctors from all causes had been reported to or discovered by the researchers. They came not only from the returns made by the registrar-general but from the General Medical Council and the British Medical Association. In this, according to Hill, "Richard had again applied his customary assiduous search to ensure a complete record. For every one of the 88 deaths attributed to cancer of the lung he had sought confirmation, and the basis of the diagnosis, from doctor, consultant or hospital. We accepted 84 as established. Once more, step by step, we jointly analysed these data and built up the statistical picture."[3]

This watershed study appeared in the *British Medical Journal*, and its simple arithmetical logic and biological sense confirmed the strength of the association.

> From the retrospective studies... we concluded that if large groups of persons of different smoking habits were observed for a number of years they would reveal distinct differences in their rates of mortality from lung cancer. They would show, we believed, (1) a higher mortality in smokers than in non-smokers, (2) a higher mortality in heavy smokers than in light smokers, (3) a higher mortality in cigarette smokers than in pipe smokers, and (4) a higher mortality in those who continued to smoke than in those who gave it up. In each case the expected result has appeared in this prospective inquiry.[4]

Their evidence suggested that one in eight lifelong heavy smokers died of lung cancer, against one in 300 of non-smokers. Smoking was thus established as a major cause of preventable disease. Yet this conclusion had not been universally accepted, as the evidence was observational and unconfirmed by experiment. One argument against accepting a causative connection between smoking and lung cancer derives from the old axiom that correlation does not mean causation. Even Doll and Hill were reluctant wholeheartedly to embrace the idea that statistical evidence provided *proof* of a direct link between smoking and lung cancer. In 1956 they wrote: "In scientific work it is never possible to exclude entirely an alternative explanation of the observations ... But we ourselves believe that the accumulated evidence to-day is such as to denote a cause-and-effect relationship.[5]

Different people gave different meaning to *cause*. What was undeniable was that some unlucky people, who did not smoke, got lung cancer. Therefore, in the philosophical sense, cigarette smoking was neither *necessary* nor *sufficient* for the cause of any form of cancer, but Hill and Doll were able to show that prolonged smoking resulted in a rare disease becoming ten times as common as it would have in the absence of the habit.

Doll believed that the accumulation of statistical knowledge from both case-control and cohort pointed in the direction of proof that smoking was a cause of bronchial carcinoma. No proof is, however, absolute—all are susceptible to greater or smaller degrees of confidence. "It is only by further experiment, by testing the hypothesis under fresh conditions, that confidence can be gradually increased until finally its truth is unquestioned."[6] At the same time as the research in Britain, Hammond and Horn in the US, in a very large study of almost 200,000 people, found that regular cigarette smoking caused an increase in the incidence of lung cancer and a correlation with coronary thrombosis in men and women.[7] Hill and Doll's expertise in developing and expanding epidemiological techniques to understand old and new medical problems helped to weaken the intellectual thought-barrier which existed within established medical science. However, the acceptance was not universal and indeed opposition to their scientific findings emanated from a variety of motivations: some subjective in origin, some scientific, while others reflected an emotional outpouring of libertarian free will. Indeed, it was analogous to the opposition which John Snow's statistical and epidemiological observations encountered a century earlier. He too could only offer inductive reasoning for the measures that were responsible for the control of the cholera. The fact that no carcinogen had been identified in tobacco smoke did not invalidate the evidence; as the recognition of the risk run by chimney-sweeps and tar workers came many years before the carcinogenic polycyclic hydrocarbons were isolated.

Doll and Hill's work was criticised by the tobacco companies for being "unscientific", and when the government's cancer standing advisory committee met in March 1956 it decided that nothing had happened to cause the committee to modify or strengthen its advice even in the light of the new evidence.

For Snow a century earlier, denial and disbelief were joined in righteous exultation by the *Times* when it rejoiced over the fall of the first general board of health. "Aesculapius and Chiron have been deposed, and we prefer to take our chance of cholera and the rest than be bullied into health." The writer did indeed take his chance of cholera, which was rampant in London within a month. But the chance was not to persist much longer. On the advice of the medical profession, led by Sir John Simon, who said, "the neglect... of those laws of healthy existence with the consideration of which the science of public health professes to deal," the last major cholera epidemic in Britain was brought under control in 1866—seventeen years before Koch isolated the cholera vibrio.

Doll and Hill having rejected all other possible causes of the lung cancer epidemic were left with inductive reasoning based on purely statistical and epidemiological observations. If the control of cholera was brought about by these techniques, how long would it take to overcome the sceptics before public health steps would be taken to end the rapid increase in mortality from lung cancer?

Harold Macmillan's Conservative government was now facing two unenviable political possibilities. Either tobacco was responsible for providing both the greatest amount of money to the treasury in revenue and the greatest threat to the nation's health, or atmospheric pollution, which was still viewed by some as a major cause of the disease, was denuding the nation of its citizens. (Doll and Hill had noted in their 1952 study that the risk of developing lung cancer was lower in the countryside than in the larger towns, although the differences were small and not statistically significant.)

The acute effects of the 1952 smog, which caused an estimated extra 4,000 deaths and led to the Clean Air Act of 1956, were not evidently due to any new types of pollution. What made the 1952 smog unique was its longevity. For five days Europe's largest city was engulfed in a noxious miasma of dense smog. The act itself dealt only with domestic use of coal, not with the greater levels of pollution coming from industry. The legislation was seen by one historian as showing that "although the government was wary about the smoking and lung cancer case as a policy issue, it was infinitely preferable to air pollution. That was an issue that the government did not want reopened."[8]

For some statisticians, arithmetic is the best morality. After five years' research, the tobacco industry's statistician Geoffrey Todd became convinced that Doll and Hill had found the true carcinogen. Todd then advised the cigarette industry that on the basis of their investigation he was convinced that cigarettes were the principal cause of the disease. He told the Imperial Tobacco Company and the Tobacco Research Council, which the industry had set up, that unless they accepted the conclusion that smoking caused lung cancer he could not work for them any longer. So they sacked him. Six weeks later he was reinstated and the industry had taken him back on his conditions.*

From then on, for some years, Doll had what he described as

a very good relationship with the tobacco industry in Britain.
They agreed that they would not say anything to imply that smoking

---

* Doll believed that it was largely at Todd's instigation that the Imperial Tobacco Company agreed "not to say smoking did not cause lung cancer," a double negative that was nevertheless a huge concession.

did not cause lung cancer or some other diseases, but they would continue to take the view that as people enjoyed smoking, they would continue to provide them with tobacco. So our relationship with the tobacco industry in Britain was initially good and all our contacts were polite.[9]

Doll and Hill's 1956 study of British doctors—the first major prospective study of smoking and death in the world[10]—and Himsworth's unwavering support led to a change in the climate of acceptance. In June 1957 the MRC issued its long-awaited special report on smoking and lung cancer. It was the first national institution in the world to formally accept the evidence that tobacco is a major cause of death.[11] At this point, doubts within the Ministry of Health disappeared, and the parliamentary secretary expressed in the House of Commons unambiguous support for the conclusions reached by Doll and Hill in 1950. For the first time the government also accepted a responsibility to make this information available "to all those with responsibility for health education".[12] Two days later, on 29 June 1957, the *British Medical Journal* published a leading article entitled "The Dangers of Cigarette Smoking".[13] The article was a vindication of Doll and Hill's work, and the epidemiological techniques they pioneered. It marked the beginning of a public health campaign against the dangers of smoking, in the country where the lung cancer rates were the highest in the world.

The *BMJ's* opening paragraph was unequivocal. "The Medical Research Council has now advised the government that a direct causal connection exists between tobacco-smoking and lung cancer." The article went on to alert its readers to the role played by tobacco in causing coronary thrombosis, chronic bronchitis, cancer of the mouth and oropharynx, and "some would add, a delusion that smoking is harmless." Relying heavily on Doll and Hill's findings, the leader outlined the accumulated knowledge that had been gathered from nineteen inquiries published in six countries. It also supported the need for continued research and noted that RA Fisher had agreed to become a scientific consultant to the tobacco manufacturers' standing committee, which was set up "to assist research into smoking and health questions, to keep in touch with scientists and others working in the UK and abroad, and to make information available to scientific workers and the public."

The closing paragraph highlighted the fact that 18,000 people died of lung cancer in 1956 and that "it is incumbent on doctors to do all that they can to dissuade the young from acquiring a habit so deleterious to health. Smoking is a widespread and pleasurable social habit, and unfortunately the appetite for it grows with what it feeds upon. But the hazards to life are undeniable, hazards which must be brought home to the public with all the modern devices of publicity..."

Doll and Hill did not use the article, which extolled their work, to build a public health campaign against the smoking addiction that was killing ever increasing numbers of people whom the NHS was pledged to protect. On Hill's advice, Doll decided neither to get involved in public education—nor to become emotional about the subject. Their role was to remain objective and produce reliable information, not to campaign on the basis of that evidence; that was for others to do.

Originally, Doll and Hill envisaged the British doctors study ending after five years. However, the findings were so unexpected—revealing other fatal diseases caused by tobacco, and showing the possible beneficial effects of quitting smoking—that in 1957 it was decided to extend the investigation of the 34,439 British male doctors. Marie Kidd was one of twelve graduates who started work on the new data in 1957 at the London School of Hygiene and Tropical Medicine. Kidd recalled that when the group first met, Doll took a straw poll. "How many are smokers?" What was interesting was that Doll was not anti-smoking. "He improved the lot of the common man—but like that initial straw poll he didn't tell us to stop. And at lunch people would smoke."[14]

This tolerance towards smoking was not recognised by another of Doll's colleagues at the LSHTM, Walter Holland. Holland, who became a professor of social medicine in London, thought that after 1950 Doll was vehemently anti-smoking and "would scowl at people who lit up in front of him." This, according to Holland, was in marked contrast to Hill— and perhaps it shows how indelibly the cigarette culture had permeated

British culture—who kept a box of cigarettes in his desk drawer. When Holland first worked for him in the 1950s, Hill opened the drawer of his desk, took out the box of cigarettes and offered him one. "No thank you," replied Holland, "I smoke a pipe." To some of his junior colleagues, a visit to Hill's office became an ordeal where they would be put to the tobacco test. Eventually, Holland asked about the box of cigarettes? Tony replied, "Well, it's polite, isn't it?"[15]

It was initially in the US, and later in Britain, that the scientific controversy between the advocates of public health and the tobacco industry entered the public arena. In the US, the tobacco industry research committee dedicated itself to undermining epidemiological studies on the hazards of cigarette smoking. On 4 January 1954 the committee released its notorious Frank Statement to Cigarette Smokers. Published in more than 400 newspapers across the continent, the Frank Statement assured addicted customers that their health was the tobacco industry's overriding concern. It highlighted the lack of consensus among scientists as to what constituted "proof" of the correlation between smoking and lung cancer. The statement, predicting the scientific storm that was to surround Doll and Hill, assured American smokers: "Indeed, the validity of the statistics themselves is questioned by numerous scientists."

That Doll and Hill's work aroused accusations from the tobacco industry of being "unscientific" was understandable, even inevitable; that it attracted scepticism from a predominantly innumerate political establishment was predictable. However, what was not foreseen was the *casus belli* declared on their work by RA Fisher. Statistician, evolutionary biologist, mathematician and geneticist, Fisher was the Darwinian creator of the intellectual foundations of modern statistical science. What had triggered the wrath of the world's leading theoretical statistician against Doll and Hill's statistical observations?

The leading article in the *British Medical Journal* in 1957 had aroused Fisher's naturally disputatious nature. He felt it went beyond the evidence and, assuming smoking had been proven to be the cause of lung cancer, led to "the almost shrill conclusion that it was necessary that every device of modern publicity should be employed to bring home to the world at large this terrible danger."[16] This was abhorrent to Fisher, reminding him of the unscrupulous use of such devices in the Second World War. The campaign against smoking thus announced violated the whole trend of Fisher's philosophy for it contradicted one of his sacred shibboleths of scientific inference. Correlation must not be accepted as proof of causation.

Fisher was a highly complex and contradictory man. A libertarian and "inveterate pipe smoker", [17] he was capable of being a sincere friend, but not a generous enemy. Indeed his biographer—and, as his daughter, she must have known him more thoroughly than most—wrote: "He seemed inhuman in his lack of consideration for the feelings of others. Capable of rough handling those who opposed him with ready-made arguments that he treated with contempt. He was sometimes arbitrary and disagreeable and he was recalcitrant to any form of coercion."[18]

Fisher acknowledged that statistics had gained a place of modest usefulness in medical research but did "not relish the prospect of this science being now discredited by a catastrophic and conspicuous howler."[19] In the beginning, Fisher's criticisms were scientific in origin. In their 1950 case-control study Doll and Hill reported that smokers with lung cancer reported inhaling less often than smokers without the disease (62 per cent against 67 per cent).[20] This led Fisher to write: "There is nothing to stop those who greatly desire it from believing that lung cancer is caused by smoking cigarettes. They should also believe that inhaling cigarette smoke is a protection. To believe either is, however, to run the risk of failing to recognise, and therefore failing to prevent, other and more genuine causes."[21]

In addition to the inhaling anomaly, Fisher cited three further criticisms of the observational evidence. Firstly, that the secular changes in smoking habits could not be related to the increase in lung cancer since "lung cancer has been increasing more rapidly in men relatively to women," while "it is notorious, and conspicuous in the memory of most of us, that over the last fifty years the increase of smoking among women has been great, and that among men (even if positive) certainly small."[22] Secondly, that it was possible that the association between smoking and lung cancer could have arisen because lung cancer caused smoking rather than the other way round, if, as he suggested, the development of the disease was preceded by malignant changes that caused irritation that was relieved by smoking. Thirdly, there might be some common factor responsible both for the individual's smoking habits and the risk of developing the disease. His last point was addressed by Doll: "This he postulated could be genetic and he supported his hypothesis by showing that the smoking habits of pairs of monozygous (one egg) twins were more similar than those of dizygous (two egg) twins irrespective of whether they had been raised together or apart."[23]

The lung cancer inhaling anomaly not only created a scientific dispute, it transcended the accepted parameters of statistical interpretation into the realm of personal integrity. The leading actors in the drama that was unfolding were Hill and Fisher. Though Doll had done most of the day-to-day statistical analysis, he readily acknowledged Hill's dominant role in establishing the arithmetic of proof: "in origin, design, and execution".[24] Fisher and Hill were great scientists; they represented august institutions, and for most of their professional lives were on good terms. Indeed, Fisher even offered Hill a post at the Rothamsted Experimental Station in the 1930s. Hill, while flattered by the offer ("I thanked him warmly"[25]), was more interested in the application of statistics to medicine than agriculture—and opted to make his career at the LSHTM.

By the late 1950s, however, the fraternal relationship had degenerated into suspicion and accusation. Hill, like Fisher, was a fellow of the Royal Society, and was revered for the clarity of his teaching and thinking—but he did not possess Fisher's mathematical brilliance. Few, if anyone, did. Nevertheless, Doll believed that Fisher resented the status that Hill had attained as a medical statistician. "Fisher was the world's leading theoretical statistician, and renowned in applying genetics to agriculture, but he didn't really have any knowledge of clinical medicine."[26]

Fisher's thesis that "inhaling cigarette smoke was a practice of considerable prophylactic value in preventing the disease" was based on his interpretation of the 647 males and 41 females with cancer of the lung. To build his case against causation based on *a simple association* Fisher wrote to Hill for a copy of the data he had used. By then Doll and Hill had data on almost 1,400 people with cancer of the lung, based on their 1952 retrospective inquiry. When Doll and Hill offered Fisher the complete data set, Fisher refused the offer and demanded the original 1950 findings. At the time, the difficulty for chest physicians and epidemiologists lay in predicting, without direct observation, where the smoke droplets were deposited on the lung. In their 1952 survey Doll and Hill found that "while inhaling was associated with a diminished risk of cancer of the large bronchi, it was associated with an increased risk of developing cancer in the periphery of the lung which would make biological sense."[27] This was slightly different to the 1950 study, which led Fisher to the conclusion that inhaling would prevent lung cancer.*

On several occasions Doll and Hill offered Fisher the unified data and on each occasion he refused. This impasse led to what Doll termed a "nasty" sequence of events between the two camps. "That's when he accused us of suppressing data. It wasn't because we were refusing to give him the 1950 data—it was because we thought it less appropriate than the completed survey of 1,400 people with cancer of the lung."[28] Doll recalled reading Fisher's accusation of their intentional suppression of information and urged Hill to sue for libel. Hill's natural caution—and probably his lawyer brother's advice—led him away from litigation, opting instead for confrontation.

---

* The principal site for carcinoma is the epithelium of the main bronchi. Doll and Hill in 1952 found that a higher proportion of smokers with peripheral lung cancers said that they inhaled compared with smokers having central tumours (63 per cent to 52 per cent)—a statistically significant difference, although there was no significant difference in cigarette consumption. This led Professor Nicholas Wald to observe: "What was once seen as an objection to smoking as a cause of lung cancer can be explained and is consistent with smoking being a cause of the disease."

On 30 October 1958 Hill wrote Fisher a letter:

Dear Fisher

I do not normally take notice of hearsay but I have recently been told
on good authority that you are suggesting that Doll and I are deliberately "concealing" some of the data which we gathered about inhaling
in our retrospective study of patients with lung cancer. That would be
an extremely serious accusation, and, of course, utterly untrue. We published six years ago what we considered to be of value and interest in
that inquiry and since then we have provided any further information
that could be extracted from the data whenever the request has come
from a reputable scientist. If you yourself require further information I
would expect you to follow that customary procedure of reputable scientists, namely to specify what it is that you require and to ask me
whether it is or could be made available. I shall await that request.
Meanwhile I am reluctant to believe that such hearsay has any foundation in fact.[29]

By return of post Fisher's emotional and statistical views were given vivid
expression:

Dear Bradford Hill

What a stuffy letter! I thought I had given the impression that you were
rather honest, though mistaken. However, if you are willing to give the
data on which the results in the *BMJ* September 30 1950 were based, I
am sure it will remove any impression of concealment... What is
wanted, and what I asked Doll for nearly a year ago, is the breakdown
showing how many... declared themselves to be inhalers...[30]

In the autumn of 1958, when Doll and Fisher* spoke at the
Cambridge University Medical Society on the subject of smoking and carcinoma of the lung, Fisher did not confront Doll on the issue of the sup-

---

* The title of Fisher's address was "Combustion and the Products Formed".

posed concealment. In fact, Fisher left the lecture theatre after making his formal address, refusing to take part in the programmed open debate.[31] When the information was finally handed over, the punch cards from the 1950 study had worn out, and Doll and Hill had to make the tabulation specifically for Fisher. Hill then passed the two sets of data separately to Fisher but "he only used the London one [1950], which suited his bill, because the other one didn't suit it so much; he left that out. And I thought that was a bit crooked."[32]

The friendship and co-operation that had once been hallmarks of the relationship between Hill and Fisher was now replaced with mistrust, and in Fisher's case, malevolence. Peter Armitage witnessed the decomposition of the scientific respect between the two men. "I was present at a meeting of the National Institute of Health in the late 1950s in which [Fisher] gave a seminar on smoking and lung cancer, among other things... He actually said there that Bradford Hill did not deserve to have been made a fellow of the Royal Society. That [seemed] an incredibly vicious remark to me."[33] Fuelled by misanthropic contempt, it led to an incident of biology overtaking science. Fisher did not like people having so much respect for Hill because he felt Hill did not have his abilities, which was true, but Hill had other abilities, a sort of common sense which Fisher sometimes lacked.

Fisher's scientific interests continually confronted him with the basic problem of statistics, how to make inferences from the particular to the general. To scientific problems he could bring to bear one of the greatest intellects of his generation, and he was not unconscious of the fact that he possessed a superior brain. But it was the manner in which he imposed his views that left so much human debris in his wake. Hill and Doll were not the first scientists to incur his opprobrium and it seemed that this capacity was part of his nature. Walter Bodmer was among the last of Fisher's students and disciples and while venerating his mentor as an extraordinary scientist, he also acknowledged the complexity of his personality. "Fisher was a proud man in addition to his sensitivity, and this undoubtedly explained some of the antagonistic interactions he developed with scientific colleagues."[34]

In his disquisition *Smoking: the Cancer Controversy*, Fisher, while discussing the inhaling anomaly, wrote: "It has taken some years, therefore, to elicit the tables below which are a reconstruction of the original observations."[35] As Peter Armitage observed, this was a mischievous misrepresentation of the facts.[36] Clearly Fisher was talking from his heart not his head and, and as the years went by, it became increasingly important to determine which organ prevailed.

But what of Fisher's other criticisms of Doll and Hill with which he was "teasing" the British Medical Association and being "deliberately provocative"? Could cancer cause a person to smoke? This did not seem biologically plausible to Doll and Hill as most patients in their survey had begun smoking some forty years before the development of the disease. As for the evidence of secular changes, Fisher had ignored the effects by which the risks among successive cohorts are determined not merely by their recent smoking history, but by the accumulated risk evolving from the distant past. As the habit of cigarette smoking became acquired by greater numbers of women for longer periods of time, the trends in the sex ratio of the disease reflected the trends in cigarette consumption over the relevant periods. If women were going to live like men—at least in terms of smoking-related diseases—they were going to die like men.

The most intellectually challenging argument put forward by Fisher was that of confounding. As Fisher saw it the researchers had merely shown a correlation, in which case there were three possibilities. "A may be the cause of B, B may be the cause of A, or something else may be the cause of both."[37] Doll was not convinced that Fisher's genetic explanation would fit quantitatively with the geographical and social distribution of the disease. This, however, did not prevent him from attempting to establish his own twin study. So in 1959 Doll took part in a television programme about the smoking epidemic and appealed for monozygotic twins who had different smoking habits to contact him. He wanted to examine Fisher's constitutional hypothesis. Britain at the time did not have a twin register, and Doll's efforts failed, as only five sets of twins came forward. "I'm afraid the appeal fell on deaf ears."[38] Doll never took Fisher's genetic view of a "common cause" seriously. What he did take seriously was some people's reaction to it,* in particular the media who publicised it, with the encouragement of the tobacco industry. It took another twenty years before Doll could demonstrate Fisher's genetic hypothesis to be nonsensical.

In his twenty-year follow up of the British doctors' smoking habits, Doll discovered that when some doctors gave up, the risk of lung cancer in the whole population of doctors fell relative to that of the general population.[39] Fisher, on the other hand, had said that it would not make any difference because people who gave up were those who were not susceptible to developing the disease. So for Doll "that demonstrated that the hypothesis could not be correct."[40] With the passage of time more epidemiological evidence emerged contradicting Fisher's findings in monozygotic twins with different smoking habits.[41]

As we have seen, Britain in the 1950s was a society in which smoking was deeply entrenched. This, in some ways, explains the resistance to the idea that it was such a dangerous habit. Doll's 1953 prediction that smoking-related deaths would increase steeply over the next twenty years was an ingenious calculation and one that had a degree of influence on scientists, and doctors, but none at all on the general population. This can in part be explained by what psychologists term cognitive dissonance; a collective

---

* "In Australia," Fisher's biographer wrote, "his lectures on the subject were frankly intended to raise questions... Audiences were quick to laugh when he pointed out the negative correlation between lung cancer and inhaling; and there were other anomalies: the positive correlation between smoking habit and genotype, the lack of success at that time in isolating any carcinogenic substance from tobacco, the difference in incidence of cancer between smokers of cigarettes and smokers of tobacco in other forms, between people in different environments, between the sexes... If he seemed to some the devil's advocate, his reasonableness, good-humour and wit were hard to resist. His talks were generally well received."

refusal to acknowledge the reality of a hazard. To permeate this society-wide resistance, a campaign would be required using "all the modern devices of publicity". This, the media of the time was not prepared to make. Deliberately eschewing a public health role, Doll did not zealously walk around pulling cigarettes out of the mouths of smokers, as some doctors did. Doll was subtle in his advocacy. He wanted people to know the risks involved with the habit and then to make up their own minds on the basis of the best information available. "It's their decision and their life, not mine."

Risk and how people perceive it is intriguing and complex. It is possible for people to understand the concept of "chance" and the "odds" of something happening while "risk" is open to more abstract interpretation, particularly when measured against the dangers associated with smoking cigarettes. This is because harm of a new sort or of an unfamiliar origin is often considered worse than harm that is familiar. Risks that are endured by choice are of less concern to people than those that are suffered involuntarily. British society in the early 1950s was more concerned with nuclear annihilation, the curtain coming down on the British Empire, and food rationing than it was about the hazards of smoking. As Jeremy Bentham pointed out a century earlier, the deterrent effect of a punishment not only depends on its probability and its severity, but also on what he called its "propinquity"—that is, how soon one is likely to suffer the consequences of one's own actions. Thus, the universality of the smoking habit, the emerging nature of the epidemic and the long gestation period of the disease combined to obscure the sense that tobacco might be a major threat to the nation's health.

Fisher thought that Britain should be concerned about the epidemic of lung cancer; he just did not see "the mild and soothing weed" as being its cause. As the 1950s came to a close the forces of resistance to Doll and Hill's research were manifest. Smoking rates were still on the increase, the government remained reluctant to take up the cause of public health and tobacco advertising stressed the life-enhancing qualities of the cigarette. In this atmosphere it seems paradoxical that Fisher felt alienated for holding dissenting views that contravened accepted orthodoxy. Joan

Fisher Box struck a religious chord in describing his crusade. "The emotional tone of the first as of succeeding campaigns against smoking was one of religious fervour; it was mounted on simple absolutism and any agnosticism appeared as moral turpitude. No ambiguity, no doubt was permissible."[42]

Fisher had, however, left himself open to accusations of venality, when in 1956 he had accepted the invitation of the tobacco manufacturers' standing committee to be their scientific consultant. Hill suspected that the attack upon him and Doll arose out of this relationship but also that Fisher's ego would disabuse people of this correlation. According to Hill, "He was vain enough to think that people wouldn't connect that with him."[43]

Fisher was both a scientist and a libertarian. He did not see any dichotomy in receiving payment from an organisation and giving expert advice. He wrote of this falsely perceived moral dilemma: "I am free under our agreement to say what I like, however much financial damage it may do the interests of the tobacco companies."[44] Yates and Mather made an attempt in their 1962 Royal Society memoir of Fisher to explain the psychology determining his behaviour:

> It has been suggested that the fact that Fisher was employed as consultant by the tobacco firms in this controversy casts doubt on the value of his arguments. This is to misjudge the man. He was not above accepting financial reward for his labours, but the reason for his interest was undoubtedly his dislike and mistrust of puritanical tendencies of all kinds; and perhaps also the personal solace he had always found in tobacco.[45]

Fisher was no ordinary critic. His intellect was feared and revered throughout the scientific world. *Smoking: the Cancer Controversy*, his polemical battering ram against Doll and Hill, read like a legal document and was convincing to an uninformed reader. Its style was a mixture of vexation against the lack of clear thinking, of moral outrage against the excesses of political involvement in the life of the individual; and, of course, it advocated the primacy of randomisation. Fisher placed paramount emphasis on the need for randomisation in order to obtain valid estimates of error. This was the centre of his mathematical universe, and his Achilles' heel in interpreting *cause* and *proof* in clinical medicine. He wrote: "It is not the fault of Hill or Doll or Hammond that they cannot produce evidence in which a thousand children of teen age have been laid under a ban that they shall never smoke, and a thousand more chosen at random from the same age group have been under compulsion to smoke at least thirty cigarettes a day. If that type of experiment could be done, there would be no difficulty."[46]

Fisher underestimated the accuracy of non-randomised evidence in the art of examining observational data. This was a grave confusion of thought. He had voiced his concerns that a generation of intelligent and highly trained statisticians were being sent out "with a dense fog in the place where their brains ought to be".[47] But if anyone was impeding a national effort to discover and prevent disease it was Fisher with his "erroneous numbers" and supposedly "fair minded" assessment of the value of the statistical evidence relating to the incidence of lung cancer.

For Walter Bodmer, Fisher's antagonism to the data on smoking and lung cancer developed as a response to deductive reasoning from observational facts and to the inferences which those facts warrant. "He thus sought common causes such as genetic factors, but without at the time really being aware of the strength of the association and the unlikelihood of it being due to a common cause rather than a direct effect."[48]

If the world's greatest statistician refused to acknowledge the direct effect from the interpretation of epidemiological observations, others did not. Jerry Morris's classic work *Uses of Epidemiology* (1957) extolled Doll and Hill's epidemiological techniques. Politically, Morris and Doll were uneasy bedfellows, but this was not an impediment to the respect in which they held each other's scientific work. In 1958 the barometer of acceptance rose further when the eleventh edition of Jameson's medical encyclopaedia *Synopsis* fully reflected developments since the last edition of 1952, which had reserved only one sentence for the work of Doll and Hill.[49]

For all his advocacy of "clear thinking" and "deductive reasoning"

Fisher did not cease to speak out in opposition to the epidemiological evidence. Even his most dedicated supporters cite the 1957 *BMJ* editorial (that every effort should be made to discourage people from smoking) as the contagious germ that infected his thinking. In 2003 Bodmer acknowledged its decisive impact. "That was actually the ticket to his antagonism. The other arguments developed subsequently."[50]

Early in 1960 Fisher visited the United States at the invitation of a legal firm representing an American tobacco company whose case was brought to trial in April of that year. Other suits were either not brought to trial or were unsuccessful, and the legal pressure on tobacco companies was relieved for a time. Later that year while in Australia giving lectures on the negative correlation between lung cancer and inhaling, Fisher took comfort from letters he had received. He felt exonerated that "opinion in England has been somewhat softened up and several of my points seem to be taken seriously."[51]

Facts are stubborn things. At the end of his life even Fisher's critical intelligence began to see beyond the weakness of his "common cause" hypothesis and the corresponding strengths of Doll and Hill's dose-response relationship. By the time of his death in 1962, it is believed that Fisher had come to accept smoking was a "co-factor" in the cause of the lung cancer.[52] Not a true apostasy. It seemed that the recantation was only partial; yet this was merely semantics: in epidemiology a co-factor is a factor.

For Doll, however, the damage had been done.[53] Fisher's opposition had an international significance and it provided the tobacco industry with a defence that the smoking/lung cancer link was controversial. Mental endeavour, the clash of personality and rigorous argument are all aids to thought in the discovery of scientific truth. This, alas, was not such an occasion. Fisher delayed the acceptance that tobacco causes cancer, together with the urgent public health campaign that was needed to mitigate or prevent the consequences for smokers. What Fisher did not understand and Doll and Hill did was that if people started smoking when young and continued the habit there was a fifty per cent chance that it would kill them prematurely.

Forty-one years after the publication of his landmark paper on smoking, Wynder, who in 1950 co-authored a paper identifying the dangers of tobacco, could see that sound judgement, so elemental a part of Fisher's scientific personality, had been missing in his bitter dispute with Doll and Hill.

> ... with respect to the relation between cigarette smoking and lung cancer, we can now state with certainty that Fisher erred; more importantly, we know that scientific truth prevailed, and this has given us the opportunity for intervention... Clearly, in the absence of cigarette smoking, lung cancer mortality will be significantly reduced. As more and more adults have stopped smoking, lung cancer rates have begun to decline in the younger age groups, as we predicted according to Koch's postulates. The chain of evidence for causality has thus been closed.[54]

One simple observation can be made from this anatomy of a scientific dispute. That is the importance of character and how it forms a relationship with science and between scientists. Fisher may well be the greatest of all Darwin's disciples, and his exhorted status as an evolutionary biologist is permanent and deserved; but he too was both a product and a casualty of the slow evolutionary scale of human psychology.

Chapter 12
The Agnostic Adoption Society

"Once more the storm is howling, and half hid
Under this cradle-hood and coverlid
My child sleeps on."

WB Yeats

By the early 1950s it became apparent that Joan Faulkner and Richard Doll were not going to be able to have a baby of their own although Joan, of course, had her son, Tim, from her marriage to Hugh Faulkner.

There are many possible explanations as to why Doll and Joan did not have children of their own but what is undeniable is that gonorrhoea can cause infertility, and that Joan had caught gonorrhoea from Faulkner. When Doll was asked how he felt about his genes not being handed onto another generation, his reply was characteristically rational. "If something's impossible, I tend not to worry about it." In place of disappointment the couple turned their thoughts to adoption. At the time, however, the adoption service was dominated by religious orthodoxy and required Christian commitment. This reality immediately placed the Dolls in a moral dilemma as both were atheists.

Prior to any formal contact with an adoption society Doll sought the support of his boss Tony Bradford Hill. Scientifically, the men were as one, but in other respects they were separated by a moral universe even though they had known each other since 1947 and Hill had asked Doll to join his staff. When Doll asked him if he would write a reference in support of the application to adopt, the answer was as hurtful as it was truthful. "Hill thought for a moment and then said, 'I don't think communists should have children. It wouldn't be right.' I thought to myself, 'Bugger you, I've got other friends.' I only asked him once. He knew it was important to Joan and me, but that was his answer. I think I forgave him for it—eventually."[1]

The formal adoption agencies all required a reference from their own members or those of other religious organisations, and at the very least obliged prospective parents to attend church services for a period of some months. For the Dolls such pretence was unacceptable.

Fortunately, in the early 1950s the Dolls had a friend who worked in an obstetric clinic and before long they were put in contact with an unmarried pregnant woman who wanted her child adopted. The Dolls then visited the woman in a nursing home off London's Sloane Street and she confirmed her wish to have them adopt her daughter. Within a few weeks the excited couple were looking after the "dear little thing" and they very quickly bonded with her. So it came as a disabling shock when, three months later, the woman wanted her baby back and of course they had to comply. They were devastated, but then another woman from the nursing home came to their salvation. The woman had been in a relationship with a man who was away deep-sea diving when his son was born—and although, on his return, she hoped he would embrace his parental role he did not, and she now wanted her son to be adopted. The child (he was named Nicholas by the Dolls) was only a few weeks old and quickly made himself part of the family.

Joan and Doll were able to dedicate themselves to their new responsibility with the help of a professional children's nurse, and this was how family and professional life progressed for almost a year. The preliminary legal procedures were completed and all that remained was for the mother to sign one last form when suddenly she decided she wanted the boy returned to her care. The Dolls' solicitor, Alan Oliver, advised that there was not much chance of success but that they should take the case to court. Joan was too fearful to attend the hearing; Doll went along with the nurse and Nicholas. The judge ruled that the mother had the right to demand the child back, and Doll left the court alone.

Richard and Joan could not remember how they survived the next 24 hours. The following day the phone rang—it was Nicholas's natural mother saying that the baby had cried continuously and she could not stand it any longer. Doll was not a man prone to excitement or overt displays of affection, but as he waited for the nurse to bring Nicholas home he realised his life had changed. "It was about ten o'clock that she brought him home. When I opened the door, Nicholas, who was by now just quietly whimpering, stopped crying, held out his arms to me, and lay contently against my shoulder. It was one of the most marvellous moments of my life." The next day Doll called on Nicholas's natural mother with the final legal document. After exchanging pleasantries, and for once dropping his English reserve, he slammed the form on to the table and said "Sign it!"

Some fifteen months later they set out to adopt again, and through a medical colleague they were put in contact with a young woman who had just given birth to a baby girl and wanted to have her adopted. They took charge of Catherine when she was about six weeks old and employed Shirley Davies, a professional nanny, and an Italian au pair to help with the care of the children. All the formalities went smoothly, except that the child's mother did think about changing her mind. Nothing came of it, however, and after they were visited by a social worker to satisfy the local authority that they were responsible parents, the adoption was legalised.

The whole experience had been traumatic for the couple, and their sensibilities so disturbed that they decided that they would try and do something to diminish the suffering of other humanist couples who wanted to provide a loving home for children.

The Dolls were in no doubt that there was a need for a formal adoption society that would not judge the suitability of prospective adopting parents by their religious affiliations, and they approached the Humanist Society about their willingness to sponsor an adoption society. They were not prepared to do so officially, but they agreed to give informal support and some initial finance. With the guidance of members of the society, the Dolls set up the Agnostic Adoption Society and employed a social worker to work for them. An early policy statement setting out the aims of the society indicates their advanced thinking and still stands today: "To help would-be adopters from minority as well as majority groups, people from all religions or none, and not to turn away any child who it is within our power to help. Babies which other agencies have classified as difficult we accept gladly."

The society's social worker, Jayne Dunbar, recalled that the first meeting of the Agnostic Adoption Society took place on the dining table of the Dolls' home at 24 Lansdowne Road in the early summer of 1965. "It was just the three of us." In July 1965 the Adoption Society got their first premises on East Street, Walworth, in south-east London, and Dunbar was soon confronted by more than 2,000 letters from hopeful applicants, while cheques and postal orders came from well-wishers and many letters from pregnant women. During the first early months order was slowly created out of chaos and the society began to work. By the end of 1966 nine babies (three girls and six boys) had been adopted in part as a result of the efforts of Dunbar, who "threaded her way through London and the Home Counties interviewing potential adopters, consoling young mothers, finding foster homes and fetching babies out of hospital," according to Mary James, who worked for the society. The society did not insist on agnosticism as a criterion for adoption. On the contrary, it ruled that religion was a private matter, which was irrelevant to the suitability of prospective adoptive parents.

The society's survival was the result of a remarkable effort made by all those associated with it (Jayne Dunbar's salary came from the generosity of the Dolls and their friends). The society had two committees, a management committee, chaired by Richard Doll, which was responsible for raising funds and general policy, and a case committee that Joan Faulkner chaired, which considered individual applications. After two years, however, the society found that it was having problems with the adoption of mixed race infants.

Then an offer was made that some on the management committee thought might ease the obstacle to the adoption of non-white babies and at the same time remove a mounting financial crisis. The society was offered a large sum of money from an anonymous donor—which would be sufficient to pay for another social worker—on the condition that it was used for the adoption of "British babies", which everyone, including the Dolls, understood to mean white babies. The management committee decided, on Richard Doll's advice, to accept the money on the grounds that it would free Jayne Dunbar to specialise in the adoption of babies of mixed parentage and so enable the society to provide for many more such adoptions than they had been able to do previously. With the existing financial structure enhanced by the anonymous donation the society felt it could grow to fulfil the wishes of humanists who wanted to adopt.

Was this a naive belief? The management committee accepted the money and its overtones of segregation, the justification being the need for financial consolidation. It may have been one of those rare occasions when Doll allowed his heart to rule his head, but for both the Dolls this decision marked a nadir in their lives. Even though the acceptance of the money allowed the adoption of greater numbers of both white and non-white children, those opposed to the benefaction led a revolt on the committees. The Dolls were accused of racism, and the next few months were for Richard Doll "among the most psychologically distressing of my life". Articles were written in *Private Eye* describing the society as racist, singling out Doll in particular for attack, and a letter was published in the *New Statesman*, which at the time was obligatory reading for most of the Dolls' friends and colleagues.

Laura Sproule, a social worker, was one of their most vociferous critics. This was particularly hurtful for Doll as she was a friend and guardian to Nicholas. Jayne Dunbar spent 27 years working for the society and saw the internecine dispute as a defining event. "It was a terrible time when the Dolls were accused of racism, but if it hadn't been for the donation we'd have gone to the wall." The majority of the management committee, however, remained supportive and gradually the vilification died away.

In 1969, 54 babies were placed with new families; eighteen of them came from a variety of ethnic backgrounds, including Chinese and Afro-Caribbean. That same year, as the requirement for religious affiliation was gradually dropped by most social service departments, the relevance of "Agnostic" in the title diminished, and at a general meeting of the society its name was changed in 1969 to the Independent Adoption Society. Bram Oppenheim, an academic at the London School of Economics, attended the meeting: "The word 'agnostic' had a rather antiseptic smell about it. Not every adopted parent cared to be called 'agnostic', but independent was okay." This also marked the end of the Dolls' direct involvement in the society, its destiny moving the custodianship to another generation committed to humanitarian ideals.

For many years the Independent Adoption Society had the reputation for carrying out the most responsible and most liberal adoption service in the country. In December 2005 the society celebrated its 40th anniversary. Attending the historic meeting were some members of a remarkable group: the men and women who were adopted as a result of the Dolls' abhorrence of hypocrisy and their dedication to social justice.

Chapter 13

The End of the Communist Dream

"Stalin was not a Marxist. He wiped out all that is sacred in a human being."

Nikita Khrushchev

In 1956 politics filled the air. On 25 February, Nikita Khrushchev, general-secretary of the Communist Party of the Soviet Union, made his famous speech* to the 20th Congress of the Communist Party in which he accused Stalin of creating a personality cult. Having distanced himself from Stalin's excesses, he then sent Soviet tanks to crush the popular uprising in Hungary in October, the same month that Anthony Eden ordered the invasion of Port Said. The Suez Crisis ended Britain's illusion that it was a world power of the first order, and it also had the unforeseen consequence of deflecting the attention of the international community away from the Soviet atrocity. It seemed an appropriate metaphor for the times that John Osborne's play *Look Back in Anger* was being performed at the Royal Court Theatre.

The news of the repression in Hungary was a hammer blow to the communist movement in Britain. At 16 King Street, known as "the glass-bricked bastion of truth"[1] and the headquarters of the Communist Party of Great Britain, the atmosphere was one of emotional atrophy. Stalin, the great war leader, had been demythologised, and his political successors had shown themselves to be inflexible autocrats with unrepressed totalitarian tendencies.

The day after the Soviet invasion of Hungary, Shirley Davies, the Doll children's nanny, started work at 8.00 am, as normal. Entering 24

---

* The speech debunked the myth of Stalin as "the disciple of Lenin": in fact, under the guise of fighting the "enemies of the people" Stalin had eliminated Lenin's closest associates. It was reported that thirty of the 1,600 delegates fainted during or after Khrushchev's speech.

Lansdowne Road she realised something was wrong: Doll and Joan seemed deeply troubled. They were in a state of shock, mystified by the actions of a government they had lionised, believed in and loyally served for a quarter of a century. Left-wing politics was the milieu in which they lived their lives. It was the nexus of their friendships, it informed the way they saw their role in society: the Communist Party had been their lifeblood.

The Soviet repression in Hungary caused a mass exodus from the British Communist Party. Doll did not leave in this first expression of revolt, but his discontent, which had been mounting since the early 1950s, was becoming unendurable. His disaffection had begun at meetings of the Seigerist Society, the CP doctors' forum, over the claims made by Trofim Lysenko, Stalin's dictator of Soviet biology, who claimed that it was possible to change the inherited characteristics of plants by altering their environmental conditions. The atmosphere around this issue was oppressive and Doll objected to Angus McPherson who ran the society: "He held a rigid Stalinist interpretation and accepted the claims but I couldn't be persuaded by it."[2] JBS Haldane, the renowned geneticist, also at one time tried to justify Lysenko's assertion. Eventually, however, the contradictions became too much for Haldane* and in 1957 he left for India and the life of a Brahmin.

Doll had admired the work and political commitment both of Haldane and of another scientific giant of the age, JD Bernal. Many intellectuals of Doll's generation had been swept into the Communist Party and the "Bernal view of science" in the 1930s.** Bernal was a molecular

---

* When Haldane was diagnosed with cancer he sought a second opinion from Doll, his friend and former comrade. Having talked to his doctors Doll was able to tell Haldane the prognosis: "They think you've got six months." Haldane replied: "Six months! What good is six months to me?" He died on 1 December 1964.

** In 1939, Bernal published *The Social Function of Science*. He was chairman of the World Peace Council from 1959 until 1965, and was awarded the Lenin Peace Prize in 1953.

physicist, an indefatigable campaigner for peace, and a communist scholar. He played a vital role in the dynamic "red science" movement, which linked science's importance to society. "Ideas," according to the statistician David Cox, "just flowed out of him."[3] Bernal was firmly convinced that science should serve society and not only pursue knowledge for its own sake, and in 1951 he founded Scientists for Peace. Yet even Bernal's acknowledged genius was dulled by his political allegiance to the Soviet Union, which led to his endorsement of Lysenkoism. Doll came to recognise that the Lysenko doctrine must have been sanctioned by the highest authority and that an organisation of lies had descended on the party.

By 1956 Doll's idealism, which had been forged visiting the Bolshevik Park of Culture and Rest in Moscow, walking with "Red Ellen" Wilkinson, MP for Jarrow, on the Hunger March of 1936, fighting fascism and writing *Humanise our Hospitals* with Joan, was being eroded by the Kremlin. It was still possible, according to Julian Tudor Hart, to be "a good communist" by holding up placards protesting "Hands off Korea" and listening with admiration to Comrade Harry Pollitt, the party's leader in Britain, but many, after the Lysenko affair in 1948, had become disillusioned.

The Dolls were members of the Norland ward of the Communist Party of Great Britain in North Kensington. Lying within the borders of Notting Dale, and economically poorer than Notting Hill, it was active in agitational work, and its members dutifully sold copies of the *Daily Worker* on Saturday afternoons on Portobello Road. At that time, the Communist Party's main function was to act as a pressure group keeping the idea of socialism alive within the Labour Party, which was ideologically fractured and in the political wilderness. Branch meetings were held once a month and Tudor Hart, also a Norland ward activist, remembered that the Dolls turned up occasionally to help with money and sometimes to give a hand with jumble sales.[4]

Even at this stage, Doll had lost none of the idealism that had inspired him to join the Inter-Hospitals Socialist Society, the Communist Party and the Medical Association for the Prevention of War. But what had changed was the authoritarian bite that was snapping at the heels of former comrades. So in May 1957, at a meeting of the Norland ward, Doll resigned from the Communist Party. Retaining his own political integrity and directing the ideological failings up the chain of command, Doll told Chris Birch, the ward secretary, of his departure with a declaration redolent of Leon Trotsky. "I haven't left the Communist Party—the Communist Party has left me."[5] According to Birch, the cause of Doll's self-declared excommunication was the issue of "inner party democracy".[6] This phrase related to the response within the party to the former members who had left in October 1956. Doll's refusal to denounce those who had gone before him was equalled by his resistance to renouncing those who remained after he had gone.

Doll's resignation from the Communist Party did not mark the end of his involvement in direct political action. In the late 1950s, like other former communists, he joined the Labour Party in the hope of keeping socialism alive in the years of Tory domination. The Labour Party was suspicious of this influx of communists "smuggled" into their midst disguised as loyalists, but after a bitter debate by the North Kensington Labour Party executive, his membership was accepted. Doll had a conscious radical intent. True to form, he set up a housing inquiry that looked into the exploitation by Rachman-type* landlords of the many local "stub-end" lease houses which were then opened up for multiple occupation by immigrant families and shown to be a major component of the race riots and tensions in the area.[7]

While the political stance of communist doctors like Julian Tudor Hart and Tony Ryle did not directly affect their careers—both were going into general practice where they could be "their own masters"—this was not a possibility for Doll. He had to work within the political status quo of medical research. In the same year that Doll resigned from the Communist Party he succeeded, by examination, in becoming a fellow of the Royal College of Physicians.

---

* The eponymous Peter Rachman (1920-62) was an exploitative landlord who bought up slums to fill with immigrants at extortionate rents. He owned a property empire in the area around Notting Hill and Westbourne Park Road. Ben Parkin, MP for North Paddington, coined the phrase "Rachmanism."

Harold Macmillan's historic phrase of 1960 "the wind of change is blowing through this continent" recognised the shifting relationship of Europe's nation states with Africa. The diplomatic move reflected a retreat from the acquisitions of nineteenth-century imperialism; and an acknowledgement of the nationalist struggles in Africa for self-determination. This was the political background to another occasion when Doll's communism counted against him. Harold Himsworth, secretary of the Medical Research Council, wanted him to go to east Africa and investigate reports about variations in heart disease in Kenya. This was the apex of the Cold War, and in the aftermath of the Mau-Mau uprising the authorities were determined to prevent any potential *agents provocateurs* entering into the equation. Doll was told he was not allowed to go to "sensitive colonies".[8]

The "national unity", which William Beveridge regarded as one of the great social achievements of the Second World War, was also breaking down on the streets of North Kensington. In the late 1950s Britain was undergoing a social transformation. The years of rationing and austerity had given way to a booming economy; and a flourishing youth culture was moving to the rhythm of rock'n'roll. The Conservative government's need to keep the economy growing encouraged immigrants from the West Indies to come to Britain to fill labour shortages, and Notting Hill was one of the few inexpensive places they could find accommodation. It was a combustible confrontation, for Notting Hill was also the location for two openly violent racial nationalist groups: the White Defence League and the National Labour Party. These "Keep Britain White" groups with their nodding admiration of Nazism created a violent mood on the streets around Notting Hill, and reached an explosive climax in 1958 when four days of rioting broke out in west London.

For Doll, the talk of racial superiority and forced repatriation was repugnant. There was, however, no denying the racial tension between blacks and whites in the area around Ladbroke Grove and Portobello Road. He recalled the atmosphere becoming unpleasant to the point that people would cross the road to avoid walking past someone of a different skin colour. The situation grew so tense, and fighting seemed so likely to break out that Doll went to the local police station and volunteered to be a special constable if any were required. They were not. Then, on 17 May 1959, Kelso Cochrane, a 32-year-old carpenter from Antigua, was stabbed to death by a group of six white men in Notting Hill. No one was ever convicted. It was widely believed that white racists in the area were responsible for the murder, but people were afraid to come forward for fear of retribution. On the day of Cochrane's funeral, more than 1,000 people, black and white, joined in a procession in shared recognition of the young man's sacrifice. For Doll: "It was as if everyone agreed that things had gone too far. I joined the funeral procession and found myself next to a black woman with a child and a baby in her arms. I offered to carry the baby and was allowed to, and walked with it in my arms up Ladbroke Grove to our destination."[9]

The sympathetic social response to Kelso Cochrane's murder was not universal, and reaction against black immigration had been the dominant theme of the White Defence League. In the autumn of 1959 Prime Minister Harold Macmillan called a general election, and Sir Oswald Mosley was invited by the Keep Britain White movement to stand for election in the North Kensington constituency. Doll and Mosley had shared the political firmament from opposing positions. In 1957 Doll had left the communist camp, never to return; but what he never lost, or was reticent to discuss, was the compulsion he felt to join in the fight against fascism. He no longer wanted to change society towards a communist model—he now sought an egalitarian one. The arc of Doll's idealism and his objectives for medical science reflected the impulse of post-war reconstruction and a sense of social solidarity. He saw Mosley as a dangerous anachronism and joined in the opposition that poured onto the streets of Kensington. However, on 8 October, the day of the election, people remained unexcited by Mosley's racist appeal. Showing no redemptive grace, he finished bottom of the poll at North Kensington with eight per cent of the vote and lost his deposit.[10]

Joan and Richard Doll were intellectuals caught up in the medical and political battles of the day. Their whole lives had been dominated by political ideology. In 1959, while attending a conference in Vienna, Doll and Philip D'Arcy Hart* discussed the changed landscape of their political age. Doll asked D'Arcy Hart the question that had convulsed all "good communists": "Do you think Stalin was right about everything?"[11] Doll valued his membership of the Communist Party, perhaps more than anyone would have expected when he later became, in the words of Richard Bayliss, a colleague at St Thomas's, "about as established as the Bank of England". Doll was not ambivalent about his "card-carrying" past; even if he had suffered for it. The criticism of Doll's failure to adhere to his radical antecedents comes partially from the "puritanical"[12] gradations with which former communists measured political commitment; and partly from the perception he gave to people that the past should remain closed.[13] What was undeniable was his acceptance of the impracticality and undesirability of command economies to satisfy the material needs of society.

The quarter of a century that defined Doll's political principles also witnessed a medical revolution. In his early adult life, while trying "to find a place in the world", Doll had wholeheartedly embraced the humanist belief of DH Lawrence: "Find your deepest impulse, and follow that."

The choice between idealism and pragmatism had been made by Doll. Over the coming decades, under his leadership, epidemiology contributed more than any other branch of science to society's knowledge of the causes of cancer. John Osborne had complained in *Look Back in Anger* that there were no more "great good causes". Doll's dispassionate scientific mind had found one.

---

* Doll wanted Philip D'Arcy Hart to join the Communist Party. "I remained on the fringe of the movement, but my wife Ruth was a member. Everybody was in the CP who was against Germany. They thought and believed it was going to do something. Richard was a very honourable man."

Chapter 14

Epidemiology and the Atomic Age

"It was a queer, sultry summer, the summer they electrocuted the Rosenbergs..."

Sylvia Plath

The testing of the *Bravo* hydrogen bomb in 1954 had triggered Doll's medical interest in the carcinogenic effects of world-wide radioactive fallout.[1] The explosion had altered the perspective of governments and their scientific advisors throughout the globe and a scientific understanding of the quantitative effect of small doses of radiation became a burning issue.[2]

Ominously, national mortality statistics of England and Wales showed an almost unbroken rise in the annual death rate from leukaemia, from 17 per million in living persons of both sexes in 1931 to 49 per million in 1954.[3] This near tripling of the death rate was thought by some to be due to improved diagnostic procedures; but others feared the increase might be due to mounting exposure of the population to ionising radiations through diagnostic and therapeutic radiology and fallout from nuclear tests. The subject was medically an embryonic field; politically the issue was radioactive.

In December 1954 the increased deaths from leukaemia so concerned scientists that the Medical Research Council held a conference to consider its possible causes. On 29 March 1955 Prime Minister Winston Churchill turned to the MRC for enlightenment and, if at all possible, an ethical panacea. Under the chairmanship of Sir Harold Himsworth, a special committee of the MRC was asked to review "the existing scientific evidence on the medical aspects of nuclear and allied radiations."[4] The government's request came as a result of "the widespread public concern about the long-term effects of nuclear weapon testing".[5]

One of the main questions the committee had to consider was the long-term effects of small doses of radiation, but very little evidence was available to enable them to assess this risk. Auspiciously, some innovative work on the relationship had been carried out by a radiobiologist called Dr Michael Court-Brown. Born in 1918, Court-Brown was one of the most productive medical research workers of his generation. Initially interested in the acute effects of radiation, he sought to find a biological explanation for the sickness and vomiting which was often a distressing concomitant of radiotherapy. Reports from the Atomic Bomb Casualty Commission (ABCC), set up in the United States in 1948, provided evidence of increased mortality from leukaemia among the survivors of the atomic bomb explosions at Hiroshima and Nagasaki, and Court-Brown had shown some evidence of a similar increase following the use of X-rays for the treatment of ankylosing spondylitis (a crippling and extreme form of rheumatism). At the time, most scientists thought that the production of leukaemia and other forms of cancer required exposure to large amounts of radiation and that there was a minimum dose below which serious effects were not produced. There was, however, no real evidence that this was so, and it became increasingly important to be sure as the nuclear nations added to the radioactivity in the atmosphere by exploding hydrogen bombs.*

Court-Brown's early results indicated a higher rate of leukaemia among the irradiated spondylitic patients than in the rest of the population. The finding, which Himsworth believed was an "explosive one",[6] had been established without statistical expertise and the MRC thought it advisable that if the study were to be enlarged, for greater scientific accuracy, then an epidemiologist skilled in the subtleties of measurement and meaning should join the investigation. Accordingly, Himsworth asked Court-Brown to collaborate with Doll in the planning and execution of a study "as a matter of urgency" into the incidence of leukaemia among patients irradiated for the treatment of ankylosing spondylitis.

---

* For eighteen years, between 1945 and 1963, the world's population was exposed to unregulated radioactive fallout from bombs tested by the nuclear powers.

The MRC wanted to know if it was possible to determine a dose-response relationship for cancer and ionising radiation. The attraction of the spondylitic patients for Doll and Court-Brown was that these were people who had been irradiated for a benign condition. If they had been irradiated for cancer it would never be known, with confidence, whether a subsequent cancer was really a relapse of the original cancer or, indeed, what it was.

The retrospective study started in August 1955 and was completed within nine months, with a preliminary report based on 13,500 patients from 83 radiotherapy centres distributed to MRC members in January 1956.

It was a colossal undertaking, only made possible by the determination and intellectual drive of the two principal researchers. They were assisted by an unprecedented army of 100 MRC-funded personnel who were involved in locating and abstracting the radiotherapy details and follow-up notes of the patients. The results that the government and the MRC had so eagerly anticipated arrived at "about half past two on the morning"[7] of 1 January 1956. The decision was made to phone Himsworth: this audacious act, at such an unwelcome hour, was almost certainly perpetrated by Court-Brown. The researchers had found a *threshold* relationship: no effect with a small dose and then the disease suddenly mounting with increased radiation dosage. However, their estimate of the radiation dose was based on the advice of WV Mayneord, the doyen of the international medical physics community and professor of physics at the Institute of Cancer Research at the Royal Marsden Hospital. He had in mind when making his recommendation—the total mass of the body irradiated.[8]

When Doll and Court-Brown presented these results to the full MRC committee, one of the radiotherapists, Professor JS Mitchell, objected to their methodology. As Doll recalled: "He told us that our estimations were not accurate, that we 'had to measure the radiation dose in the bone marrow'."[9] So they had to start their investigation again. This time the accuracy of measurement was revolutionised by the construction of a "phantom", a human-like skeleton with implanted dosimeters allowing for patient-specific dose estimates.[10]

The study took Doll and Court-Brown all of 1956 to complete and they published their classic report in April 1957*. The main findings of the study confirmed a highly significant excess risk of deaths from leukaemia and aplastic anaemia, the numbers observed being more than ten times the expected numbers within the general population. Furthermore, the excess cancer mortality rate was largely confined to those sites that were likely to have been directly in the radiation beams. Most importantly, they noted that "for low doses the incidence of leukaemia bears a simple *proportional* relationship to the dose of radiation and that there is no threshold dose for the induction of the disease".[11]

Doll and Court-Brown had such confidence in the accuracy of the investigation that they advanced a dose-response prediction: "Calculations based on this hypothesis and on the data for the incidence of leukaemia among men given only spinal irradiation lead to the conclusion that the dose to the whole marrow which would have doubled the expected incidence of leukaemia may lie within the range 30 to 50 r. for irradiation with X-rays of the same average energy as those used for the treatment of ankylosing spondylitis."[12] This approximation is remarkably close to the value that is accepted today.

From this study a quantitative relationship was deduced which was used internationally as a basis for determining the acceptable levels for industrial and medical exposure. It also made a major contribution to knowledge of the long-term effects of radiation exposure. As an investigation into somatic (not inherited) illness it expanded the discipline of non-infectious disease epidemiology, and a new era was opened up. Radio-epidemiology moved from the wings to centre stage.

In the development of epidemiological methodology Court-Brown and Doll's innovative work made three indelible contributions. Firstly,

---

* Court-Brown WM and Doll R, *Leukaemia and aplastic anaemia in patients irradiated for ankylosing spondylitis*, Medical Research Council Special Report Series No 295 (HMSO, 1957).

the researchers were tracing people who had been radiated as far back as 1935. A follow-up of some patients was difficult because they might have moved or their record of irradiation history had been lost. To circumvent this difficulty the registrar general agreed to provide the death certificates for all persons dying in the UK with leukaemia or aplastic anaemia for the duration of the follow-up period.* The names of the patients in the series were then looked for on the leukaemia death certificates.

Another innovation was the use of a sample of one in six of the whole study population to abstract radiotherapy information necessary to estimate the radiation dose delivered to the bone marrow and to collect, for comparison, similar radiotherapy data for all patients who developed leukaemia. "This," according to Peter Smith—who later worked with both Doll and Court-Brown—"was essentially an application of the 'case-cohort' approach that was later 're-invented' by other investigators and became very widely used in epidemiological cohort studies."[13] A third intriguing aspect of the investigation was the far-sightedness of the researchers by including in the study around 1,000 patients who were diagnosed with ankylosing spondylitis but who were not treated with X-rays. These patients were treated with either physiotherapy or drug treatment. When these patients were followed up, no deaths from leukaemia or aplastic anaemia were found.

From the beginning of 1956 the Dolls' home at 24 Lansdowne Road echoed to the rhythm of human industry. In the dining room Doll was working on his investigation while in the kitchen Joan stayed up late into the night writing the main report for Himsworth. As a member of the report's secretariat, Joan was responsible "for co-ordinating the work of

---

* The initial report dealt with mortality from leukaemia up until 1956. The follow-up later extended to 1960 and the numbers of deaths from leukaemia and other specific causes were compared with the numbers that would have been expected had the patients died at the same rate as the general population of England and Wales (Court-Brown and Doll, 1965). Remarkably, 98 per cent of all patients in the series were followed up.

the panels and the various special inquiries that we had initiated."[14] Joan Faulkner was a powerful scientific administrator, according to Barbara Hafner, a member of Doll's staff. "She had an aura of being in charge. She was very bright."[15] She wanted to make her mark and did so with radiation.[16]

As the title implied, the report was about the hazards to humans of ionising radiations from all sources—"natural, medical, industrial and military". But what Prime Minister Anthony Eden, who had succeeded Churchill in April 1955, urgently wanted was its views on weapons tests. On this point the report concluded: "The present and foreseeable hazards from *external* radiation due to fall-out from the test explosions of nuclear weapons, fired at the present rate and in the present proportion of the different kinds, are negligible." Lorna Arnold, the historian of Britain's nuclear industry, believed that the MRC report gave the government "if not the green light, then the amber light"[17] for the H-bomb trials, codenamed *Grapple* that took place in the Pacific in 1957 and 1958.

Such considerations may have been far from the minds of Court-Brown and Doll as they excavated patient records in subterranean repositories in forty hospitals across Scotland. Peter Smith worked on follow-up studies of this population and found "an extraordinary high proportion of either Doll or Court-Brown's handwriting on the radio-therapy record cards. Today this would be done by a clerk, but they did the work themselves."[18]

Both men were notorious for their intellectual self-discipline. Court-Brown, according to Doll, "did not suffer fools gladly… and was not always an easy taskmaster."[19] That made two of them. If Doll had few interests outside science, the same was true of Court-Brown. They shared a dynamism few could equal; the greater the demands, the more they achieved. They shared the same utterly meticulous approach to research, the same let us get out there and do it ourselves attitude. Barbara Hafner began her career as an administrator at Gower Street in 1951 where Court-Brown often went for meetings, and she remembered him as being: "Gorgeous. Tall and so bad tempered. He was never nice to you," while she found Doll "much more humane even if he was busy."[20] While at the

London School of Hygiene and Tropical Medicine, Hafner was one of a team of five women working on the doctors' study, and in a light-hearted break from the rigours of arithmetic, the women made a blackboard drawing entitled: "The Doll's House". They thought it was lovely and amusing. Doll, however, did not, and he made them remove it.

So great were the political pressures being exerted by the government on the MRC that Joan Faulkner was seconded to work on the study with Doll and Court-Brown. What should have created a productive scientific synthesis instead provoked an emotional hiatus when Court-Brown envisaged an amorous relationship with Joan. After long hours of concentration the three investigators would go to a bar in whichever town they happened to be and although the drinking was not excessive Court-Brown could not hold his alcohol,[21] and later he stopped drinking completely. Joan was not an alluring woman in the conventional sense but her cleverness, an infectious laugh, her wit and vitality captivated Court-Brown.

After making a failed attempt to seduce Joan, Court-Brown then made the daring—and for the mid-1950s somewhat culturally adventurous—offer to Doll of a wife swap. There is no record of what Joan thought of this idea, but Doll's response was almost an uxorious one. "I didn't want to. I wasn't attracted to his wife at all. She was a rather cold Scot." That Court-Brown could find himself attracted to Joan was understandable, given the unusual circumstances he found himself in, but what was altogether less comprehensible was his reaction to Doll's rejection of his sexually liberated offer. He accused Doll of being a "homosexual",[22] an intentionally cruel epithet said with asperity. Doll deeply resented this. In the wake of this episode there was a breakdown in their cordial relationship; even so, their scientific collaboration continued for a further decade and their relationship had been restored by the time of Court-Brown's death in 1968.

In 1958 Doll published the first paper in another long-running study on the mortality from cancer and other causes among British radiologists.[23] The study found an increased risk of cancer mortality among radiologists who entered the profession before 1921, the year in which radiation protection standards had been significantly tightened, but not among those who started work later in the twentieth century. These investigations into the long-term carcinogenic effects of radiation helped expand scientific knowledge and established their reputations in the vanguard of radiation epidemiology.

Great minds do not always think alike. Court-Brown and Doll were visionary and inspiring scientists. Yet through a combination of professional training, scientific experience and intellectual disposition they represented contrasting philosophies of the causes of cancer. Court-Brown's background in radiobiology led him to study the effects of radiation on individual cells. Groundbreaking methods for displaying chromosomes were just being developed and he immediately introduced them into his work. By 1956 Court-Brown was director of a new MRC unit at the Western General Hospital in Edinburgh that had been set up to examine the clinical effects of radiation exposure. He exploited the emerging field of human cytogenetics with his colleague Patricia Jacobs, a zoologist from St Andrews (who later became his partner), and together they established the new science of human population cytogenetics. Discoveries followed one another with breathtaking rapidity, the most notable being that Klinefelter's syndrome was due to the presence of three sex chromosomes in each cell (X,X, and Y) instead of two (X and X, or X and Y). This discovery showed for the first time that the Y chromosome was the determinant of maleness in mammals and that human disease could be due to an abnormal complement of chromosomes. In 1960, when it became possible to examine chromosomes from blood,[24] the way was open for large-scale surveys.

For Doll, environment and lifestyle were the main determinants of disease and epidemiological science was the study of "disease distribution in man in relation to the environment to which he is exposed". Genetics or environment—these were the schools of thought represented by Court-Brown and Doll. The primacy of the discussion is as relevant today as it was in the middle of the twentieth century. In the early days of her career, Patricia Jacobs had a debate with Doll about the causes of cancer:

We were having a conversation when I was very young, and he insisted that cancer was not genetic, and I insisted it was—what a cheek I had because I didn't know anything about it at all—and he said: "Well if you say so." That's why I can remember it—he was extremely sarcastic. I was sort of right, and he was right too. There is everything from a very strong environmental component to a very strong genetic component.[25]

Doll was influenced by Henry Sigerist who stated that the history and geography of disease were the foundation for all medical historical work and that historians could not fully understand medical theory and practice unless they were familiar with the common disease problems of the relevant period and place. The realisation that the incidence of common cancers varied materially with place, social environment and time grew only slowly. Gradually, attitudes changed, expedited in the UK by Percy Stocks's graphical demonstration in 1936 of the substantial variation in age-standardised mortality rates of the major cancers throughout the country. By the 1950s it had come to be accepted that most of the differences reported between populations were not only real, but also provided potentially important clues to the cause of the disease. Strong supporting evidence for Doll's environmental theory had been found in the disease patterns of the Japanese who migrated to the US. These people carried the same genes as those who remained in Japan but they had very different cancer histories when they changed their lifestyles.

In 1957 Court-Brown and Doll's place in the iconography of radiation epidemiology was acknowledged with an invitation to visit the ABCC study in Hiroshima. They were the first non-military foreign scientists to do so. Doll was still in a self-confessed "anti-American phase" and he objected to having his finger prints taken or to answer questions about his political beliefs. To enable him to enter the country (the flight was via the

---

* Sam Shuster had left the Communist Party before visiting America but that did not prevent him facing a political inquisition. "When I filled in my visa forms in the early 1960s, in London, I told the lady in the embassy that I had a problem with completing three questions: 1. Did I have, or had I had a venereal disease? I said

US mainland and Hawaii) "unmolested"* by American immigration, Harold Himsworth secured him a waiver. Upon their return both Court-Brown and Doll were awarded an OBE in recognition of their work on the leukaemogenic effects of radiation. That same year, Doll, who had been a founder member the Society of Social Medicine, attended the inaugural meeting of the International Epidemiological Association (then called the International Corresponding Club) in Holland. Doll's epidemiological approach and mathematical techniques that were once the preserve of statisticians were, by the 1950s, spreading geographically and medically into clinical research and consequently into clinical practice.

Perhaps Court-Brown had some knowledge of a genetic predisposition because "he expected to die young"[26] and this happened at the age of fifty from a coronary thrombosis. Doll had stopped smoking as a result of his own research on the life-shortening hazards of the habit; Court-Brown had not. Whether it was lifestyle or genetic susceptibility that was responsible for his fatal heart attack we do not know. What we do know is how Doll evaluated Court-Brown's scientific contribution for posterity: "He was unusually free from scientific jealousy... his standards of excellence and honesty, both scientific and personal, were impeccable. Among the circle of his immediate colleagues he inspired intense loyalty and affection."[27]

In 2003, approaching the end of his career and now in his 91st year, Doll was asked what he thought was his most underappreciated work. "My favourite paper is the one with Michael Court-Brown deriving the dose-response relationship between radiation and leukaemia... In many ways it was the best-designed study I have ever participated in and possibly my best work."[28]

What may have contributed to the relative neglect of a study he viewed

---

impossible to say till the incubation period was over. 2. Was I or had I ever been insane? I said I was the wrong person to ask that question. But it was question 3, the one about membership of the CP that really made them stroppy."

as representing the pinnacle of his science was that the 1957 investigation was published in an MRC special report and not in a widely circulated journal. When compared to his other formative scientific collaborations, the one with Court-Brown, while full of emotive force and scientific enlightenment, was comparatively short. And while, psychologically, the men were polarised—Court-Brown was outward-looking and emotional, while Doll was inward-looking, and controlled—scientifically they complemented one another, alchemising into a collaborative endeavour that gave both men a sense of excitement as they discovered truths about the natural world while helping to protect society from carcinogens.

Much reliable information on the long-term effects of radiation exposure in peace and war came as a result of the determination and ingenuity of the two prodigious researchers united in a common cause. Doll did not speak with unequivocal admiration of many scientists; he did of Dr WM Court-Brown.

Chapter 15
The Royal College of Physicians Report

"Of course, we had long discussions on the analysis, and we made, no doubt, many adjustments, in the ways of presentation to meet our individual viewpoints. But ultimately, as I recall we never, over the whole ten years, had a serious difference of opinion."

Austin Bradford Hill

Doll had been lucky when Hill chose him to assist on the lung cancer study—but over the years Doll established himself as a leading figure in cancer epidemiology. Thus it came as no surprise when, in 1959, Hill invited him to become deputy director of the Medical Research Council's statistical research unit. Theirs had been a monumental alliance, and with the years the asymmetry of the original relationship had matured into a collaboration of equals. Together they redefined the parameters of epidemiological inquiry and their unemotional presentation of scientific findings persuaded some powerful groups within society of an inescapable conclusion: smoking kills.

At this time Doll would spend his evenings in Lansdowne Road working the "final shift" of the day. Starting after dinner, it was often his most creative period of writing and thought. Being in the same room as Joan as she listened to music and read, and breathing the same air, gave him a feeling of contentment and purpose. Joan, according to Michael Ashley Miller, her colleague at the MRC, "gave Richard the freedom to concentrate, she allowed him to be what he wanted to be: a one hundred per cent scientist." One of the secrets of his success, according to Francis Avery Jones, was "his great ability to organise his time".[1] A colleague at the MRC believed that "his qualities were hard work, and he probably never switched off,"[2] while Hill had noted the "obsessive" dedication to even the most exacting of tasks. Doll believed that intellectual ability while young is defining, but that with age organisational ability can count for more.

This rich period of fulfilment, however, came temporarily to an end for the lean, ascetic-looking Doll, when in 1959, at the age of forty-seven, he began to lose his productivity and power. He could no longer work in the evenings—invigoration had given way to incapacitation. Progressively he became moribund with lethargy. Earlier, his professional and personal good fortune had been attenuated by the loss of a kidney and his life almost lost to tuberculosis. This may have gone some way to explaining his perception that there was never a time in his life when he was not frightened of something.[3] This time his malady was diagnosed by his gastroenterological colleagues at the Central Middlesex Hospital as celiac disease* in which a hypersensitivity to gluten in the small intestine causes a chronic failure to digest food. The disease had little effect on Doll's subsequent life, and he came to enjoy a gluten-free gastronomy.

Political life, too, had affected the Dolls' domestic life. George Bernard Shaw's precept that "socialism takes a terrible toll on your evenings" was becoming true for the Dolls. By this time both had risen to positions of power and responsibility, and for the continued smooth running of their professional and family lives it was decided to employ a housekeeper. Joan Doll advertised the post in the *Evening Standard*, the *New Statesman* and *The Lady*.[4] Early in 1961, Isabelle Sutherland read the advertisement in *The Lady* and applied for the position. A scion of Scotland, she was an antidote to idleness. During the war one of her jobs had been to test parachutes. With a failed marriage and an unsuccessful business venture in the motor industry behind her, "Steve", as she would forever be known, sought stability and peace in a world about which she knew little—the mysterious atmosphere of left-wing intellectual life. Anne

---

* Gluten enteropathy: a condition in which the small intestine fails to digest and absorb food. Affecting 0.1-0.2% of the population, it is due to a permanent sensitivity of the intestinal lining to the protein gliadin, which is contained in gluten in the germ of wheat and rye and causes atrophy of the digestive and absorptive cells of the intestine. Symptoms include stunted growth and distended abdomen.

Hamilton, a family friend of the Dolls in Kensington, remembered that the advertisement sought someone who could "cook, clean and drive a car." At her interview Steve said, "I know nothing about the other two, but I can strip an engine down for you." It may have been her prowess behind the wheel that swung it for Steve and she started working for the Dolls on 16 January 1961. "It was a difficult thing to go and live in someone's house. For the first six months I thought 'This is not for me'—fortunately that feeling passed."[5]

Steve lived with Joan and Richard Doll, under the same roof, for the next forty years. It could not have been easy for her to work for two such powerful people. One of their friends thought she was a "servant" in the old fashioned sense of the word.[6] Joan, who was very comfortable in Steve's company, was able to say that "She's really now part of the family."[7] The same warmth was never evident from Doll. Joan was very fond of Steve and it is probably true that Steve grew to love Joan; but it is a remarkable achievement of emotional disguise that after forty years Steve could say with utter honesty, "I would never know what Richard [thought] of me. It doesn't worry me. He had absolute integrity, but—this was cutting—right from 1961, to the end, if there were visitors he said, 'This is Steve, or Mrs Sutherland, my housekeeper.' We were never friends."[8]

In the same year that Steve joined the Doll family, Austin Bradford Hill decided to retire early. Under his inspiring and arithmetically clear-thinking leadership, non-infectious disease epidemiology had metastasised into an irreplaceable speciality within medical science. He now thought that the time was right for the subject's future development to pass to the next generation. As a result, Donald Reid became head of the department of medical statistics and epidemiology, Peter Armitage was appointed to the university chair of medical statistics and, as Hill put it, "Richard, to my pleasure and great content" [9] was appointed director of the statistical research unit. It is a measure of the man's status that it took three people of outstanding ability to replace him.

At the age of 49 Doll had the opportunity to build on the achievements of Pearson, Greenwood and Hill. It marked a turning point in his scientific development. In his new role Doll looked around the London

School of Hygiene and Tropical Medicine and felt there was too much epidemiology in one institution. He had always been a semi-detached member of the Keppel Street intelligentsia, and he wanted to create a unit of like-minded scientists dedicated to research. After failing to find rooms at the Middlesex and the Hammersmith hospitals,* Doll's salvation came from Sir Max Rosenheim at University College Hospital (UCH). Rosenheim was very interested in people—he had such a wide circle of friends that he started writing his Christmas cards on 1 July. The two men shared a passion for public health medicine and their subsequent alliance in the Royal College of Physicians would help change the health of the nation.

In 1962 the statistical research unit moved to UCH, and in the same year Doll won the United Nations Gold Medal for cancer research. There, Sir Thomas Lewis was one of the most innovative, if intimidating, medical scientists, and his belief that nothing is too much trouble to get it right became a guiding principle of Doll's unit and his own scientific philosophy.

Despite the compelling scientific evidence of the dangers of cigarette smoking from retrospective and prospective studies, cigarette consumption in Britain remained endemic. Among men the peak in consumption was reached in 1941 (4,420 cigarettes per adult male) and did not mate-

---

* The equilibrium of dislike between Doll and Sir John McMichael of the department of medicine at the Royal Postgraduate Medical School, Hammersmith, was still evident. "'Oh yes,' he smiled 'we'd love you here; the only thing is we've got absolutely no room whatsoever, but all you need to do is get permission from the London County Council (LCC) to build out onto a bit of land on Wormwood Scrubs Prison.' As that boundary was absolutely sacrosanct the LCC wasn't going to allow the post-graduate school to expand: so that was as good as a 'Fuck off'— which I did."

rially change until 1973 (2,980). Among women the zenith of consumption was reached in 1974 (2,630 per adult female per year) and declined to 2,050 in 1982.[10] So great was the frustration felt by George Godber, the chief medical officer, and others at the lack of interest shown within the Ministry of Health to the dangers of smoking that they decided to act unilaterally. As Godber explained: "We wanted to come up with a plan to offset the influence of the commercial sector in trying to keep people smoking after the scientific breakthrough brought about by Doll and Hill."[11]

Godber was joined in his cause by Charles Fletcher. They were a formidable team: persuasive, well-connected and united in a shared objective. Fletcher (the son of Sir Morley Fletcher, physiologist and the first secretary of the MRC) had built his reputation in public health when he was appointed by the MRC to the newly formed pneumoconiosis research unit in South Wales. They both believed that if they could produce a report from an institution that was "above suspicion",[12] they might be able to persuade the Ministry of Health to take some action.

In 1958 Russell Brain, a neurologist with a career-defining nomenclature, was superseded as president of the Royal College of Physicians by Robert Platt. This change in the power structure presented an opportunity for Godber and Fletcher to act. Platt was an enigmatic figure in the history of the college: a humanist and socialist, he was decisive in redirecting its interest towards preventive medicine. When Platt was approached with the idea that the college should produce a report for the general public on the dangers of smoking based on Doll and Hill's research he responded with "alacrity".[13] This was a courageous stance for the college to adopt and one that no other institution was willing to make at the time. Unable to make a frontal assault on the epidemic of lung cancer, the College of Physicians volunteered to make a covert bid to alert the nation to the risks of smoking tobacco.

Jerry Morris attended the first meeting of the committee in the old college building in Pall Mall, and looking around the august gathering, he realised that a link in the chain of persuasion was missing. "We didn't have a medical officer of health (MOH), and we couldn't write a report without one!"[14] Collectively the most enlightened physicians in the country could not think of one MOH who was interested in doing something about smoking. Eventually they appointed John Scott, a concerned MOH on the London County Council. Almost a decade after Doll and Hill helped set off the big bang in understanding the hazards of tobacco, it was difficult to find a MOH who actively campaigned against the dangers of a habit that led to a 25-fold increase in lung cancer. The college committee, chaired by Robert Platt, took two and a half years to complete the work, which was written by Fletcher.* The report was presented and approved by a meeting of the full college in July 1961.

The report was aimed at the interested layperson, and a bold step was taken to publish 10,000 copies, one of which was sent to Geoffrey Todd, secretary of the tobacco advisory committee. The report was published on Ash Wednesday 1962, with Platt asking the reporters at the press conference if they would fly with an airline if one in eight of their planes crashed every decade. This momentous report on *Smoking and Health*** was the first official report specifying the dangers of smoking.[15] As the driving force of public information began to move towards prevention, Doll did not lobby*** politically for the changes that his epidemiological work had dictated as being essential for the improvement of people's health. He was not metaphorically running away from his scientific discoveries. Rather, he still adhered to Hill's scientific doctrine that his role was to be a neutral dispassionate scientist describing the relationship and leaving the public and physicians to draw their inevitable conclusions.

---

* Charles Fletcher had also instigated the 1959 MRC bronchitis survey, which provided the first detailed evidence of the respiratory benefits of stopping smoking.
** Royal College of Physicians, *Smoking and Health* (Pitman Medical, 1962).
*** On the publication of the forty years' observation on male British doctors, when the true hazards of really prolonged smoking had been reliably assessed Doll said, "In the last ten years I've actively supported programmes for discouraging smoking. I think it would after forty years have been silly not to. But I wouldn't have done that in the first ten years."

The impact of the 1962 report was enormous at the time and in retrospect it marked a decisive moment in the development of non-infectious disease epidemiology. All of the 10,000 copies of the report were
sold within days, and for the first time in the modern history of tobacco
addiction in Britain there was a significant (12.5 per cent), if ephemeral,
decrease in 1962 in the consumption of cigarettes.* The report drew par-
allels between the epidemic of lung cancer and those of tuberculosis and
the plague. Newspapers were evangelistic, with front pages carrying the
headline "Doctors Say Smoking Dangerous."

The Royal College of Physicians report also had an historic impact in
the United States, the world's biggest tobacco market. Twenty thousand
copies were sent to the US Cancer Society and distributed nationwide to
its members. The report was one of the factors that led President John
Kennedy to ask the surgeon-general to prepare the first of their opinion-
forming reports on the health consequences of smoking in 1964.**

The adversarial relationship between the medical profession and the
tobacco industry was heightened by the report. Anti-smoking propaganda
in schools had never been more than half-hearted, and it only began on
any scale after 1962. The opposition to the anti-smoking campaign was,
however, more formidable than ever before. Television propagated the
values of smoking, and independent television emerged as a powerful
vehicle for the advertisement of tobacco. The advertising media used pervasive and sophisticated techniques to send out subliminal messages on
the lifestyle enhancing qualities of cigarettes. It was not until 1962 that
the television advertisers made their first token concession by agreeing to
alter their advertisements so that they would appeal less to the young.[16]
That year also saw the opening of the nation's first Stop Smoking clinic

---

*   *British Medical Journal*, 1962; volume 2, p. 1457
** US Public Health Service, *Smoking and Health. Report of the Advisory Committee
to the Surgeon General* (US Government Printing Office, 1964).

which Dr Howard Williams ran for 25 years.* He believed that to "choose smoking was like playing Russian roulette with your life."[17] The Royal College of Physicians report shattered the chimera that smoking was harmless: yet the government retained a laissez-faire attitude to the addiction and failed to mobilise a public health campaign within the NHS.

Fortunately Doll and Hill were soon able to scientifically reinforce the RCP's historic report. In 1964 Hill, by now formally retired, made his final and enduring contribution to the prospective study of smoking and British doctors.** Doll and Hill's first report in 1954 had indicated strong associations between smoking and death, not only from lung cancer but also from vascular disease, particularly heart attacks. Their 1964 report marked a methodological advance in non-infectious epidemiology for not only did their study inform society of the hazards of smoking on health, it also showed how these life-threatening dangers could be avoided. Among the doctors who took part in the survey, the cigarette smokers had a total mortality which was twenty per cent greater than the non-smokers. Chief among the causes of death related to smoking was lung cancer.

Doll and Hill showed the increase in mortality as linearly related to cigarette consumption, with no threshold below which there was no risk from cigarettes. Of other cancers, only those affecting the upper respiratory tract and oesophagus were found to be significantly related to smoking and to the quantity smoked. They also found a relationship between smoking and cancer of the bladder and prostate, peptic ulcer, cirrhosis of the liver and alcoholism. These causes of death which were related to smoking differed from unrelated causes in two different ways.

---

*   In 1987 Williams wrote a book *Giving Up for Good*. The foreword by Lord Ennals, formerly secretary of state at the Department of Health and Social Security, described it as "a very significant contribution to final victory" in the campaign to bring about a total ban on smoking.
** Doll R and Hill AB, 'Mortality in Relation to Smoking: ten years' observation of British doctors', *British Medical Journal*, 1964; volume 1, pp. 1399-410, 1460-67.

The first is that the risk is related to the amount smoked. The second is that the risk falls after stopping. This is most dramatic with lung cancer. Doll and Hill reported: "Between 1952 and 1961 the death rate from cancer of the lung in all men aged 25 years and over in England and Wales increased by 22 per cent. In the doctors here studied it had slightly declined (seven per cent) between 1951-56 and 1956-61, and this fall can be attributed to the concurrent change in their smoking habits. Many have given up smoking and many have reduced their consumption."[18]

The mortality rate was shown to be almost halved after stopping for five years, and after 15 years it was only twice the very low rate of non-smokers. For lung cancer they found overwhelming evidence that the association was due to cause and effect: and the effect of stopping smoking was particularly persuasive.* Another finding that was innovatory was the effect of inhaling on pathological changes in the bronchi of smokers rather than in those of non-smokers.

Doll and Hill's statistical study brought dramatic attention to the tragic effect that smoking was having on health, estimating that cigarette smoking was killing 6,500 men under the age of 55 each year: "If the excess deaths in smokers under the age of 65 years from (a) cancer of the lung, (b) chronic bronchitis and emphysema, and (c) coronary thrombosis without hypertension be taken as attributable to their cigarette smoking, then the total mortality from all causes at ages 45-64 years is increased thereby by approximately 50 per cent."[19]

They concluded their study with a dispassionate observation and a public health message for the prevention of a fatal epidemic yet to reach its peak. "One of the striking characteristics of British mortality in the last

---

* RA Fisher had suggested that smokers inherit a susceptibility to lung cancer together with a desire to smoke cigarettes and that both the susceptibility and the desire may be less in those who give up smoking than in those who continue. Among doctors it was seen that large numbers of them gave up smoking because of new knowledge of its dangers and not because they had inherited a reduced desire to smoke.

half-century has been the lack of improvement in the death rate of men in middle life. In cigarette smoking may lie one prominent cause."[20]

The Royal College of Physicians report, the first official report specifying the dangers of smoking, and the study of smoking among British doctors had a transforming effect: although in retrospect they underestimated the dangers of prolonged smoking.

The finding that cigarette smoking killed thousands of men and women every year drew an immediate proselytising response from the columns of the *British Medical Journal*.[21] It called for legislative, educational and evangelical action. It urged a reluctant government to wake up to the smoking catastrophe, and supported calls for legislation to control the advertising of cigarettes. Firmer government action was advocated including "forbidding smoking in all public places and instituting a far more vigorous educational campaign than the posters which have so far been put out by the Ministry of Health." It ended with a clarion call to its readers to become inspired with a great humanitarian vocation. "Doctors have started to take the necessary prevention steps for themselves. We must continue this abstinence and see that the laity follow our example."

This undeniably became one of the unintended benefits of the study. Doctors saw the results on themselves or on their colleagues and gave up smoking much more quickly than the general public. Jerry Morris,* for example, had admired the clarity of Doll and Hill's work on smoking and found their logic so persuasive that he had given up cigarettes as early as 1950.[22]

British doctors became conscious of the dangers of smoking long before doctors in other countries. Spanish doctors, for example, continued to be heavier smokers than their national population for many decades following the survey of their British counterparts. In another sense, cigarette smoking represented a great failure in public health—for over-

---

* Morris left the Socialist Medical Association soon after the war because it had been infiltrated and taken over by members of the Communist Party—an event that Doll was proud of.

whelmingly the prevention of lung cancer means the prevention of smoking. In 1964, after all of Doll and Hill's logic, clarity and meticulous calculations, still only one in three smokers believed that smoking caused cancer.[23]

Chapter 16

Cancer Prevention: Pointers from Epidemiology

"The creation of the Institute of Social Medicine in Oxford and the leadership of its director, Professor John Ryle, were largely responsible for arousing my own interest in epidemiology and my purpose in preparing this monograph is epitomised in the second of the Institute's three purposes: 'to investigate the influence of social, genetic, environmental and domestic factors on the incidence of disease and morbidity'."

Richard Doll

"Richard Doll," according to Lady Joan Avery Jones, who knew Doll at the Central Middlesex Hospital, "wanted to use statistics for the common good." From his predecessors in British epidemiology, Doll formulated a new way of thinking about causality in medicine which led to programmes of disease prevention at home and abroad. He was aware of being part of a great collective medical endeavour: understanding the causes of cancer.

More than any other cancer epidemiologist, Doll was to show—like the incidence of infectious diseases in the nineteenth century—that much cancer comes from external causes and that the disease is no more an inevitable part of human existence than the infectious diseases had been. Moreover, he demonstrated that it was possible to find a cause of lung cancer, and advocate a programme of prevention, without understanding the exact biological mechanism of the disease. (In fact, there are so many cancer-causing compounds in tobacco smoke that we still do not fully understand the mechanisms that cause lung cancer.)

If the majority of fatal cancers could not be cured, then prevention had to be the objective. One way of preventing the disease was to gain an understanding of its causes. To help in this search might there be some rigorous, philosophically found guidelines to follow in establishing "the meaning of causality"? But, as Doll wrote:

> Whether epidemiology alone can, in strict logic, ever prove causality, even in this modern sense, may be questioned, but the same must also be said of laboratory experiments in animals. What can be achieved, even sometimes on epidemiological evidence alone is proof beyond reasonable doubt, which in a court of law is sufficient to condemn the accused to the utmost penalty and which in society is sufficient to justify action to reduce risk.[1] ·

Doll and Hill had shown how the association between smoking and cancer was causal and could not be explained by chance or methodological bias in their investigation. Their balanced assessment of the evidence in the British doctors study played a major part in convincing public health agencies across the world of a causal relationship, and subsequently changed smoking habits. However, another historical outcome of their work, stemming from the initial opposition it provoked, was the formulation of Hill's widely used guides* for causality. These were the first codification of guidelines used in medicine to determine cause and effect based on epidemiological data. Hill's groundbreaking work reflected the displacement of Koch's postulates, which were not relevant to chronic disease aetiology where a lot of different factors could be interacting with

---

* "Our observations reveal an association between two variables, perfectly clear-cut and beyond what we would care to attribute to the play of chance. What aspects of that association should we especially consider before deciding that the most likely interpretation of it is causation?" Hill cited nine elements: strength, consistency, specificity, temporality, biological gradient, plausibility, coherence, experiment and analogy. "Here then are nine different viewpoints from all of which we should study association before we cry causation... None of my nine viewpoints can bring indisputable evidence for or against the cause-and-effect hypothesis and none can be required as a *sine qua non*. What they can do, with greater or less strength, is to help us to make up our minds on the fundamental question—is there any other answer equally, or more, likely, than cause and effect?"

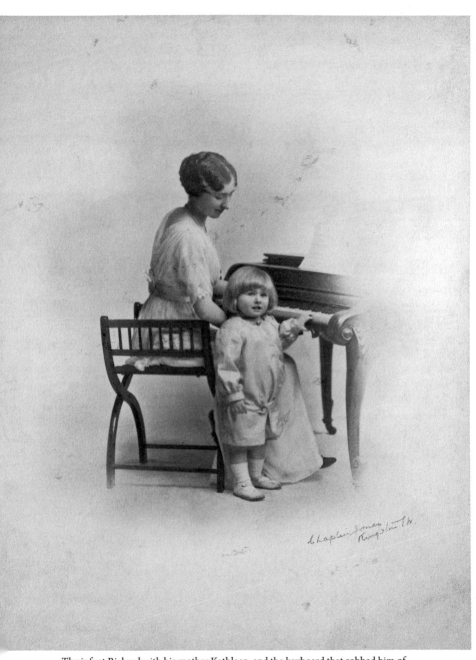

The infant Richard with his mother Kathleen, and the keyboard that robbed him of
maternal love.

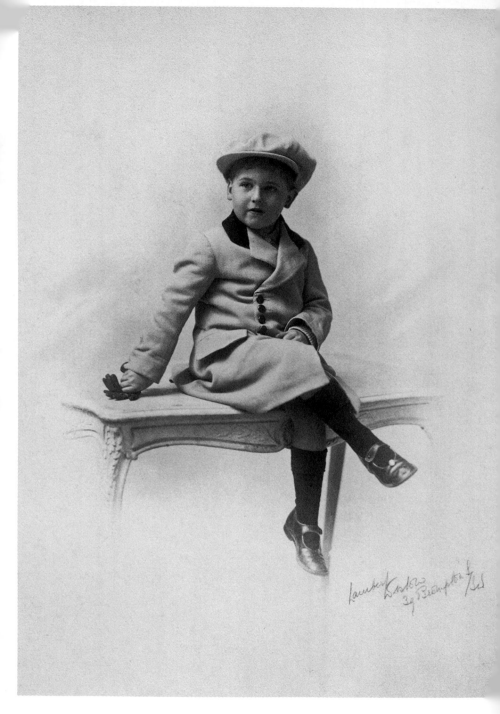

An Edwardian childhood pose: the young Richard.

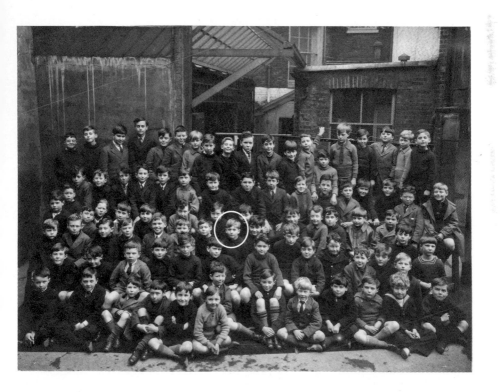

One of the masses: Doll (ringed) at Gibbs's Preparatory School, 134 Sloane Street.

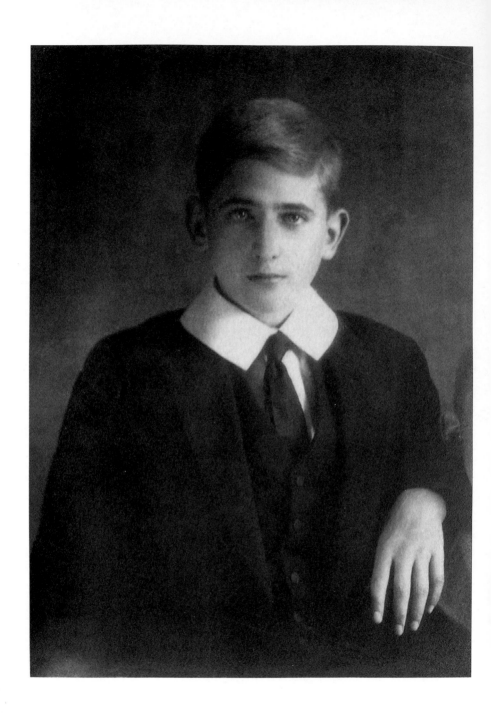

Westminster School and the trademark Eton collar.

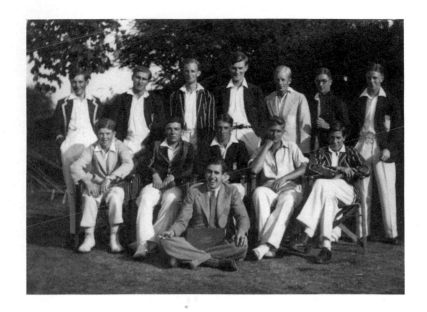

On the playing fields of England: the communist Doll as cricketing gentleman (1st row seated, 2nd from right) with "the Triflers". (above)

London Medical Schools' hockey team: Doll is 5th from left. (below)

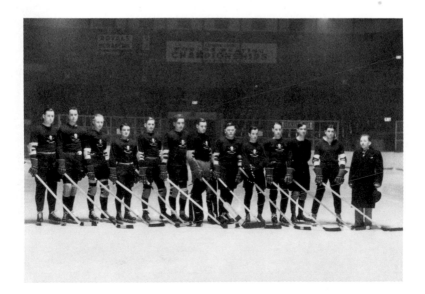

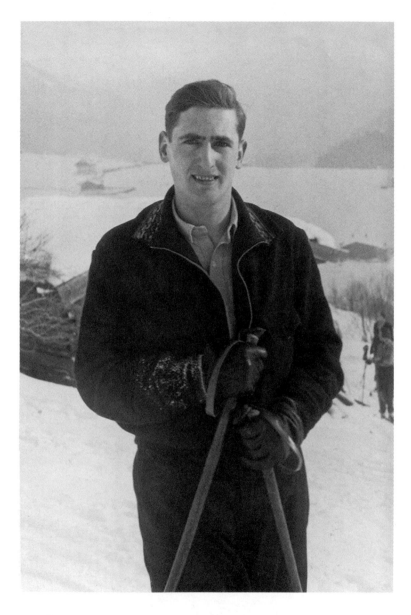

Doll skiing in Austria, c. 1936. He broke his ankle on the slopes and was dancing that same evening.

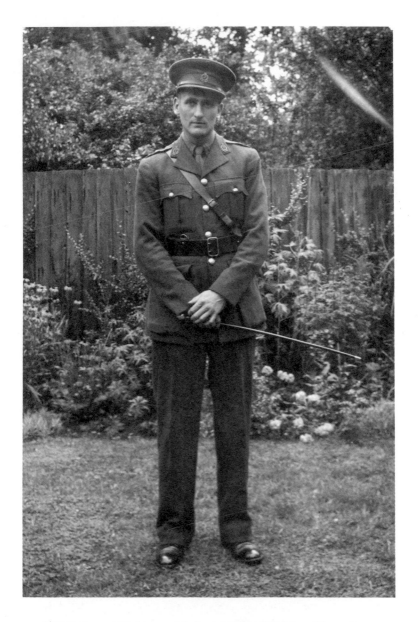

1939: Doll on a visit to his parents before joining the British Expeditionary Force.

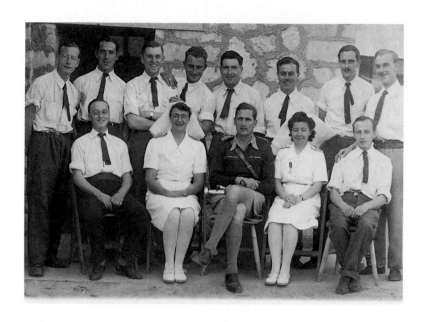

Major Richard Doll and his medical colleagues in Cairo, 1942. (above)

The first meeting of the International Corresponding Club, Holland, September 1957. Doll is the only male figure not in jacket and tie. (below)

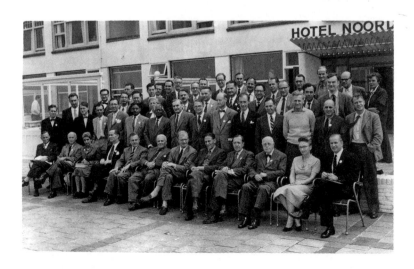

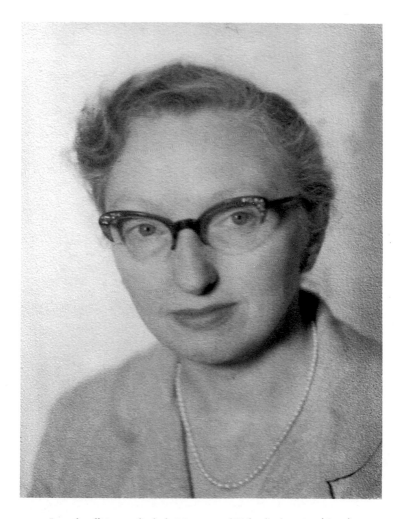

Joan, the efficient medical administrator and Richard's champion.(above)

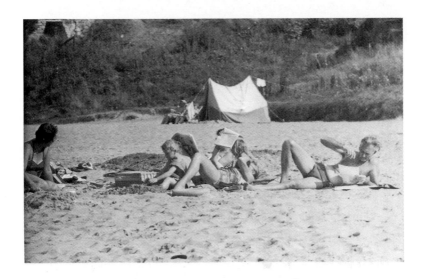

Doll on a family holiday—but still absorbed by his work. (above)
The joke that backfired: a tribute from the Gower Street women. (below)

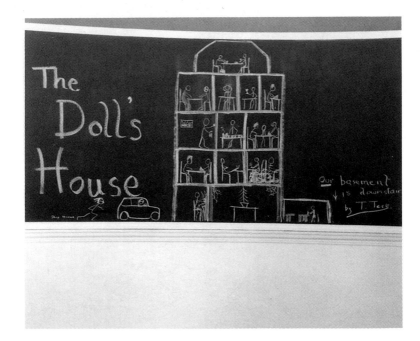

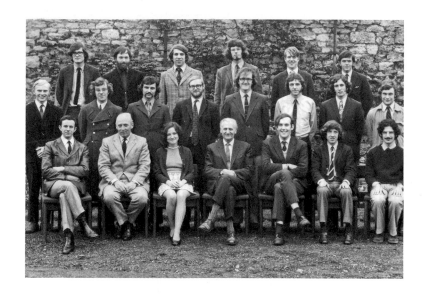

The expanding clinical student intake under Doll's stewardship, April 1972 (above) and April 1975 (below).

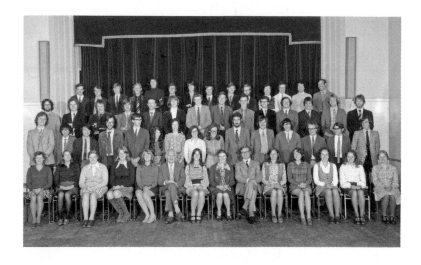

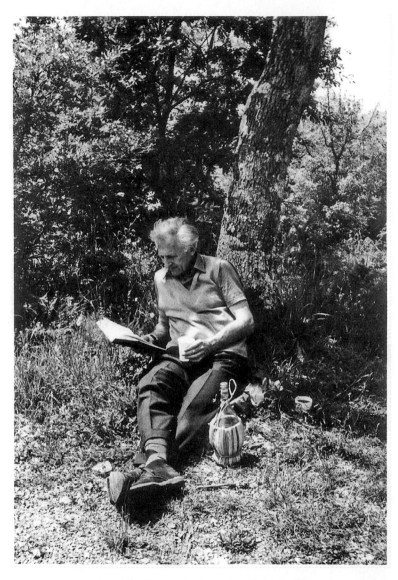

One for the heart: Doll enjoys a glass of wine in Italy.

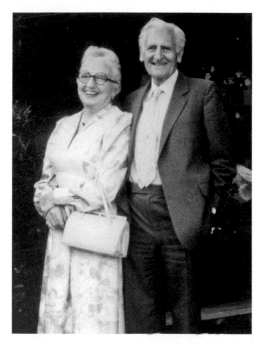

Joan and Richard, Green College, 1982.

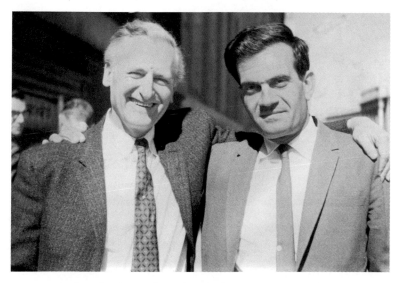

Ernst Wynder and Richard Doll; Winder published a paper in 1950 with his superior
Graham while only 23 years of age and still a medical student.

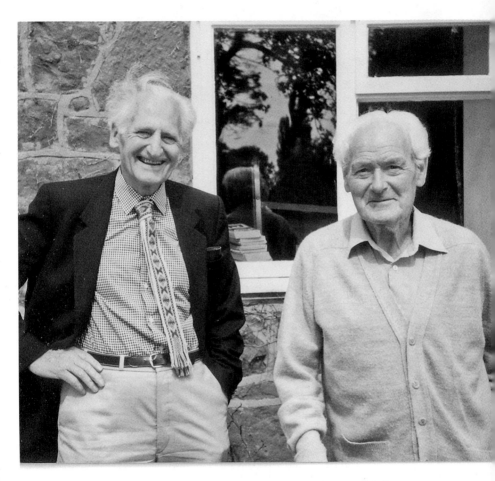

Richard (left) with his great mentor Austin Bradford "Tony" Hill.

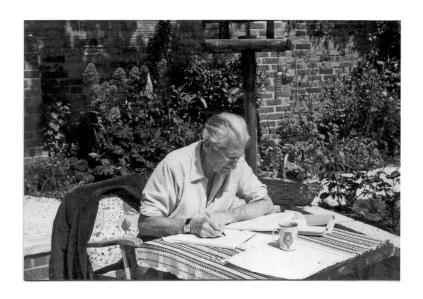

Doll in his beloved garden, 12 Rawlinson Road, Oxford. (above)

The Regius Professor of Medicine leaves his home at 13 Norham Gardens for an academic meeting, c. 1972. (below)

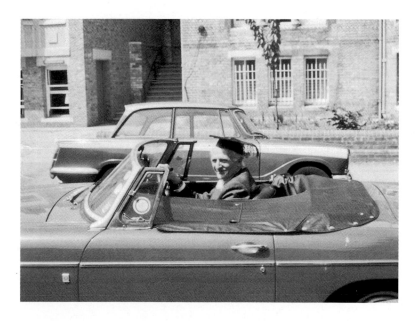

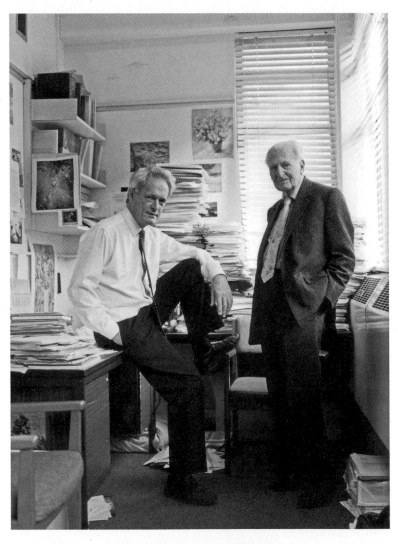

Sir Richard Peto and Sir Richard Doll in Peto's office, Oxford, 2002, surrounded by the inevitable sea of paper.

each other in the causation of disease. Hill's 1965 article *The Environment and Disease: Association or Causation* reflected the intellectual journey he and Doll had been on since the publication of their 1950 paper on smoking. Then they had found a large relative risk greater than 20:1 which could not be explained by bias or attributed to chance. Yet even this seemingly incontrovertible evidence was doubted. In medicine such examples of clarity in the marked causal relationship are rare: often, relative risks are 2:1 or less, and here the problems of eliminating bias and confounding are immense. Hill's "guidelines" on causation have transcended the field of medicine, forming a subject of expert debate in legal trials across the world.[2]

The study of smoking in doctors and its initial focus on lung cancer mortality set the stage for much of Doll's subsequent work for it showed that what was to become the most common fatal cancer had external causes, and that ninety per cent of the risk of getting the disease was something that people had personal control over. Before Doll, it was thought that cancer was one unified disease and that it was inescapable. What he did was to show that while there are numerous types and hundreds of subtypes of cancer, a few predominate in each country and the varieties that dominate in different countries may differ. Gradually, it began to be accepted that the incidence of cancers that were at all common varied significantly with place, social environment and time.

By the 1960s it came to be acknowledged that most of the differences reported between populations were not only real, but also provided potentially important clues to the cause of the disease. Epidemiological studies had shown that cancer incidence is far more dependent on the conditions of a person's life than had previously been supposed. That lifestyle and environment may be responsible for many of the common fatal cancers led the World Health Organisation (WHO) in 1964 to set out a theory of prevention:

> The potential scope of cancer prevention is limited by the proportion
> of human cancers in which extrinsic factors are responsible. These
> include all environmental carcinogens ... The categories of cancer that

are thus influenced, directly or indirectly, by extrinsic factors include many tumours of the skin and mouth, the respiratory, gastrointestinal and urinary tracts, hormone dependent organs (such as the breast, thyroid and uterus), haematopoietic and lymphopoietic systems, which, collectively, account for more than three-quarters of human cancers. It would seem, therefore, that the majority of human cancer is potentially preventable.[3]

Doll was a metonym for epidemiology not statistics and he liked to have a big-brained statistician close at hand. In 1963, Malcolm Pike, a dynamic bearded South African, had just completed a doctorate at Aberdeen University. He applied for a post at the London School of Hygiene and Tropical Medicine with Peter Armitage and attended the interview wearing his only suit. When he came out, Doll was waiting for him in the corridor. "You didn't get the job. I think you should come and work for me instead."[4] Pike was leftwing, an opponent of apartheid and eager to make his mark in an evolving science. He became the first of Doll's scientific apostles at 115 Gower Street. As part of his mission to develop empirical knowledge of the causes of cancer, Doll sought to compare the frequency with which the disease occurred in different communities, in different geographical areas and at different times. Yet his wish to support tropical epidemiology in the field had been prevented by the authorities because he was seen as being politically dangerous: Doll's past never stopped following him around. This was another contributory factor in the recruitment of Pike, for as well as collaborating with Doll on the epidemiology of smoking he also worked on Burkitt's lymphoma in Africa.[5]

Doll had affection for the people and culture of the African continent, but for apartheid in South Africa he had only antipathy. In 1965 when his friend Geoffrey Dean, another fellow of the Royal College of Physicians, was arrested in South Africa after writing a letter to the *South African Medical Journal* about injury to prisoners in jail, Doll mobilised a defence. He organised an influential group, including the president of the college, to speak on Dean's behalf at his trial, an initiative that may well have been decisive in the charge being dropped by the authorities.

Cancer Prevention: Pointers from Epidemiology

What is epidemiological evidence telling us about cancer? In 1936 Stocks had shown a substantial geographical variation in age-standardised mortality rates of the major cancers throughout Britain.* If these pointers could be interpreted successfully, then the next step was, where possible, to eliminate the environmental causes, or at least reduce them to socially acceptable levels. In his study of lung cancer Doll had found that the incidence of the disease had changed over time. What had been a very rare disease in Britain in 1920 had become a fatal epidemic by 1970. This temporal understanding of cancer increased dramatically in Europe and other parts of the world with the expansion of medical services, improvements in diagnosis and the use of reliable statistical techniques.

Just when mortality statistics had begun to prove their reliability as a reflection of cancer occurrence, treatments began to improve, in some respects dramatically, and the need for reliable incidence data also became acute.[6] At a 1964 meeting of the International Union Against Cancer (UICC) in Mexico, it was decided to bring together in one book data from 32 cancer registries in 24 countries from 39 scientists supplying figures in a standard way. Building on the achievements of this meeting, Doll co-edited *Cancer Incidence in Five Continents* in 1966. The object of the book was "to bring together the available cancer incidence data in one place and to present them all in the same way, so that the research worker can make

---

* In a comparison of the mortality of two populations, say those of two different countries, the crude death rates may be misleading. If the two countries have different age structures, this contrast may explain a difference in crude rates. A highly industrialised country like Britain, with a rather higher proportion of individuals at the older ages, and Uganda, a developing country with a small population of old people, provide an example—the death rates at each age (age-specific) are substantially higher for Uganda than for Britain, and yet crude death rates are higher in Britain than in Uganda.

whatever comparison between them he chooses."[7]

Doll helped to transform accepted thinking on the causes of cancer, and with the publication of *Cancer Incidence in Five Continents* he was established as the pre-eminent cancer epidemiologist in the world.[8] His status within the history of cancer registration was recognised with his appointment to a UICC committee on geographical pathology. In 1965, on the basis of its recommendations, the International Agency for Research on Cancer (IARC)* was established as a specialised cancer research centre of the WHO. Doll was asked to be its first director, but the combination of Lyon, France, being chosen as its headquarters, and Joan's unwillingness to relinquish her position as the most powerful woman in the MRC led to him to decline the offer.

In 1966 any disappointment he may have felt about not going to the WHO was cushioned by his election to the Royal Society, the nation's highest scientific accolade. His citation read:

> Doll is distinguished for his researches in epidemiology and particu-
> larly the epidemiology of cancer where in the last 10 years he has
> played a prominent part in the elucidation of the causes of lung cancer

---

* In the course of his work on the committee Doll learned how the international agreement to set up the agency had been achieved. "IARC owed its origins to a public proposal by General de Gaulle to the four other allied powers—the US, the UK, Italy and the USSR that each should submit 0.5 per cent of the national defence budgets for the establishment of a major research institute to conduct a war against cancer. This was an embarrassing proposal as it was not something that either the US or the UK wanted to undertake but neither was it something that could be easily rejected in view of its public appeal. The problem was solved, or so it was thought, when a British civil servant suggested that the proposal be accepted in principle, but with such trivial funding offered that de Gaulle would reject it. The sum agreed between the British and the Americans was an annual contribution of $200,000 for each of the five states. The offer was made, but instead of rejecting it in a huff, de Gaulle said that anything was better than nothing and that they should proceed on that basis."

in industry (asbestos, nickel and coal tar workers) and more generally, in relation to cigarette smoking, and (b) in the investigation of leukaemia particularly in relation to radiation, where using the mortality of patients treated with radiotherapy he has reached a quantitative estimate of the leukaemogenic effects of such radiation. In clinical medicine he has made carefully controlled trials of treatment for gastric ulcer. He has been awarded the United Nations prize for outstanding research into the causes and control of cancer and Bisset Hawkins medal of the Royal College of Physicians for his contributions to preventive medicine.

Few medical doctors have been awarded a FRS and Doll immediately showed his enthusiasm for new initiatives by organising a meeting in 1966 in Nairobi,* with the objective of gathering data on cancer incidence in Africa. Pike had by this time established an exemplary study in Uganda— the Kampala cancer registry in conjunction with Denis Burkitt. Burkitt's epidemiological observations revealed that the lymphoma had environmental rather than genetic or racial origins as it had an equal effect on African, Asian or European children if they lived within the lymphoma belt (ten degrees either side of the equator). Burkitt's cancer incidence survey of up-country hospitals in Uganda, Kenya and Tanzania was also conducted from Doll's unit in Gower Street with the help of Paula Cook, a geographer. Pathologists and surgeons from many parts of the African continent attended the Nairobi meeting along with doctors from the remote up-country hospitals.

---

*   According to Paula Cook, after the Nairobi conference, she drove with Pike and Doll down from the highland into the Rift Valley to take a boat to Lake Naivasha. In the densely populated Western Province of Kenya they saw women walking at the roadside smoking cigarettes with the lighted end inside their mouth. They stopped to investigate and were told that the women smoked the cheaper tobacco and that it stayed alight better when shielded inside the mouth. In the interests of science, Doll and Pike experimented to see what it was like to smoke counter-culturally.

Doll used the evidence of the geographical distribution of cancer in Africa to expand his understanding of the causes of the disease and how epidemiological knowledge could be used to prevent it. In his examination of the data Doll used for the first time what he termed "truncated incidence rates" for a restricted age group (35-64), which concentrated on those most likely to be able to get to hospitals and to be properly investigated. These were important factors to be considered when comparing diseases which increase in incidence very sharply with age—as many cancers do—and where access to treatment may be variable between different regions and countries.

This aspect of comparing rates was central to Doll's thinking during the years of refining geographical comparisons.[9] His particular interest in Africa was due to the fact that life was lived closer to the physical environment where social customs that developed over generations were still intact. Differences in incidence of different cancers might reflect these patterns more clearly than in the prosperous populations of the developed world. This occurred with Burkitt's lymphoma* and changing temperature and rainfall; also with cancer of the oesophagus that was commonest among people whose staple food was maize and who drank maize beer, and showed rates of primary liver cancer a thousand times greater in Mozambique than in Europe. For Pike, Doll was "a master of using mathematical statistics to illuminate disease processes at the population level".[10]

---

* Burkitt's father, James, was a surveyor and a naturalist. He was the first to identify individual birds by ringing their legs with metal bands of different patterns. This system, formulated to identify the territorial distribution of birds around his house in Ireland, bore similarities to the approach which would be adopted years later by Denis Burkitt when identifying tumour distribution in Africa. He found a definite pattern in the distribution of the disease, as most of the tumours were contained in a band which stretched across Africa, running between 10 degrees north and 10 degrees south of the Equator. The five million square miles within this band became know as the lymphoma belt. Burkitt published his results in the *British Journal of Surgery* in 1958.

A geologically layered theory of the environmental causes of cancer crystallised in Doll's mind as a result of the fusion of his position on the scientific council of IARC and his observational experiments in Africa. In 1967 Sir Ernest Rock Carling—who had earlier obstructed the acceptance of the hazards of smoking—presented him with an opportunity (when he gave the annual Rock Carling lecture) to make an enduring contribution to our understanding of the cause and prevention of cancer. Doll's Rock Carling monograph,* *Prevention of Cancer: Pointers from Epidemiology*, can be seen as a leitmotif of his thinking, and of epidemiology's influence on medical practice today. Its eight chapters deployed Hill's nine requirements of proof, added to the accumulated knowledge Doll had synthesised over the previous two decades.

He illustrated the geographical differences in distribution of cancer with a vivid example. "In the Gurjev region [of Kazakhstan], where the rate is highest, cancer of the oesophagus is two hundred times as common as in Holland or Nigeria, and about three times as common as lung cancer is in London." He also noted that gastric cancer among ethnic Japanese in Hawaii resembled that of their host culture more closely than that of their homeland, and made a prophetic observation:

> Within countries, cancer of the breast tends to run in families, but genetic factors can not account for the principal geographical differences. Non-whites for example, have the same rate as whites in the United States, although the disease is rare among Africans in Africa, and the Japanese in Hawaii suffer a rate which is appreciably higher than that of the Japanese in Japan. Fertility and prolonged lactation are associated with lower rates, and may have a minor protective effect.

---

* His election to the Rock Carling fellowship was dependent upon the holder reviewing in a monograph a field in which Sir Ernest Rock Carling had been particularly interested. The monograph was introduced by a public lecture which Doll delivered in Rhodes House in Oxford.

Such factors, however, are inadequate to account for the eight-fold differences between communities. The very striking gradient from west to east across Europe suggests the possibility that a dietetic factor may play a part.[11]

With lung cancer and smoking he acknowledged that some believed that genetic factors may be responsible. But, he wrote, "this hypothesis is difficult to fit with the fact that the incidence of the disease fails to increase with age when smoking has been stopped, and with the rarity of the disease in non-smoking populations like the Seventh Day Adventists."

For Doll, the observational science of epidemiology could prevent cancer in three main ways. By showing:

differences in the incidence of cancer in different communities and correlating them with differences in the prevalence of a potential aetiological factor, it may be possible to suggest a new clue to its cause. Secondly, hypotheses about the cause of cancer can be tested by relating the occurrence of the disease to a personal characteristic of the affected individuals—either to their constitution or to the degree to which they have been exposed to an environmental agent. Thirdly, the reality of a causal relationship can be put to the acid test of practice, by seeing whether the disease can be prevented by changing the prevalence of the suspected agent.[12]

The majority of Doll's scientific career took place after Crick and Watson's discovery of DNA in 1953. Their work and the mushrooming of molecular biology that it inspired have found, and will find, avoidable causes of genetic diseases. Doll did not deny molecular biology's scientific ability to enlighten—but the more important issue for him was to reduce *everyone's* risk and not spend time finding the *minority* of people who were genetically predisposed to a disease. Doll was interested in the big killers. Why try to find the few that were predisposed to lung cancer when, by stopping smoking, ninety per cent of the risk would be avoided? To look for the ten per cent would detract from the public health. His objective was to understand how to prevent the big environmental causes of cancer.

In Doll's words, death in old age is inevitable but death before old age is not. The Rock Carling monograph offered a scientific way of thinking that has guided investigators around the world. One sentence gives encouragement to all and is the central pillar of Doll's general theory of carcinogenesis. "No cancer that occurs with even moderate frequency, occurs everywhere and always to the same extent." What Doll was saying, and the reason why his name will forever be linked with cancer epidemiology,[13] is that the principal causes of cancer are not genetic; they are environmental and therefore they are in principle preventable. It is a very simple line of inference indicating that wherever a particular cancer is common it need not be, and every type is rare in some parts of the world.

If it is true that the public likes doctors to give them absolution and not exhortation then Doll fulfilled the expectations of a physician. He concluded his book on the catechism of causes of the disease with a chapter entitled "Practical Steps to Prevention". His message was that most cancers are in principle preventable and many could be avoided by an appropriate choice of lifestyle and environment. More than anybody else, Doll showed how the *age-adjusted* risk of cancer could be halved, without the aid of molecular biology.*

One of Doll's principles of prevention was that "no dose of a carcinogenic agent, no matter how small, can be assumed to be safe." This led him in 1967 to call for import licences for crocidolite, that particularly dangerous type of asbestos. He supported the idea of concentrating medical attention on groups of the population who are particularly liable to develop the disease.

> It is valuable, for instance, to distinguish families with polyposis coli, since affected individuals almost invariable develop cancer of the colon if the colon is not removed prophylactically; and to distinguish individuals with red hair and fair complexion, since they are prone to

---

* Doll R, introduction to 'The Double Helix Perspective and Prospective at Forty Years', Donald A Chambers (editor), *Annals of the New York Academy of Sciences*, 1995, volume 758.

develop cancer of the skin when heavily exposed to ultra-violet light. On the whole, however, there is little to suggest that man has much inherent variation in susceptibility to most of the individual types of cancer, and he certainly possesses no important hereditary character-istics that make him either more or less susceptible to the whole range of cancers in all organs.[14]

Doll advocated the benefits of concentrating preventive measures on high-risk groups, defined by their exposure to a carcinogenic agent or by the recognition that the cancer process had already developed to a nearly malignant stage. While encouraging the prohibition of certain food addi-tives, cleaner motor engines and factories changing their methods of man-ufacture, he proposed that the most dramatic impact on the incidence of cancer was effected by measures which we can take ourselves. And that there was evidence, beyond reasonable doubt, to believe in some circum-stances the step could be taken from an "observed *association* to a verdict of *causation*".[15] He wrote: "Exposure of the skin to sunlight, the chewing of tobacco, betel and lime, the smoking of tobacco, the consumption of alcohol, sexual intercourse, and lack of physical cleanliness are all, in one way or another, related to the development of cancer and the choice between gratification and avoidance of risk is one the individual can make."[16]

This appeal did not, of course, absolve local and national govern-ments of responsibility. As in the nineteenth century, certain freedoms needed to be constrained for other liberties to prevail, and public educa-tion would be used as a form of inoculation against harmful choices of lifestyle and environment. The precedent of government action in the field of public health had long been accepted and with tobacco responsible for 12 per cent of all male deaths between the ages of 45 and 64 years, Doll believed that intervention was justified. He sought to reconcile the effects of tobacco on the expectation of life with the claim that advertising did not encourage the desire to smoke. "The fact that so much effort is expended on preventing individuals from having access to marijuana while, at the same time, exhortations to smoke cigarettes continue to appear on public hoardings may well come to be regarded as one of the more remarkable inconsistencies of our age."

Doll set out to understand the world we live and die in. His objective was to help as many people as possible to achieve their natural expectation of life. In 1967 Doll was optimistic and thought that it might be possible to prevent "about 40 per cent of the cancer deaths that occur annually in men in Britain, and a somewhat smaller proportion—about ten per cent—in women. In addition, there is good reason to believe that a large proportion of the remaining types is, in principle, preventable, and with continued research we may learn how to prevent them within the next two or three decades."[17]

Infectious diseases had been brought under control through the combined efforts of government, medical science and a programme of public health. The prevention of cancer had come to mean the avoidance of one of the principal causes of death in childhood and middle age. *The Prevention of Cancer: Pointers from Epidemiology* indicated that this was an achievable aim.

Doll's hypothesis was not universally accepted. His former collaborator Court-Brown stated in a review of the monograph that the study was scientifically flawed—in failing to recognise the influence of genetics on the cause of disease. He reinforced his point with an analogy from their work in radiation:

> We know enough about the effects of X-ray exposure to know that if we give therapeutic doses of X-rays to the whole length of the spinal column for the treatment of ankylosing spondylitis, then about ten times as many men will die of leukaemia than would have been the case had they not been irradiated. We have no understanding at all why one man gets the disease and not another, although both may have been irradiated under apparently identical conditions, both of the same age, both in the same occupation and both with the same social habits. Is it just the play of chance or is there something about the man developing leukaemia which, given the same amount of environmental carcinogen, placed him at a greater risk than the other?[18]

Doll and Court-Brown were heavyweight proponents of counter-vailing ideas of disease causation. Court-Brown indicated that Doll down-played genetic susceptibility because to do otherwise would encourage the belief among the uninformed that cancer was incurable. His review went on: "Despite the imbalance in its arguments about genetic suscepti-bility Dr Doll's monograph should be read by all and for at least two reasons. First, it is an expression of opinion about cancer prevention by a master craftsman in the use of the epidemiological technique, and, sec-ondly, the monograph does give insight into the limitations of this tech-nique."

Public health, guided by epidemiology, had been transformed. Its concerns changed: from the control of infection, to control of environ-mental pollution, and then to education about personal behaviour. Doll rejected the notion that society should mollycoddle or that doctors should "advise people to live their lives as invalids in order to die healthy."[19] While he avoided public campaigns over what actions to take about particular results, he strongly believed in bringing scientific findings to the public and in combating misconceptions. Most people are frightened by death but for the wrong reasons. Many people fear murder more than they feared bronchitis: yet, for example, in 1979 there were about 500 murders in England and Wales while chronic bronchitis killed 25,000. For Doll, people should be treated as adults and should be told the facts. He gave people reliable information that enabled them to take control of their own destiny.

Chapter 17

Leaving London

"He was a seeker of truth which will never be attained without strife and sacrifice."

ES Anderson

It can be argued with some confidence that no smaller thing has ever made a bigger difference than the contraceptive pill. Oral contraceptives were first approved for general use in the United States in 1959. A year later, when "the pill" was introduced into the UK it became widely used, and it seemed obvious to Doll that an epidemiological study would be essential to identify and follow up a cohort of oral contraceptive users to assess their wellbeing. This, however, was not the way the Medical Research Council thought. They established a committee to analyse the effects consisting entirely of gynaecologists, endocrinologists and biochemists. This annoyed Doll but he decided to let the MRC "stew in its own juice" and to do nothing about it.

With the passage of time and the lack of evidence to support the MRC's concerns about a possible hazard of diabetes mellitus, interest began to be aroused in the possibility that some of the oral contraceptives might cause venous thrombosis and a risk of fatal pulmonary embolism. In 1966 a general practitioner in East Anglia reported the occurrence of a case and shortly afterwards the Food and Drug Administration in the US noted that most of the reported deaths from thromboembolic disease associated with the use of oral contraceptives occurred within the first four months of use.[1] But it was also pointed out that this might well have been due to the differential reporting of events which occur soon after a new drug is prescribed.

Doll realised that a proper epidemiological study was necessary to evaluate the effect of oral contraceptives on the cardiovascular system. To this end he carried out a pilot study at the Central Middlesex in 1966 where he held an honorary consultant appointment as a research physician attached to Francis Avery Jones's department of gastroenterology. Examination of the discharge diagnosis in the records department showed that every year a few women were discharged with a diagnosis of pulmonary embolism or deep-vein thrombosis, and examination of notes of women discharged with either of these diagnoses over the previous three years showed that the cause of the condition was not always known.

The number of such cases was, however, too few for any one hospital to provide worthwhile information, but Doll believed that a reliable answer might be obtained if he could use the records of all the hospitals under the control of one of the 14 regional hospital boards of the NHS. In 1966 he obtained permission to seek information about relevant patients admitted to hospitals under the north-west metropolitan regional board.

Just at this time Doll was asked by Max Rosenheim if he could find a position in his unit for a young doctor called Martin Vessey who had impressed him while a student at University College Hospital. Vessey had gone on to work in statistics and wanted to apply what he had learned to medical research. The recommendation came just at the right time for Doll. He persuaded the MRC to give the young doctor a trial appointment and asked him to carry out a case-control study of all the women discharged from the regional board hospitals with a diagnosis of idiopathic deep-vein thrombosis or pulmonary thrombosis over the previous three years. Doll had found his second disciple.

In May 1967 a subcommittee of the MRC, of which Doll was a member, reviewed the preliminary results of three inquiries into the risks of thromboembolic disease in women taking oral contraceptives.[2] Their findings* all pointed to the existence of a hazard of venous thrombosis

---

* The Oxford Family Planning Association study eventually involved determining all material illnesses in 17,000 married women initially aged 25-34 years over a period of 25 years and provided the first detailed assessment of the overall health effects of all the main forms of contraception and of the many factors that affect women's fertility. The most important findings were, however, the quantification of the many risks and benefits caused by the use of the various forms of contraceptives. In a paper commemorating the 30th anniversary of the study in 1998 it

and were reported together in the same issue of the *British Medical Journal*.[3] Vessey and Doll's paper[4] marked the beginning of a collaboration that continued for more than three decades. It formed the bedrock of Vessey's career in epidemiology and is rightfully celebrated as part of an unbroken sequence of studies aimed at effective contraception, free of risk, and psychologically acceptable.

Vessey and Doll found that 45 per cent (26 out of 58) of patients admitted to hospital with deep-vein thrombosis or pulmonary embolism had recently been taking oral contraceptives, while only nine per cent of controls who were admitted for reasons other than thromboembolism were taking the drugs—a figure very close to the national average for the proportion of the female population at risk of pregnancy who took them. They found that about one in every 2,000 women using oral contraceptives were admitted to hospital each year with "idiopathic" venous thromboembolism in comparison with about one in every 20,000 not using them... "and it is concluded that oral contraceptives are a cause of the disease."[5]

The *British Medical Journal* found Vessey and Doll's investigation to be "correct" and that the occurrence of the disease "in one out of every 2,000 women on the pill each year is disquieting."[6] Yet like Doll, the *BMJ* wanted to put the risks to women's health in perspective. Other forms of contraception—apart from sterilisation—had high failure rates. Also the risk of death in pregnancy, even from thrombosis alone, was greater than that of taking oral contraceptives for the same length of time. As an arbiter of risks Doll always sought to "weigh the evidence" of benefits against

was found that the overall effect of their use in terms of years of disability is probably beneficial, as it certainly is if the woman is a non-smoker, for the effect on the risk of myocardial infarction and stroke interact with those of smoking and in the absence of smoking are very small.

dangers. From his position on the committee on the safety of medicines he was able to measure and report on the pharmacological advances in oral contraceptives.*

It was unavoidable that big changes in medicinal practice would encounter reaction, and it arrived with Pope Paul VI's anti-contraceptive encyclical of 1968. But for Doll, the threat of unwanted pregnancy had historically encumbered women with anxieties that did not weigh on men in the same way; those taking the pill could enter relationships on more equal terms than before. As an epidemiologist he saw his role as looking at the rare side-effects such as thrombosis and the possibility of a greater risk of diabetes or other diseases; and the fact that "the Pill may actually improve health by reducing the risk of some kinds of breast disease."[7] Six years after his observation with Vessey, Doll concluded in a further report that the Pill was on balance beneficial to women's health. As was customary, his analysis of the benefits and hazards of oral contraceptives to the health of women was given with simple analogy. "One must say that the risks of bad side effects are extremely low— something between the risk of being killed by a motor car as a pedestrian and being killed travelling inside a car—and these are risks we take every day."[8]

In 1967 Doll received a letter from the statistician David Cox at Imperial College London. He is reputed to have written that he had a very bright student called Richard Peto who had just completed an MSc in statistics and would be either brilliant or a total disaster. Peto had studied natural sciences at Trinity College Cambridge, and been under-whelmed by the teaching he had received. Upon finishing his first degree he was not sure if he "even wanted to work or not", and when he went for the interview at Gower Street he had "never heard of Richard Doll or epidemiology".[9] Doll spent most of the interview inspiring Peto with his

---

*   In 1976 Vessey and Doll wrote an article: 'Is "the pill" safe enough to continue using?' (*Procedures of the Royal Society*) B. 195: pp. 69-80, in which they concluded that "the medical and social benefits that many women obtain with oral contraceptives use outweigh the hazards, and that 'the pill' can continue to be used."

thoughts on science, the unit's statistical projects and epidemiology's capacity to change clinical practice and hence clinical medicine. Doll must have experienced some kind of scientific alchemy with the 24-year-old sitting in front of him that day, for as with Sigmund Freud's concept of the "golden seed", he planted an idea in Peto's mind and saw a potential in him that Peto himself had not perceived.

This demonstration of belief—and confidence in not yet realised abilities—had a profound effect on medical science. From that moment on Peto immersed himself in looking for solutions to the mathematical problems of trying to link causes to disease and effects to treatment. Peto was an enchanter of numbers and Doll had found more than a disciple: he had a protégé. Peto was an English intellectual with what the lawyer Martyn Day described as "the brain of a giant"[10] and possessing, in the words of John Cairns, "colossal powers of speed of mind and boundless energy".[11] Politically the men had much in common. Peto's parents held meetings of the Southampton branch of the Communist Party in their front room, and this shared background led to Peto being "recruited into the family". Within a short time he showed himself to be the final component in one of the rare intellectual dynasties in British medical science. The apostolic succession from Pearson, Greenwood, Hill and Doll was now complete.

Like Austin Bradford Hill, Peto was not medically qualified, which may explain their shared passion for prevention. His status in modern epidemiology is assured because he has saved so many lives by being more interested in the medicine than the statistical techniques which enable him to obtain an answer. From being ambivalent about embracing a work ethic Peto became the acme of productivity. As Hill had got Doll "obsessed" with epidemiology, the process was repeated with Doll and Peto. Now there was only time for work, and it became his universe. "You suddenly realise that results on paper can save lives in the real world."[12]

Theirs was a father and son relationship. Their intellects were in harness, both were idealistic and they had a shared objective: preventing premature death. Peto succeeded Hill as Doll's collaborator on the British doctors study and he brought to the research a crusading zeal. Charismatic

and charming as he is, there is no diplomacy with Peto, which is com-
mendable when dealing with tobacco companies, and he thought nothing
of humiliating people if they were wrong.[13] Peto did not ride off, as he had
once contemplated, into a hippie sunset on his Triumph motorcycle in
1967. Instead he became a scientist on a mission, interested in medical
problems on a world scale— their collaboration made an enduring contribution to the health of the global community and continued uninter-
rupted until Doll's death.

As a scientist Doll was used to living with uncertainties. Joan had been
"feeling seedy for some time" and, in 1966 after a debilitating attack, Doll
asked Avery Jones to visit her at Lansdowne Road. After an examination
she was taken to St Mark's Hospital where colon cancer was diagnosed.
Every operation carries its risks, and Doll knew only too well what they
were for such a major procedure. As he walked through the hospital's corridors he became conscious of the beauty and brevity of life: Joan was 52.
The operation, however, was successful, and within weeks she was back
working at the MRC and at the centre of family life in Lansdowne Road.
Doll was reunited with "his best friend".[14]

With the arrival of the children and particularly since Steve had
become part of their lives, the Dolls felt it was essential to get out of
London at the weekend. Initially they rented a house in Wales, and in the
early 1960s they bought what Joan had once described as a "rural slum" in
Herefordshire. This primitive, idyllic home, set in four bucolic acres,
became a place of adventure and detachment for the family. Washing was
done under an outside pump, nature was embraced, time seemed limitless,
and for everyone but Doll the pressures of life could be forgotten. When
asked if he was a "family man", Joan replied, "No. Richard likes his family,
but he's very busy with his work."[15] Doll suffered the irreconcilable
demands of a scientist with responsibilities to his work as well as to his
family and friends, and he spent much of his scientific life disproving the
fallacy that you can only do one thing at a time. Within that highly regu-

lated allocation of a scarce resource—his time—it was his family life that was sacrificed.

It was common for Doll to bring an academic paper or some mathematical data with him to the picnic rug, or while being physically present on a beach holiday he would be spiritually absent, absorbed in some graphs of an esoteric statistical confounder. Steve recognised that Doll was one of those exceptional individuals who catalyse and define history but that it was those closest to home who bore the burden. "He wasn't a good Dad. He was never there. He would stand up and be counted when it mattered, but he didn't play with the children or go to school sports days."[16] His daughter Cathy called him "Richard" and not "Dad", which he disliked, but in her early life she did not think that he was a real dad to her.[17] He did, however, read JRR Tolkien's three-volume *The Lord of the Rings* four times during his life, twice out loud to the children. This may have been more to do with his admiration for the work of high fiction than any canvassing for Tolkien by Cathy or Nick. Nor was Doll the kind of man to take his children to the bakery in Notting Hill on a Saturday morning, or for a swim in a Herefordshire stream—there was no time for that. He was fair with the children but it was not until much later in their lives that he succeeded in resolving the uneasy relationship between responsibilities to public health and the wellbeing of his family.

The MRC statistical unit at 115 Gower Street was a synonym for Doll's philosophy of epidemiological science. Attracting equal numbers of statisticians and doctors, he inspired investigations into occupational and environmentally related solid cancers and leukaemia, clinical trials in the treatment of tuberculosis and peptic ulcers and research into the role of infectious agents on a wide variety of other chronic diseases. The unit's *raison d'être* was to understand the nature of disease, and then to determine what action could be taken on the basis of that knowledge to reduce human suffering. The kudos of Doll's unit was such that the most ambitious and brightest were attracted to its doors. Doll had introduced many of Hill's working practices; foremost among these was the management style of creating an atmosphere where researchers could pursue their work with encouragement and without obstruction. The door to Doll's office was always ajar and through it walked a continuous stream of scientists with research papers in various stages of completion. Usually, within 24 hours, they would be returned, covered with arrows redirecting the text, voluminous paragraphs in his inimitable spidery handwriting, together with a recommendation as to which journal might prove the best destination for the paper.

In 1966 a young American called Frank Speizer joined Doll's unit. He was immediately set to work on a study of asthma deaths in young people in England. This study[18] showed that the excess of mortality in such individuals was attributable in large part to overuse of pressurised aerosols of sympathomimetics by young asthmatics. Speizer later wrote, "The results of this series of studies led to public health warnings that were subsequently estimated to have saved the lives of over 3,500 children."[19] While working with Doll, Speizer had the idea of contacting the wives of Doll and Peto's 34,439 British male doctors to study their patterns of disease and mortality. The results gave him encouragement. Upon returning to the United States in 1968, his mind turned to the idea of setting up a prospective study within the American nursing profession. This became the nurses health study of 121,000 women followed for 25 years, which generated some of the most important epidemiological findings in the fields of cancer and overall public health.

After working for twenty years in Africa, Denis Burkitt came back to London and Doll gave him a desk in his MRC unit. In 1967 Doll introduced Burkitt to the retired naval physician, Captain Surgeon TL "Peter" Cleave. This meeting opened up a whole new area of research and endeavour for Burkitt,* which would become for him even more important than the discovery of the lymphoma.

---

*   Burkitt began collecting masses of information about the distribution of disease in the Third World which would help substantiate Cleave's claims. During his travels in 1969, he met Alec Walker in Johannesburg. Walker had studied several very different ethnic groups and had found that they all had different disease patterns and that they consumed different foods. Walker had accumulated a vast

Cleave had visited Doll one day in the early 1960s and tried to interest him in his book *The Saccharine Disease*, which he had published privately. Cleave had formed the opinion during his travels round the world that some diseases such as myocardial infarction, duodenal ulcer and diseases of the large bowel, which were very common in the UK, Western Europe and North America but rare in many parts of Africa and Asia, were due to an excess consumption of sugar. He was intending to produce a second edition and, knowing of Doll's interest in the geographical distribution of disease and its value as a clue to aetiology, he asked Doll if he would write a preface. Doll agreed, not because he was convinced of the theory (which did not attract him) but because he thought Cleave's experience of the variation in the incidence of disease was of interest and could be a good source of ideas for the aetiology of diseases of then unknown causes.

Cleave's views had been ridiculed by the establishment and he was often dismissed as a food crank. As a consequence he had failed to make any significant progress in getting his ideas accepted widely. As director of the statistical unit, and later with the increase of his scientific influence, Doll was reluctant to campaign in support of either his own discoveries or on behalf what became collectively known as "environmental issues". What he would accede to, even if it resulted in his reputation as an unbiased arbitrator of a scientific theory being impugned, was to support ideas

---

amount of information on bowel transit times and stool weights of individuals on different diets. Burkitt began his own studies on bowel behaviour and his observations were eventually published together with those of Walker and other colleagues in *The Lancet* in 1972 and in the *Journal of the American Medical Association* in 1973. On the basis of his research Burkitt believed that he had substantiated Walker's claim that fibre could provide protection against bowel cancer. He published a paper on this subject in *Cancer* in 1971, entitled 'Epidemiology of cancer of the colon and rectum'. In 1979 he published a book entitled *Don't Forget Fibre in Your Diet*, which was directed at the layperson. It was an immediate success and by the time the first few editions had appeared, over 200,000 copies had been sold around the world.

that were innovative or worthy of further inquiry.

In the foreword to the second edition of Cleave's book which was entitled *Diabetes, Coronary Thrombosis and the Saccharine Disease,** Doll wrote:

> Whether the predictions that Surgeon Captain Cleave and Dr Campbell make in this book will prove to be correct remains to be seen; but if only a small part of them do, the authors will have made a bigger contribution to medicine than most university departments or medical research units make in the course of a generation. Many of the observations of the distribution of disease under the extreme conditions of war and in the rapidly changing African environment are of outstanding interest and may well provide clues to the causation of the common diseases of European civilisation. In short, this is not an ordinary book and no one who finds the time to read it will fail to gain something from it.

Julian Tudor Hart, who was critical of Doll's later refusal to lend his authoritative weight to populist campaigns about suspected industrial pollutants, was impressed with Doll's courage in writing the foreword. "It gave the book credibility and Cleave [and Campbell] dignity."[20-]

Much of the political criticism that Doll encountered later came from his refusal to give open support to the "environmentalist movement". His strength as a scientist was that he only responded to the evidence. He did not campaign on it, he presented it. Richard Peto felt that Doll wrote the foreword because it might stimulate fresh thinking and renewed experiment. "Richard believed that you should encourage people to come up with ideas and hypothesis. It makes people think and engage a problem, not barmy ideas, but people who think unconventionally, and there seems to be something in what he wrote."[21]

---

*   Cleave TL and Campbell GD, *Diabetes, Coronary Thrombosis and the Saccharine Disease* (John Wright and Sons, 1966).

Doll was a natural leader and by the late 1960s he had recruited a stable of people who helped put Britain in the forefront of non-communicable disease epidemiology. He handed on knowledge and a philosophy of science to Pike, Vessey, Peter Smith and Richard Peto. In Doll's *Who's Who* entry under interests he listed "conversation", but for the thirty years after 1960 he had little time for it. To engage in it would have involved obfuscation; it would have taken time, and diluted the intellectual and spiritual capital he invested in his scientific work. It was a diversion neither taken nor contemplated. He would put himself out to help both individuals and causes where he saw an injustice, but otherwise he showed little interest in other people's personal lives. Doll was not a cold man, but he was reserved, enigmatic. He was quite warm underneath but he had to limit the consequences of this, so that he could concentrate on his science. Avis Hutt knew Doll for much of his adult life, from the years of political activism to the era of his professional omnipotence, and had observed an innate emotional continuity. "Richard's attitude was always a detached one. He was a private person and that's what made him the man he was. Respected and part feared."

Some people found Doll "daunting" and when the occasion demanded he could be formidable, particularly when faced with persistent woolly thinking.[22] While being courteous and kind, he suffered fools badly. Primarily Doll was preternaturally busy. He gave the impression that every five minutes of his day was accounted for.

As a result, a professional meeting with Doll was both a memorable, and for the unprepared, an unnerving encounter. He was not deliberately unkind like Howard Florey, responsible for the clinical discovery of penicillin, who upon meeting a less able scientist would ask, "Still going backwards, are we?" Nevertheless Doll's office was not the place to ruminate on the universe. After a courteous knock on the always open door you would enter his office, and his fountain pen would stop mid-sentence. He would look up believing—in hope—that the reason for the interruption would be a compelling one. Compared to almost any other person, the unforgettable aspect of a conversation with Doll was that he really listened. For people not accustomed to this, it could lead to nervousness and stultified thinking, neither of which would endear the visitor to him. But if the thinking was clear, then ideas would be exchanged, a strategy designed and inspiration would be distilled. When he thought the discussion had covered the relevant ground he would look at his watch and you knew your time was up. The visitor would leave, Doll's head would turn back to the desk, and the fountain pen would find its place and the spidery writing would set off and finish the interrupted sentence.

From 1949 under Sir Harold Himsworth's leadership, the MRC continued to expand its empire. The opportunity to build a new clinical research centre on the same site as a district hospital—and to integrate both institutions at Northwick Park in west London—was seized upon as the future of clinical practice. John Squire, a pupil of Sir Thomas Lewis, was appointed the first director of the projected centre. However, in January 1966, during a visit to London, Squire, a heavy smoker, developed chest pain. He went to University College Hospital, his *alma mater*, for treatment and died there two hours later. He was 52. His obituary notice was fulsome, according him "a magnificent brain, dynamic energy, and unflagging enthusiasm". It continued, "It is tritely said that 'no one is irreplaceable,' but it will take a great many very able men to do all the work that Squire discharged so splendidly, graciously, and unostentatiously."[23]

The MRC decided to replace Squire[24] with a director and deputy director. GM (later Sir Graham) Bull was appointed director, and Doll, after lengthy persuasion from Himsworth, was appointed his deputy. Doll was to have directed the epidemiology and health care unit at Northwick Park, but he soon felt that the project was underfinanced and he was "forced to take people who were not of the highest order."[25] Northwick Park was due to open in 1970, but Doll was ambivalent about the project; he was not attracted to being second in command, to anyone. He was at a crossroads in his career. He had shown himself to be a worthy successor to Hill, and in 1969 he was a famous scientist who had nurtured a new generation of epidemiologists whose contributions to science and health would be lasting. Out of loyalty to Himsworth he had turned his great intellectual and administrative qualities to building an institution that he did not fully believe in.

Leaving London

Then, in the summer of 1969, Doll, the quintessential metropolitan and life-long Londoner, received a telephone call from Michael Dunnill, a pathologist in Oxford. Out of the dark blue, Doll was asked if he would be interested in becoming the Regius Professor of Medicine at Oxford University. He was 56 years old and eager for a new challenge. It was with much interest and some contentment that Doll replaced the receiver.

Part Three 1969-1984

The Academic Revolution
Oxford and the Wider World

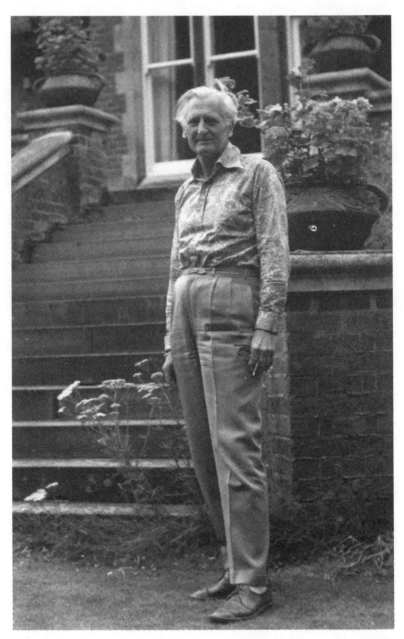

Doll as Regius, 13 Norham Gardens, 1974

Chapter 18

Oxford: The Regius Professor of Medicine

"Doll is a man who makes history. He has plans and he sees they are carried out."

TDR Hockaday

The Regius Professorship of Medicine at Oxford University was a crown appointment under the patronage secretary of the Cabinet. With Doll's predecessors as was customary, two names were put forward and the prime minister, on advice, chose one.[1] Doll's appointment broke with this tradition.

Sir George Pickering, Doll's predecessor as Regius from 1956-68, was a medical scientist and made significant contributions to our understanding of cardiovascular disease; but it was his influence on education that was his greatest contribution to the world of medicine. Largely as a result of Pickering's foresight and determination, the independent departments of postgraduate medicine that had been set up under the Nuffield benefaction were brought together to become the central focus of the rapidly expanding clinical school. Pickering had a vision for the Oxford Medical School in which university staff would do clinical medicine and NHS staff would do research. He cultivated an ethos of experimental science among his clinical recruits, offering them a bench in his laboratory, technical support and research expenses.

This concern for his staff had brought him widespread admiration, except, that is from the surgical team. Joe Smith, Oxford's first urologist, remembered that Pickering "was virulently opposed to surgery in all of its forms."[2] Anthony Steadman "Tim" Till, a renowned thyroid surgeon, was also conscious of his professor's contradictions. "Pickering didn't like surgeons, but he had a lot to be thankful of them for, he had his hip and his colon done. He was mad about research, although he hadn't done much himself."[3] One important feature of Pickering's appointment was that it formed a continuity with contemporary history. Dating back to Sir William Osler at the turn of the twentieth century, there had been a series of very clinically orientated professors of medicine. In 1968, when Pickering announced that he was leaving to become master of Pembroke College, there was immense interest in who was going to succeed him.

According to Jim Holt, a clear favourite emerged with a "huge swell of opinion behind Paul Beeson, the Nuffield professor of medicine".[4] For his part Beeson was anxious to get the job, seeing himself as a natural successor to Osler with whom he shared a medical background at McGill and Johns Hopkins. This, however, was not universally welcomed; the greatest obstacle for Beeson was that he was not British—he was an American—and it would have required an act of Parliament to change the constitution of the Regius chair dating from the reign of Queen Anne. And that was not going to happen. There then followed a period of confusion and jockeying for position, while the clear advice that Downing Street sought was absent. Michael Dunnill, the director of clinical studies at Oxford, was anxious to resolve the impasse and when he heard from Charles Whitty, a neurologist at the Radcliffe Infirmary, that Doll might be looking for a change of direction he decided to phone 115 Gower Street.

Ironically, only a year before, Doll had met Dunnill in London to offer him a post at Northwick Park, which Dunnill declined. When the latter entertained Doll at Merton College he had the unmistakable feeling that "Doll wanted to get away from Bull and Northwick Park."[5] He then reported back to his committee, which included the movers and shakers in Oxford medical science, and in 1969 they collectively wrote to the patronage secretary recommending one name: Richard Doll. Sir John Habakkuk, who was vice chancellor for most of the time Doll was Regius, remembered: "He was an unusual appointment. Because Pickering was a very hands on doctor and he cured a lot of people. But it was Doll who saved my life. I remember reading his paper in 1950 and it made me stop smoking."[6]

"You can't go to that hidebound institution" was Harold Himsworth's response to the prospect of losing his director of the MRC's statistical research unit. The Yorkshireman was partly correct. In 1969 Oxford medical science was divided internally, and antagonistic to Doll's appointment. Jim Holt was Beeson's first Oxford registrar in 1963, and believed the initial hostility to Doll was because he was not a proper doctor—he would not take over Pickering's ward with his firm—and this was resented. "When Doll came he came to a climate of hostility."[7]

Throughout his life Doll loved to accept a challenge but he knew very little about the Oxford Medical School when he took up the appointment in July 1969. At the time the school had no dean and the Regius had many of the responsibilities normally associated with the deanship serving as the connecting link with the pre-clinical departments, and being technically in charge of overseeing their examinations; while the director of clinical studies was responsible for the organisation of the clinical curriculum and the allocation of work to the individual clinical students.

The pre-clinical school at the time was thriving, having developed progressively since the middle of the nineteenth century, when during Sir Henry Acland's tenure of the Regius chair the policy was adopted of preparing pre-clinical students to the highest scientific standards and then directing them for their clinical studies to one of the London teaching hospitals. The clinical school, in contrast, was relatively new, having been reestablished only from the outbreak of the Second World War when the government sought to redistribute the many clinical students taking Oxford, Cambridge or London degrees away from the capital. During this time the school flourished, but after 1945 it continued in a desultory way with an annual intake of students limited to 32 and sometimes as few as eight.

The situation was transformed by Pickering in 1957 when he undertook clinical work at the Radcliffe Infirmary, had six university appointments in medicine associated with him, and had a small department built for his personal research and that of this academic juniors. The annual intake of students rose to fifty, and an additional professorship had been established in neurology. The pervading spirit was one of optimism for the future and the conduct of research.

In 1969, however, Doll found that the university could not have been less interested in medicine. He was also conscious of the machinations surrounding his appointment but admitted that he had definite attractions to the existing status quo. "I'm quite certain that I was offered the appointment because I had an FRS and this made me respectable to the basic scientists, the biochemists and biologists, who regarded clinical medicine as a trade rather than a science."[8] He also found Oxford had too many gastroenterologists, like himself, and as he was not needed as a clinician he decided administration would be enough. There was a lot to do and he took it seriously. He also questioned whether he would ever conduct original research again.

As the 23rd Regius Professor of Medicine at Oxford University Doll's only demand when appointed was that he be awarded a DM,[9] believing it would be incongruous for him to award the DM to others if he did not have one himself. John Ledingham was an NHS consultant in 1969 in Oxford and he found Doll's arrival contentious and politically unsettling:

> Clinical doctors were the apex; all others were dust beneath our chariot wheels. What good is having a Regius Professor of Medicine if he's going to be in the statistics department, if he can't use a stethoscope, he'll be no good teaching students, and no damn good round the bedside. We have a communist who lives in great luxury in Norham Gardens who's got original paintings of the sort that most communists would feel were the things that only the rich should have. What the hell are we having him for? That was very much the view.[10]

Doll brought with him the nucleus of his MRC staff: Pike, Vessey, Peter Smith, Paula Cook, Barbara Hafner, Diana Bull, and early in 1970 Richard Peto joined him in "Piccadilly"—the offices of the Regius in the Radcliffe Infirmary. The hospital where Charles Fletcher had given the first injection of penicillin in 1941 proved to be an inspiring location for medical research. Doll's team only had half the space on the third floor of the hospital; the rest was reserved for Pickering's lab-based staff, led by John Honour. Barbara Hafner thought that there was an uneasy "feeling" between the two groups initially and that Doll was very generous to his predecessor's animal experimental staff.

If Doll's appointment had caused disquiet among the clinicians this was not the response among Oxford's existing cadre of epidemiologists. For Leo Kinlen, the appointment of an epidemiologist to this post was so unusual that it brought a spotlight to bear both on his department and on the subject more generally. "With Malcolm Pike as his dynamic first assistant, the department in Oxford was a hive of activity—with a constant stream of visitors from all over the world. They were heady days. If our leader had found the cause of the most common fatal cancer, might not any of us be lucky with a less common cancer?"[11]

With the venerable office of Regius came attendant privileges. William Osler had bequeathed his huge Victorian house, 13 Norham Gardens, for the use of his successors. Set in the heart of Fabian-minded, academic North Oxford, the house was home to the Dolls for the next decade. For visiting scholars like Frank Speizer* it was where "discussions were held late into the night on issues such as relations among Britain, the US, and Russia as well as health care reform in the United States." Michael Gelder was the professor of psychiatry when Doll arrived in 1969 and he recalled the joyous New Year's Eve parties there which helped to create a "sense of community and team spirit". When Barbara Hafner was first shown around Norham Gardens by Doll, he said proudly, "'This is the kind of house I've always wanted—isn't it great?' So he did like the good life and so did Joan."[12] For Joan, too, Oxford marked a new and unexpected chapter in their life. She continued to commute between her career at the MRC and the comparatively somnambulant life of Oxford academe. She found it all very parochial and did not want to live in a city where people introduced themselves at dinner parties by saying "I saw you coming out of the hairdressers on Saturday morning." As she wrote: "I used to recoil, thinking, there's no privacy in Oxford."[13] Joan did not move

---

*   Jonathan M Samet and Frank E Speizer, Obituary of Sir Richard Doll 1912-2005, *American Journal of Epidemiology*, 2006; volume 164, number 1, pp. 95-100.

permanently until 1979, eventually becoming, in the words of her MRC colleague, "an Oxford grande dame".

Doll had the instincts of a politician. He made it clear that his job as Regius was as head of the medical school, and it was a complex organisation encompassing both a clinical and pre-clinical side. As a political navigator with a vision of what was going to be needed in the future, Doll soon realised that the Nuffield committee would be inadequate for the needs of a rapidly advancing science. Much needed to be done. Early in 1970 he established a working party on the development of the clinical school* set up jointly by the medicine board and the Nuffield committee, which issued a preliminary report after nine meetings in May 1970. A final report followed a year later after a total of 29 meetings, mostly held at 8.00am on Saturday mornings at Norham Gardens. The ground had been prepared by Pickering and Beeson; and Doll took full advantage of it. It was a trait of Doll's that having identified what was possible, he went for it, and achieved it.

Together with Peter Garnham, the secretary of the medical school, Doll wound up the Nuffield committee and a new clinical medicine board was introduced. The working party assumed that all clinical students would be graduates and hoped that about half would come from Oxford and half from other universities. It was hoped that the excellence of the science departments and the general intellectual environment would provide an opportunity for the school to aim at training teachers and research workers while continuing to provide a broad education allowing its newly qualified doctors to enter any branch of the profession. With the completion of the new John Radcliffe Hospital in Headington the annual intake of students was recommended to rise to eighty and more. In these

---

*   Members: Doll (Chair) Professors Paul Beeson and A Crampton Smith and Dr M Dunnill (Director of Clinical Studies) nominated by the Nuffield committee, and Professors M Gelder and W Paton and Dr J Potter nominated by the medical board, Dr R Franklin co-opted from the general board, and Dr D Hodgson co-opted from the NHS planning committee.

circumstances it was essential that the school be expanded and new professorships financed.

Doll's mission to develop the medical school was given invaluable help by Rosemary Rue,* the senior administrative medical officer of the Oxford region. They formed a unique axis of influence: Rue the clever and purposeful NHS figure, and Doll the most powerful medical academic in Oxford. Together they financed the new chairs and supported other individuals without too much bureaucracy. Rue had been interested in Doll's work on smoking and was frustrated by the government's failure to get involved in a meaningful public health campaign to combat it. Also, as a member of the clinical medicine board sitting with elected professorial departments and the vice chancellor, she had seen Doll smoothing the opposition from people who had only witnessed the establishment of perhaps one new chair in the university in the previous forty years.

Doll was determined to develop the medical school and make it grow; in Rue he had a formidable ally with access to finance. "Richard was scouring the academic field all round the world, trying to persuade people to come and do good teaching and research. We worked very well together. The clinical school was one of his great achievements at Oxford."[14] With Rue on the clinical medicine board, he was able to persuade the university

---

* Rosemary Rue trained at the Oxford Medical School where there were so few students that she used to do a ward round alone with Professor Leslie Witts, the Nuffield professor of medicine. Unfortunately in 1954 Rue contracted polio from a patient, becoming the last person in Oxford to get the disease. She surmounted great difficulties to live a prodigious life, dedicated to the NHS and the people it served. In 1957 Doll and Hill wrote a paper entitled 'Deaths from poliomyelitis among British doctors (*British Medical Journal*) 1957; 1: 372. They found that in male doctors (using 34,494 medically qualified men) the evidence suggested that men between the ages of 25 and 45 who were practising medicine in Great Britain were at special risk of dying of poliomyelitis. "The actual number of deaths recorded (eight) is small in relation to the number of men at risk, but at the rates of the general population not more than one death would have been expected to occur."

that the expanded medical school would not "swamp the university"—but no one before had ever imagined such a revolutionary enlargement of a university faculty.

During Doll's tenure he brought to the medical school and negotiated finance for five new chairs: clinical biochemistry, morbid anatomy, paediatrics, clinical biochemistry and social medicine. Within a short period of time the medical school, which had an intake of eight when Rosemary Rue was a student, was attracting 100 students and, as the *Oxford University Gazette* reported the new chairs were "an indispensable part of the planned expansion".[15] Most importantly for the success of the school, outstanding candidates were obtained for all the new posts, as well as the old posts that fell vacant and research programmes of the highest scientific standards were quickly developed. This underpinning of the academic foundations of the clinical school had led within a decade to it being generally accepted as the leading institution of its kind in the country.

Doll had come to a medical school that did not want him and within the clinical community of physicians and surgeons they thought: who is this man and what is he going to bring? John Ledingham had been in the vanguard of the critical reception but the evidence had changed his mind. "To Doll's great credit, within two years everybody thought that his appointment was the right decision."[16] The uneasy relationship that had existed between the pre-clinical and clinical school had been removed by separating the two into distinct academic faculties. The clinical school germinated an ethos of research and excellence, attained a mark of distinction and came to attract more money into the university than any other faculty. From being disparaged, clinical medicine became a crucial financial life-support system of wellbeing.

In 1971 smoking became a headline issue with a second report from the Royal College of Physicians. Like the famous 1962 report it concentrated on the damage being done by tobacco. Chaired by Sir Max Rosenheim, it captured the imagination of the media and the public in a way that the first report had not. The Conservative secretary of state, Sir Keith Joseph, was impressed by the strongly worded report, describing it as "a lobby which could not be resisted," but his actions, though more vigorous than those of Enoch Powell nine years before, fell far short of the actions the report had demanded. For example, warnings about the dangers of smoking were put on cigarette packets, but they were much weaker and less prominent than had been recommended, and the grant for health education was increased but still negligible in comparison with resources spent by the tobacco industry on advertising.

To Doll it was of paramount importance still to be seen as a neutral observer who described a relationship and left the public and physicians to draw the inevitable conclusions. This political distancing from scientific findings seemed to work on the puritanical Joseph, who said in Parliament: "It was the Doll and Hill experiment which totally convinced me that cigarette smoking inflicts very grave and avoidable suffering on large numbers of our fellow countrymen." Doll did directly support the work of Action on Smoking and Health (ASH), but it was his reputation for independence and scientific honesty that convinced journalists that the topic was newsworthy.

Of course, the most important influence on the level of smoking in Britain at the time was still exerted by the Chancellor of the Exchequer. By increasing the duty on tobacco—for health reasons—at last a megaphone was being put in the hands of public health. For the first time in modern British social history there was a reduction in the levels of smoking—primarily as a result of the media coverage of its hazards.

Institutions can change individuals. Westminster School, St Thomas's Hospital and the Royal Society (where he was vice president from 1970-71) were formative influences on both Doll himself, and on how he was perceived in the world he occupied. His position as the doyen of British epidemiology was confirmed in 1971 when he was knighted. The Regius chair came with an attachment to Christ Church, the most aristocratic of all Oxford's colleges, yet to many of his left-wing friends the acceptance of a medieval honour was both an anachronism and recognition of his status in British society. The times were changing, and so was he. He joked that he had been "forgiven" for his radicalism by an innately conservative profession, that there was something penitential about it, and that by his own admission he had changed: "I obviously became much more one of the establishment."[17]

For some of those who moved from London to Oxford with him, there had also been a discernible emotional change too. The togetherness and the scientific collaboration of the MRC unit were missing. He was bound up in university administration, busy with his own scientific work and travelling widely. For Malcolm Pike, there was a difference in Doll's Oxford persona, and if you had worked with him before then "you got a less human person". Pike missed the daily scientific collaboration and closeness of the London days. In his bones Doll was not an "old-type establishment" figure. Scientifically, he changed the establishment[18] and it became more like him. Of course he was also conventional: he loved cricket, drinking ale and working in his garden. The lawyer Martyn Day, who had the opportunity to study Doll forensically, in the drama and trauma of the witness box, thought that he was without question "establishment": "There are few experts who would ever meet his level of authority in front of a judge: now that is pretty 'establishment'. Clearly having been a radical in his past, he now pitches it at a level which says 'If I'm saying it, it's almost certain to be true.' Which means that he has had to establish himself very much at the centre: and cannot afford to be seen out on a limb in any sort of way."[19]

The Doll of the 1970s would not have dressed in the style of a political bohemian as he had done at the inaugural meeting of the International Corresponding Club in 1957, and while it is true that in his first *Who's Who* entry, under clubs he had listed The Establishment (a London nightclub famous for satire), Doll nevertheless had caused a revolution. By the early 1970s he had a world-renowned scientific reputation but Oxford gave him real power and he used it to expand epidemiology. It was a small field until the 1970s and it is notable that a high proportion of the scientists who were to dominate the subject passed through the doors of his department.

He was lucky in choosing people or they were lucky in choosing him.

To what extent he developed an environment that was so creative that everybody just improved by osmosis or whether his apostles were a very bright group it is hard to judge. But it was his achievement in advancing a scientific methodology—of bringing statistics into standard medical investigation—that helped change clinical practice. It became obvious once the tools of epidemiology and randomised clinical trials started working that big mistakes had been made by doctors in the past.[20] It was an experimental advance that was spread across the world by Doll and his academic juniors. It became the dominant ideology, and universally accepted.

On 26 June 1973, while addressing a meeting of the Medical Journalists' Association in London, it appeared that Doll's dexterity with the media had abandoned him. Speaking on the context of the 1974 reorganisation of the NHS, Doll said that its future objective was not to mount a programme to try to make everyone live to be 140. In fact, he told the story-hungry gathering that people over 65 should be prepared to accept death and should not try to preserve their life for a few more months. It was, he said, "their social responsibility to live dangerously"[21] and not to expect the NHS to spend time on research into prolonging their lives. He did, however, believe that it was "much more important to keep them happy and relieve their disabilities." Unfortunately for Doll—who was only sixty at the time*—his statement aroused more condemnation than homage among the pensionariat of the *Daily Telegraph*. Emily Harrower of Sussex wrote:

---

* This was reminiscent of the criticism that Sir William Osler suffered for his speech "The Fixed Period" given at Johns Hopkins Hospital in 1905. He claimed that "the effective, moving vitalising work of the world is done between the ages of 25 and forty" and that it was downhill from then on. He envisaged a retirement age

About living more dangerously, how should we set about this? Do more flying on the chance that the plane will crash or encourage our young drivers to go even faster than they do? No. I think that, as happened in Konigsberg when the Mongols were pouring in, cyanide should be freely available so that as many did, we could put ourselves out quietly. Alternatively perhaps Sir Richard Doll would let me have a nice pain-less pill by special request."[22]

On the other hand, David Hobman, Director of Age Concern, agreed with Doll that people should live dangerously. "This did not mean they should all try to emulate Sir Francis Chichester by sailing round the world. But it did mean they should be encouraged to keep up hobbies and pastimes, and not exist like cabbages in anticipation of living a little longer."[23]

The *Telegraph's* editorial struck a high-minded chord:

In a civilised society old people should surely be allowed to live out their lives in dignity and peace and with the respect of younger people... For most of us get old in the end; the prospect of a tranquil and happy retirement is psychologically important. Nor are people of 65 and over necessarily played out. History is full of writers, statesmen and others who did great work, in some cases their greatest work, in old age. Sir Winston Churchill was over the 65 mark when he became prime minister; so was Disraeli. At a humbler level, this is true of a lot of people. Even if this were *not* true there would still be no case for telling such people that they ought to kick the bucket. For human life is an end in itself; each one is unique and infinitely valuable.[24]

Doll was not calling for voluntary euthanasia—it was the quality of life that concerned him. Prophetically, the *Daily Telegraph* reported that "Professor Sir Richard Doll added he would be vehemently against having his own life prolonged if it meant he would be only a shadow of his former self". Doll agreed with George Bernard Shaw that you should use your

---

of 60—and his speech aroused hostility in the popular press. Attracting the head-line—"Osler recommends chloroform at sixty."

health even to the point of wearing it out. That is what it is for. Spend all you have before you die and do not outlive yourself. Do not try to live forever. You will not succeed.

Perhaps more than anybody else Doll helped demonstrate the avoidability of cancer by drawing attention to the dreadful consequence that smoking was having on mortality on men in middle age in the second half of the twentieth century.[25] The subsequent reduction in the habit greatly increased the number of ex-smokers who made it into old age. Doll, following his own advice, embraced the concept of living dangerously, and bought an MGB roadster. During the 1970s it was not uncommon to see the Regius Professor of Medicine driving through the city with his mortar board angled into the wind and his ceremonial gown billowing in the air. The image was an accurate metaphor for his life—because Doll was an extraordinarily driven person. John Stuart Mill's last words were supposed to have been, "I have done my work." For Doll work was all-encompassing, and it never really came to an end. It was probably true that epidemiology was his world and in its absence there was little remaining hinterland in his life. From the age of seventy he lived dangerously and worked continuously with enormous dedication, his ambition being "to die young as old as possible". His work came at a price to himself and his family, but Doll's investigations into avoiding and preventing premature death provided society with the knowledge of how to enjoy life more and for longer.

Doll discovered early on that the secret of doing anything in Oxford was consultation. This, however, was only after his efforts to impose his own wishes on the clinical board would be overturned by an organised rebellion.*

Two appointments in particular made during Doll's tenure as Regius had an impact on Oxford medicine and the wider world. The appoint-

---

* Jim Holt was the director of clinical studies when Beeson was leaving the Nuffield chair and Doll wanted Stan Peart from the Hammersmith as a replacement. Behind Doll's back, Holt held a dinner party for his senior colleagues all of whom were united in their desire to bring David Weatherall from Liverpool (where he

ments of the Australian transplant surgeon Peter Morris, who later became the president of the Royal College of Surgeons, and the molecular biologist David Weatherall helped transform the Oxford clinical school into an institution of national significance. Neither of the men were his first choice, but once they were in post Doll lived up to the conviction that his main duty was to create the conditions where young men and women could do their best work.

During this period of rapid expansion in Oxford medicine, Morris found Doll encouraging, good at finding money for research, and, in terms of the future, "He had his finger on the pulse—becuase the Institute of Molecular Medicine changed the whole of medicine in England. Putting molecular medicine in a clinical school was a great feat."[26] When Doll was committed to something he was like a dog with a bone. He could be hard or what others described as "ruthless"[27] and in 1974 he knew it was the beginning of a new era in which the emphasis in the study of disease was changing from patients and their organs to events at the molecular level.

When Doll arrived at Oxford in 1969, the director of the Nuffield Institute for Medical Research (NIMR) was Geoffrey Dawes, who had been appointed its first director in 1948. A gifted experimental scientist, he pioneered foetal physiology in his vertiginous laboratory housed in the eighteenth-century building known as the Tower of the Winds beside the Radcliffe Infirmary. His textbook *Fetal and Neonatal Physiology* (1968) is a tribute to his scientific innovation. By 1975 it was obvious that the Tower of the Winds* would become redundant as a research laboratory— the new John Radcliffe Hospital had moved to Headington and the

---

held the chair in haematology). Doll tended only to take on battles that he could win, and this was not one of them.

* During Rosemary Rue's final year as a medical student she took part in physiological experiments pounding up and down the staircase of the Tower of the Winds, having her blood pressure taken at the top and bottom, then receiving a shot of adrenalin and repeating the exercise. The staircase had the additional obstacles of Geoffrey Dawes's sheep that roamed around the building.

research laboratory needed to be there too—that Dawes had made an historic contribution and that it was now time to put something new on the map.

Doll called a meeting of the usual suspects at 13 Norham Gardens – the power-brokers in clinical science, who included Bill Paton, Michael Gelder, Henry Harris, Philip Randal, Peter Morris and John Ledingham. Doll began by saying, "Gentlemen, the university no longer want to fund Professor Dawes. His department will be closed down and we must look to the future". In this new climate, the influence of the NIMR began to wane. David Weatherall had been appointed Nuffield Professor of Clinical Medicine in 1974 – through his foresight that future was the establishment of the Institute of Molecular Medicine (later renamed The Weatherall Institute of Molecular Medicine). Its creation gave the Oxford clinical school an international renown.

Doll listened, and did not just pick people in his own image. Weatherall was a haematologist who educated himself in the new technology of molecular biology; he became one of the world's leading experts on the genetics of a group of inherited haematological disorders known as the thalassemias. Michael Dunnill thought that scientifically Weatherall and Doll "were violently opposed" with the former believing that old age, osteoporosis and coronary disease were genetically determined, while Doll regarded the environment as the principal factor. Weatherall felt that this philosophical divide cast a shadow across their relationship.[29] In his elegant survey of the evolution of modern medicine, *Science and the Quiet Art*,[4] Weatherall wrote:

> With the exception of a few familial forms, cancer is not a genetic disease in the usual sense of the word. Most cancers cannot be traced through families in the way that obeys Mendel's laws. However, it has become apparent over the last few years that cancer results from a series

---

*   Weatherall D, *Science and the Quiet Art: Medical Research and Patient Care* (Oxford University Press, 1995).

of events in the life of a cell that so far alter its genetic make up that it loses its ability to divide and mature in a normal manner. In this sense cancer is a genetic disease, because it is due to acquired defects in the genetic machinery of cells, defects that they pass on to their progeny.

What epidemiological evidence had shown was that tobacco was responsible for 25 per cent to 40 per cent of all cancer deaths, and that despite the obvious potential applications to medicine, the development of significant genetic advances relevant to clinical practice could take generations. Both Weatherall and Doll were eloquent exponents of their scientific philosophies regarding the causes of the intractable diseases—particularly cancer and vascular disease, which seem to reflect complex interactions between genetics and the environment. During the years that they worked together, Weatherall never felt entirely comfortable being around Doll[30] and thought he may have been ambivalent or even sceptical about the new genetics and new biology and the role they would play in the medicine of the future vis-à-vis epidemiology and the environment.

Weatherall admired Doll for his clarity of thought and analytical brain, yet allied to those qualities he found him to be "one of those people who just don't give. It isn't a coldness or shyness; I just think he doesn't give. He is a very private person. Doll's the kind of person that it's hard to get close to. Socially he is terrific, and he gives a good party, but if you want to get any deeper … "[31] Perhaps this distance was a residue of Doll's initial dispute over the appointment with the clinical board; yet he certainly supported Weatherall for a Royal Society prize so he must have been genuinely impressed with the new science's discoveries.

Epidemiology had shown how the age-specific risk of cancer could be halved, without the aid of molecular biology. Unfortunately that knowledge did not mean that people would take the steps necessary to bring it about. Doll certainly believed that molecular biology, by classifying people according to their susceptibility to particular types of cancer, would encourage the most susceptible to take appropriate steps to avoid the disease. More importantly for Doll was molecular biology's ability to show the mechanisms by which the disease is produced, allowing doctors to reduce risk by interfering with the mechanism, by specific antiviral immunisation. On the 40th anniversary of Crick and Watson's discovery of the double helix, Doll wrote:

> Cancer of the cervix provides a beautiful example, for we now know that by far the most cases are produced by the integration of certain types of human papilloma virus (HPV) into the genome of the cervical mucosa cells... * All that needs to be done is, therefore, to produce an effective method of immunisation against the specific types of HPV to reduce the risk of cervical cancer by some 80-90 per cent—which may, however, be easier said than done."[32]

Many specific causes of cancer are now known, the most important being smoking, asbestos, obesity, and a few oncogenic viruses. That, of course, still leaves the fifty per cent (of common cancers such as breast, prostate, colon and rectum) that medical science does not know how to avoid; but Doll believed that the combination of the older sciences and molecular biology would provide clear directions how it could be avoided by 2030.[33]

The development of the medical school is one of the great academic achievements at Oxford University over the last 100 years.[34] Doll's ability to recruit leading scientists, to finance five new chairs, while at the same time establishing the world's leading epidemiology unit, is a tribute to his single-mindedness. Yet, the man who could be found eating crisps in the consultants' dining room was never wholeheartedly accepted by Oxford's

---

* The most important discoveries of the past two decades in cancer epidemiology relate to the carcinogenic effects of infectious pathogens that had not been characterised twenty years ago. *Helicobacter pylori*, a chronic gastric bacterial infection that can cause gastric ulcers, is a major factor in the development of stomach cancer. About one-fifth of all human cancers worldwide arise in the stomach (nine per cent), liver (six per cent) or cervix (five per cent), and most of these would be prevented if these infections could be eradicated.

medical establishment. "Red Richard's" political past militated against an easy assimilation into the status quo. He was never in fact entirely forgiven. Perhaps it was an English reserve, but one of the unusual aspects of his character was that very few people, even his closest colleagues, had a personal relationship with him.[35] Such "keeping his own counsel" brought him respect, and allowed him the time to keep the compartments of his life under tight control. Doll spent much of his life using good manners as a means of maintaining distance. People became conscious fairly quickly that he was "a superior kind of person and used to getting his own way;"[36] this, allied to the unconscious intimidation he projected, led some to be frightened of him. There was a kindness about Doll and he was too much of a gentleman to be unpleasant, but some did tremble in front of him.[37] Whether this surprised him or not is uncertain. But what can be said without equivocation is that for those within his aegis a dressing down from Doll would have been chilling to contemplate and a catastrophe to receive.

Doll was epidemiology's guardian angel. His life was dedicated to science and finding reliable answers to nature's experiments. If his personality had not brought him reverence his methodology had. The statisticians may not have belonged to the sandal brigade but Doll had helped make them the equals of doctors at the patient's bedside. Even the most ardent diehards such as John Ledingham were converted: "He's a revolutionary. Doll is the man who pulled epidemiology from being a backroom study, to being respectable. The whole concept of evidence-based medicine really depends on people like Doll. So he has produced a revolution, a revolution in medical thinking."[38]

Chapter 19

The Truth behind the Myth: Richard Doll and Alice Stewart

"It is not the nature of things for any one man to make a sudden, violent discovery; science goes step by step and every man depends on the work of his predecessors. When you hear of a sudden unexpected discovery—a bolt from the blue—you can always be sure that it has grown up by the influence of one man or another, and it is the mutual influence which makes the enormous possibility of scientific advance. Scientists are not dependent on the ideas of a single man, but the combined wisdom of thousands of men, all thinking of the same problem and each doing his little bit to add to the great structure of knowledge which is gradually erected."

Ernest Rutherford

Rarely in the history of twentieth-century medicine have two more contrasting personalities and scientific approaches co-existed than those of Richard Doll and Alice Stewart. Their celebrated disputes about the effects of ionising radiation led to a long-lasting and, at times, bitter antagonism, which caused damaging personal and scientific fallout. Yet this problematic atmosphere would have been difficult to predict in the light of their shared political beliefs and life-long dedication to epidemiology.

Alice Stewart (née Naish) was born in Sheffield in 1906 to enlightened and socially progressive parents, both of whom were clinicians with a special interest in children's welfare. They were determined, whatever the sacrifice, to educate all of their eight children to the highest possible standard. This egalitarianism enabled Alice to excel academically, and follow her parents into medicine. However, the freedom from conventional restraints that had enriched Alice's intellectual life disappeared in the mire of bigotry she endured during her early days at Cambridge University. Reading medical sciences, where she was one of only four women in a student body of 300, she was angered and shocked by the chauvinistic behaviour of the male students: in her first lecture, she was obliged to walk right down to the front of the lecture hall, her every step accompanied by the orchestrated thunder of fists being slammed in unison on the desktops, jeering at a woman's attendance at medical lectures. This ritualised humiliation went deep, and understandably helped convince Stewart that some of the main setbacks in her later career could be attributed to sex discrimination.

In 1929 Stewart moved to London and began her clinical training at the all-female Royal Free Hospital in Hampstead. This marked the beginning of a brilliant, albeit flawed, career, and a political awakening. Brought up in Sheffield, she had seen the harsh social conditions which the city's industrial families endured, yet the poverty and daily humiliations experienced by most Londoners came as a revelation. "I had no idea how bad it was. It gave me very sharp, pro-Labour opinions. I've always wondered how anyone could do clinical medicine in the thirties and be a Conservative."[1]

The 1930s was a period of achievement and great change for the young doctor. In 1933 she married Ludovick Stewart, and managed to combine bringing up two children with building a stellar career in clinical medicine. She taught at the Royal Free in the 1930s, becoming a registrar in 1941, and it was during this period that Alice Stewart's life intertwined, if indirectly, for the first time with Richard Doll's. One of her young students was the audacious Joan Faulkner, and Stewart's enthusiasm for medicine had a great impact upon her subsequent career. According to Alice, Joan once said, "Dr Stewart taught me all the medicine I know."[2]

Within British society generally, and the medical profession specifically, a new attitude towards the nation's health was beginning to emerge. Rather than merely removing or alleviating a present pathology, the idea that medicine should be applied to the service of all society—social medicine—was being advocated. Henry Sigerist reflected that political and philosophical shift: "We have reached a time in which the physician must assume leadership in the struggle for the improvement of conditions." Stewart, like Doll, was involved in the Committee Against Malnutrition and the Socialist Medical Association, both of which were concerned with the close link between poverty and ill-health.

The Second World War weakened Alice's marriage, but not her ambition. Ludovick was sent to Bletchley Park "where someone stole him away from me,"[3] but it was a period when Stewart's career flourished. In 1941 Alice joined the staff of Dr Leslie Witts at the Radcliffe Infirmary in Oxford. It was to be a fortuitous step, and saw her eventual move from general medicine to social medicine (as non-infectious disease epidemiology was then called). Alice Stewart's first investigation in her new discipline was to assess the risk of developing jaundice or aplastic anaemia from filling shells with TNT. "So, you could say I got into social medicine because of the war—it was an accident of war. I would never have got such a position otherwise."[4]

By the time Stewart arrived in Oxford, academic medicine had just been revolutionised by philanthropy. William Morris, later Lord Nuffield, had created a vast industrial empire at his Cowley car factory, and with the persuasion of three eminent and powerful men within the university, £2,600,000 was donated to Oxford medicine via the Nuffield Benefaction in 1936. Sir Farquhar Buzzard, then the Regius Professor of Medicine, Sir Hugh Cairns, the pioneering neurosurgeon, and Sir Douglas Veale, the university registrar, were men of vision, drive and ability: together they directed Nuffield's benefaction into the establishment of a postgraduate medical school, which established chairs of medicine, surgery, obstetrics and gynaecology, orthopaedic surgery and, for the first time, anaesthesia. At the outbreak of the Second World War, the London teaching hospitals were evacuated. Buzzard invited the fifty Oxford students who had just completed their pre-clinical training and would normally have gone to London hospitals, to stay in Oxford, if they wished, for their clinical training.

A 1938 report of the registrar general on occupation mortality had drawn attention to the class basis of much illness. Using census returns, the report divided the population into five social and occupational classes and found startling discrepancies: infant mortality rates, and the death rates from many adult diseases, increased steadily with descending social scale, becoming approximately twice as high in the lowest as in the highest social class.[5]

If the structure of Oxford medicine was being changed by the war, so too was the city's sociology. In September 1939 a great army of children was evacuated from London and other metropolitan cities of Britain, to escape the anticipated bombing by the Luftwaffe. Oxford railway station was deluged with thousands of young Londoners seeking refuge with the local population. Their condition highlighted the inequality within British society and the social class differences in disease, inspiring Hugh Cairns to report his misgivings to Veale. "Evacuation has shown that the health of the people is not up to the standard that could be obtained in the present state of medical knowledge."[6]

However, Oxford's first attempt at financing an Institute of Social Medicine was unsuccessful, and the nature of the failure reflected the political realities of the day. Prior to the National Health Service, much of the nation's medical treatment was provided by charities and insurance companies. Part of the income of these institutions was set aside for medical research, and it was to this reserve fund that the Oxford hierarchy initially turned for help in setting up such an institute.

In April 1940 Veale wrote to his friend Hackford about a meeting he was due to have with representatives of the New Tabernacle Approved Society. "Could you advise me on a rather delicate matter? Buzzard and I want to see Duff, Canter, and Rockcliff before the meeting. Are they 'Reds' who would be shocked at being asked to an apolaustic capitalist abode like the Union Club or the United Universities, or would they feel at home there …?"[7] Hackford reassured Veale that a club lunch would have great appeal, but added, "You will appreciate that they will require rather careful handling and that it must not be too obvious that it is their money that you want."[8]

The university registrar was a very smooth operator. Not for nothing was the registry known as "Hotel de Veale" and there were even rumours of "Veales within Veales"[9] so his failure to secure funding from the Approved Society in 1940 probably had more to do with the financial uncertainties imposed on the insurance companies by the war than any shortcomings in persuasiveness. Nevertheless, as Britain was mobilising for total war, forces were coalescing around the demand that a healthy nation—a nation strong enough and vigorous enough to withstand the Nazi threat—must be a national goal.

In 1942 the Royal College of Physicians set up a committee to consider the need for a social as well as an individual approach to the origins of disease. This social medicine committee recommended that departments of social and preventive medicine should be established in every medical school and in July of that year the Nuffield Provincial Hospitals Trust announced that they would devote £10,000 (approximately for ten years) to the creation of a chair of social medicine at Oxford University: "It will be the first of its kind in England: and its purpose will be the prevention rather than the cure of disease."[10]

This uncharacteristically speedy reaction in Oxford was a result of Buzzard's campaigning zeal. He believed that social medicine had been unjustly neglected. "Only experience can direct the march of a progress which must in present conditions be pioneering work. The trail must be blazed. Upon the new institute at Oxford University will devolve the heavy responsibility and the high honour of blazing it. Maximum health is the national goal. Social medicine is the means of achieving this."[11]

As a consequence, in 1943 Dr John Ryle was appointed head of the new Institute of Social Medicine with the title of professor. Ryle, then 54 years of age, had had a distinguished career as a consultant physician at Guy's Hospital, where he had graduated in 1913. A brilliant diagnostician, he became the King's doctor, and established a successful Harley Street practice. His intellectual range and concern for social reform had marked him out for an academic post and it came as no surprise when, in 1935, he was appointed Regius Professor of Physic at Cambridge. More of a surprise was the fact that he never seemed to adjust to Cambridge life and, in 1939, on the outbreak of war, he returned to Guy's and three years later severed his connection with Cambridge entirely. The decision to take up the professorship at Oxford was probably due to the evangelising powers of Buzzard, and the fact that, unlike Cambridge, Oxford did have a clinical school, which might be fertilised with his ideas of the importance of what he described as social pathology.

With Ryle's arrival at the Institute in Museum Road a small staff was recruited, including WT Russell, an able statistician, and the young Alice Stewart, on a salary of £1,200. "I don't know why Ryle wanted me as his first assistant. I suspect he couldn't get anyone else. I had no statistics, no degree in mathematics—I had to sit down and learn statistics."[12] He chose the name social medicine because it "embodied the idea of medicine applied in the service of 'societas', or community of men, with a view to lowering the incidence of all preventable disease and raising the general level of human fitness."[13] The term epidemiology was rejected because at that time it was thought to involve only infectious diseases; also there was a department of epidemiology within the school of bacteriology at Oxford, with which Ryle did not want his project to be confused.

Alice was described as an exceptional "catch" for the Institute,[14] and in 1946 her status was elevated further by being made a fellow of the Royal College of Physicians, the first woman under forty ever to have received the honour.

Research, however, had not been the basis of Ryle's reputation. He had made useful observations on gastric and cardiac function in his early days at Guy's, inventing in their course a tube for the collection of gastric secretions which came to bear his name, but his reputation rested on his clinical skill, his clinical teaching and three books: *The Natural History of Disease*, published in 1936, *Fears May Be Liars* (1941) and a series of lectures emphasising the importance of environmental factors in the production of disease, subsequently published as *Changing Disciplines* in 1948. The Institute's research projects were consequently not well-planned or well-executed except for some of Stewart's work on the conditions conducive to the spread of tuberculosis. "Ryle was a lovely man, very nice, and good to work for, you knew where you stood. He accepted responsibility, but wasn't highly initiating, and [had] not too many research ideas."[15]

An understanding of Ryle's personal and professional influence on the Institute is essential, because the early years laid down the intellectual and scientific rails of ideas upon which social medicine at Oxford was to travel for the next few decades. Ryle was not universally revered within social medicine; some people viewed him as arrogant, and as being someone who did not appear to appreciate that medical and social sciences alone were unable to improve health and reduce social inequalities to the levels required.[16] Although he espoused epidemiological methods as essential to understanding the causes and distribution of disease, he failed to appreciate the development of epidemiological methods being pioneered by Major Greenwood, Richard Doll and Bradford Hill, or the methodological and conceptual contributions of Richard Titmuss and Jerry Morris. Yet these five were working on similar problems to Ryle in London between 1945 and 1950.

By 1948 Richard Doll in London and Alice Stewart in Oxford had their feet firmly planted in the embryonic subject of epidemiology. But it was Alice Stewart, standing in for John Ryle, who attended the historic meeting in 1947 at the Medical Research Council which decided to investigate the inexorable rise of lung cancer.

Stewart witnessed the moment:

> Ryle was ill and I went as his substitute. We went to hear Percy Stocks, and there were a lot of people at the meeting who thought the increase in lung cancer was caused by things other than smoking. But Stocks stuck to his guns and thought the most promising line of inquiry was smoking... I always thought that if Ryle had been well enough, that study would have come to Oxford. Because Ryle wanted it and Bradford Hill did not want it. After all the arguments had gone around the room, they hardly noticed me because I was an understudy. Mellanby, who was then head of the MRC, finally said to Bradford Hill: "Looks, Tony, as though we've got a job on our hands." He replied "Yes, we'll do it. I've got a young man, I'll put him on to it." And that was Doll. So everything hinges on that; of course he did the work, but he had it given to him on a plate. So he shouldn't be praised for having done it from the word go.[17]

This criticism of Doll by Stewart was not triggered by professional jealousy arising over the groundbreaking investigation. The beginnings of the dispute, which affected Alice all of her professional life, stemmed from the status of social medicine at Oxford in the post-Ryle years, as much as her dispute with Doll about the hazards of radiation.

In her tendentiously titled biography *The Woman Who Knew Too Much: Alice Stewart and The Secrets of Radiation*, the author, Gayle Greene, registers the startling contrast between the careers of Stewart and Doll as early as page seven: "There's a lifelong rivalry with the esteemed Sir Richard Doll... Lauded by the *New York Post* as 'one of Britain's foremost epidemiologists,' he remains to this day at the heart of cancer research in England. His is a career with a very different trajectory from Alice's."[18]

This was certainly true. The 1950s were a definitive decade for Doll. It marked the beginning of his collaboration with Bradford Hill, and a little later, with Michael Court-Brown, his pioneering epidemiological studies into the dangers of radiation. It was also the decade that witnessed Stewart's greatest contribution to medical research—recognition of the dangers to the foetus of diagnostic X-rays—an achievement made all the more remarkable because, after Ryle's death, Stewart was both personally and professionally ostracised by the Oxford medical establishment.

Alice Stewart had an indomitable fighting spirit, perhaps acquired from being one of the few women in what was very much a man's world. The shameful behaviour of the Cambridge medical students in the 1920s had had a profound effect on Stewart, and throughout her career the feeling of being discriminated against never left her. Oxford in the 1950s and 1960s changed Alice Stewart. It inspired her most substantial work, yet it made her more antagonistic, and it created a bitterness that was never forgotten or forgiven. When Richard Doll later came to Oxford as the Regius Professor of Medicine, Alice Stewart and her team knew that the status quo was about to change. However, that social medicine and Alice Stewart had survived at all in Oxford since 1950 was a testament to her courage and strength of character.

The value of the department had not impressed the clinical professors, and it would have been closed on Ryle's premature death, had not Douglas Veale, the university registrar, advised them that closure would be unwise during Lord Nuffield's lifetime. The academic department was down-graded and renamed the social medicine unit, with Alice Stewart in charge as reader, and given a minimum of financial support from the university. Ryle had been a disappointment to the Trust, and their support for the Institute of Social Medicine would end in 1953.

The tide had turned against social medicine, for although the medical faculty was expanding, the clinical and pre-clinical schools were vying with one another and Stewart's unit did not belong to either. "With Ryle's death, social medicine at Oxford fell on evil days."[19] Stewart in her redoubtable way put up a spirited defence of the Institute's achievements and did not see it as a failure[20]—its very existence inspired the establishment of other departments of social medicine throughout the country. However, this public affirmation could not conceal Stewart's sense of betrayal, and a feeling of humiliation at the change in status of social medicine in Oxford:

> But I chose to lie low. I had of course been excluded from all committees, which suited me fine. But perhaps I should have said, "Look here, you can't do this to the department, you must give it a professorship." ... As things developed they were able to ignore us... There was no money for research, so what was I to do? The terms of the job were that I was to do such teaching as the clinical professors required, but they required nothing. If I'd been that sort of person I'd have been able to sit with my feet on the mantelpiece until I retired. I think the university hoped I'd just go away.[21]

Stewart's agitation for professorial status continued for many years, but was implacably opposed by the university. KC Turpin, a university administrator, wrote on 28 September 1956: "The other question which was bothering her was that of status. Other people had departments, but she only had a unit and she felt she would like to have a department attached to her... The more I look at it the more uneasy I am about any proposal to make the social medicine unit a department."[22]

Liberated from the time-consuming duties of a teaching physician, Stewart rejected "the mantelpiece" and with her small, dedicated team turned to a problem that was causing alarm for the government and the British public: how dangerous was radiation?

Between 1931 and 1960 the number of deaths ascribed to childhood leukaemia had increased threefold—a rate of increase that had been exceeded among the major causes of death only by cancer of the lung and coronary thrombosis. Although most of the increase was due to improvements in the ability of doctors to recognise the disease (though not, at that time, to cure it), a search for avoidable causes was needed. With a grant of £1,000 from the Lady Tata Memorial Trust, Stewart designed a trial survey on the aetiology of leukaemia. She set out to get copies of the death certificates of all the children who had died of leukaemia and other malignant diseases, and designed a questionnaire to be submitted to the mothers. Beginning with approximately 500 leukaemia deaths, she matched them up with 500 deaths from other forms of cancer, and a random sample of 1,000 live children on the birth register, for the area in which the affected child had resided when he or she died. This gave her 1,000 case-control pairs, and became the foundation of the Oxford Survey of Childhood Cancer (OSCC), which was to become the largest case-control study of childhood cancer in the world, eventually encompassing over 20,000 deaths.

This first nationwide epidemiological study of childhood cancer became Stewart's greatest scientific work, and one that within just a few years substantially changed medical practice. The investigation required Stewart to visit personally all of the 203 medical officers of health in England—probably the only person ever to have done so. Through her legendary determination, Stewart persuaded the doctors to carry out interviews (using her questionnaire) on the mothers of both the dead children and the healthy children in their areas. For its scientific originality, intellectual invention, dedication, and organisation, the OSCC stands as a stunning achievement, and groundbreaking contribution—albeit at the time a controversial one—to cancer epidemiology.

When we came to tally up the findings, we made an astonishing discovery: both groups of dead children—those who had died of leukaemia and those who had died of solid tumours—had been X-rayed before birth twice as often as the live children... It was an astonishing difference. It was a shocker. They were as alike as two peas in a pod, the living and the dead; they were alike in all respects except on that score. And the dose was very small, very brief—a single diagnostic X-ray, a tiny fraction of the radiation exposure considered safe—and it wasn't repeated. It was enough to almost double the risk of an early cancer death.[23]

It was the first time the safety of diagnostic X-rays had been seriously questioned, and Stewart realised this result would have uncomfortable implications for medical practice, so she took the precaution of showing the findings to the Medical Research Council's secretary Sir Harold Himsworth:

I knew I was onto something important and I knew I was going to cause trouble... I knew Himsworth—I'd done a research project with him—and I knew Dr Joan Faulkner, who was working with him at the time, so I went round to their office... The MRC said they thought Bradford Hill ought to look at the thing, and I said "Yes, that's fine," and he took a look and asked me all sorts of questions about the research and didn't find anything wrong.[24]

When the Oxford team published their preliminary results in *The Lancet* in 1956,[25] it created shockwaves, and it was intended to. Although the study identified a very small effect—only about one in two thousand of the abdominal diagnostic X-rays caused cancer—any death brought about by medical intervention was unacceptable.

The initial reaction of the medical profession to such a novel and unexpected finding was one of suspicion, and soon suspicion turned to disbelief. Such an attitude was understandable; after all, doctors in the 1950s were revered and occupied a status in society that engendered a sense of superiority, even infallibility. There was also widespread criticism of the methodology used by Stewart's team, specifically the reliance of the research upon the mothers' memories. "The mistake [to their minds] of course was that we relied on mothers' statements. That was the big thing. You must never rely on a lay person's statement, went the rule."[26] As a scientific experiment, the results were based upon maternal interview responses only; the possibility of recall bias (mothers of dead children could well have clearer or different recall of events compared with mothers of healthy children) had to be seriously considered.

It was not totally surprising that Stewart was widely criticised but it was hurtful, and ultimately undeserved. Coming from a background of strong social conscience, with a resentment of prejudice and discrimination, she decided to continue the case-control survey, get definitive evidence and prove her doubters wrong.

The OSCC was not the only study of ionising radiation that Stewart was involved in. She was also seconded on to the historic study headed by Court-Brown and Doll on the link between therapeutic radiation and leukaemia. During the course of this original study, Court-Brown and Doll had more than one hundred people working on the investigation, visiting 81 radiotherapy centres, checking the records of over 13,000 patients. Stewart remembered one meeting:

> We were at a meeting where he and Court-Brown were telling us all the symptoms, and how we were to distinguish ankylosing spondylitis from other forms and we were told this because we were going to collect data; and I looked around the room and I thought "The people here have less than half my knowledge of medicine, why were they telling me?" And I thought "Why are we bothering? Why don't we just take all non-malignant conditions (treated by radiation)?" I put this point and was told to shut up. And that was the end of that.[27]

Privately, Doll believed the work contributed by Stewart to this collaborative study was the least well-presented,[28] lacking clarity and care—those qualities that epitomised Doll's own scientific approach.

If Doll and Stewart represented contrasting examples of the scientific mind, politically they formed a united front. Both scientists were founder members of the Society of Social Medicine, and in 1957 attended the inaugural meeting of the International Epidemiological Association (which was at first called the International Corresponding Club) in Holland. Two of the four women in the photograph of that meeting were Alice Stewart and her one-time student Joan Faulkner.

Undeterred by the accusations of recall bias that greeted her preliminary findings, Stewart added to the original series of case-control pairs. Within a three-year period the Oxford team had succeeded in tracing more than eighty per cent of all childhood cancer deaths that had occurred in England between 1953 and 1955. Even though starved of funding, the results, published in 1958,[29] represent an outstanding achievement by an unconventional and undeterred woman. Stewart "spent the next twenty years proving... that a single X-ray, a fraction of a permissible exposure, was enough to double the chance of an early cancer."[30] Again, the findings were not welcomed—doctors did not like being told they were killing patients, and as a consequence were disinclined to accept that the result was genuine and causal. This was at a time when there was a widespread belief that a threshold dose existed for radiation-induced cancer.

To test the validity of the OSCC findings, the MRC asked one of its epidemiological teams to undertake a study into the incidence of leukaemia among children known to have been exposed *in utero* to diagnostic X-ray. The prospective study of 39,000 children carried out by Court-Brown, Doll and Bradford Hill and published in the *British Medical Journal* in 1960, involved a far smaller number of cases of leukaemia than the OSCC and did not confirm the association found by Stewart, and led to a critical reappraisal of her case-control methodology.

> Among the children, nine were discovered to have died of leukaemia before the end of 1958. The expected number was estimated to have been 10.5. There is no evidence of any disproportionate occurrence of leukaemia among the children who had been most heavily irradiated nor among the children who had been irradiated early in intrauterine life. Published data on the leukaemogenic effect or irradiation *in utero*

are conflicting. It is concluded that the increase of leukaemia among children due to radiographic examination of their mother's abdomen during the relevant pregnancy is not established.[31]

Theirs was a cohort study of leukaemia among children exposed ante-natally to X-rays in hospitals in London and Edinburgh, and the findings did not support the association, whereas if the association was genuine, they should have done. Although the raised relative risk identified by the OSCC had largely been reproduced by other case-control studies, the failure of a prospective study—particularly one carried out by such eminent authors—to confirm the association had a significant impact upon the attitude of the radiological community towards the Oxford survey.

In the same edition of the *BMJ* another study carried out at Queen Charlotte's Hospital also failed to find an association between leukaemic deaths and X-rays.[32] What was even more damaging for the OSCC was an opinion-forming *BMJ* editorial favouring the methodological approach of the cohort study. "Retrospective surveys are suspect because they depend on past history, and human memory is fallible. Prospective surveys may suffer from the failure to identify some real consequences of the act inves-tigated; but in general more confidence is engendered by the prospective survey."[33]

The blow dealt to the Oxford survey's 1956 and 1958 reports by the prospective study report in 1960 angered Stewart, for as well as delaying the deserved recognition of the major contribution made by her to science, it also postponed, though by not very long, control of the risk of X-raying pregnant women. For Alice Stewart, Richard Doll increasingly symbolised the obstruction she believed to have undermined her epi-demiological work.

Stewart's failure to be accorded proper recognition within the scien-tific community ended in 1962 when Brian MacMahon carried out a study that vindicated her work. The study population consisted of 734,243 chil-dren born and discharged alive from any of 37 large maternity hospitals in and around the north-east of the United States in the years 1947-54. The frequency of intrauterine X-ray exposure in the population was determined by review of the medical records of all who developed cancer and of one per cent of those who did not. "It was estimated that cancer mortality was about 40 per cent higher in the X-rayed than in the un-X-rayed members of the study."[34]

Being based entirely upon medical records of exposure, the study not only confirmed Stewart's findings but finally settled the question of recall bias. Although it did not identify a doubling of the risk from abdominal X-ray as the Oxford team had in the 1950s, this might have been due to an improvement in the radiological machinery being used. The forty per cent increased risk of leukaemia found in the US was very similar to the levels being discovered by the OSCC in the 1960s in the UK.

The idea that such small doses—of the order of 10-20 mGy—could in fact cause cancer became generally accepted; eventually doses to the foetus were reduced and X-rays in pregnancy came to be avoided unless absolutely necessary. Over the next few years the weight of evidence swung in Stewart's favour and her conclusion was generally accepted in Britain and by most specialists abroad.

As a result, Richard Doll soon came to believe that the association first reported by Stewart was real, and represented a cause and effect relationship. Indeed, he subsequently became dissatisfied with the adequacy of the identification of the irradiated women, and when he tried to extend his 1960 prospective study some years later, he came to believe that his own results were unreliable.[35] Such a recantation was rare, but Stewart's Oxford survey remained ungarlanded by any significant prize. However, by 1967, in his definitive Rock Carling fellowship monograph* on the prevention of cancer, Doll cited Stewart and MacMahon's work as epidemi-

---

* "Direct evidence of the effect of the small doses received from these sources is available only for the cancers of childhood that follow irradiation *in utero*. This evidence ... suggests that perhaps seven per cent of all the main types of cancer in children under ten years of age have been due to this cause."

ological evidence of the carcinogenic effect of small doses of X-rays on the foetus *in utero*.

Although Stewart's findings were (from 1966 onwards) built into radiation protection standards, her unit was never awarded another MRC research grant. Yet, in 1961, with an infusion of £25,000 from the USA[36], the OSCC continued to catalogue the risk of childhood cancer from foetal irradiation. By this time the unit had moved to 8 Keble Road, an austere and sparsely-furnished neo-Gothic house. Strangely, the success of the Oxford Survey did not make Stewart a more accepted force within academic medicine; if anything, her marginalisation had increased. Donald Acheson, who was the chief medical officer throughout most of the 1980s, recalls the extent of cold-shouldering, and Alice's caustic reaction to him straying into her territory:

> I arrived [to work in Oxford] in the mid-60s, and Leslie Witts asked me to prepare five lectures on epidemiology, and Alice was furious and discharged her guns on me. But when I arrived in Oxford she had already isolated herself, and she wasn't lecturing, so I suppose that's what motivated Witts to ask me to give the lectures. Of course I knew about her work on leukaemia, but when I was in Oxford doing my pre-clinical I never came across her. But certainly, when I was approached to give the lectures it never occurred to me to ask her about it.[37]

By the late 1960s, Alice was becoming anonymous within her own subject. The treatment she had received at Cambridge in the 1920s may have been psychologically damaging, and it was clear that she was justified in feeling paranoid about the reaction of the scientific community to her work, based on her gender. The statistician John Bithell worked with Stewart on the Oxford Survey and recognised that the paranoia was to some extent understandable; but equally, that Stewart did not emanate tranquillity and harmony:

> It had to do with other aspects of her personality, the fact that she was quite good at antagonising people anyway. A certain sort of woman would have got away with it and won people's trust, but Alice was abra-

sive, and not really given to smoothing things over, and trying to get a meeting of minds. And she was rude to Doll in public, and vice versa—it was really quite embarrassing. I suppose my loyalties were more to her, but she was the less controlled one, let's put it like that. She would be more explicitly rude—but on the other hand, I think he had ways of opposing her which were quite effective and drove her to greater degrees of frustration.[38]

When in 1969 Richard Doll was appointed Regius Professor of Medicine at Oxford University, Alice was at first pleased. "I was glad when I heard about the appointment—I thought it would be a good thing. We'd never had a Regius Professor who was an epidemiologist, and a cancer epidemiologist at that. I thought he would give us a ground for flourishing. I couldn't have been more wrong."[39]

As the director of the Medical Research Council's statistical unit, Doll had been able to assemble a team of epidemiologists. With their arrival in Oxford, "the subject was given a fresh start."[40] In his paper, "The Rise of Epidemiology in Oxford", Doll had described the 19 years between the death of Ryle and his own appointment as "not a happy period for epidemiology in Oxford". He also wrote of Stewart's Oxford Survey that "This was important work that altered medical practice, but she was cold-shouldered personally and neither social medicine nor epidemiology was given any place in the clinical curriculum." Alice Stewart had been downgraded and shunned by the university for two decades.[41] When Doll arrived, he pressed for her to be allowed to give lectures each year; however, upon attending one, he found it "frankly so bad I didn't pursue it—by then she wasn't lecturing well."[42]

Peter Smith, who had joined Doll's research staff in London and followed him to Oxford in the early 1970s, saw at first hand some of the interchanges between the two scientists:

Richard had been on the other side of the fence from many of the proponents of large effects of radiation on cancer induction, people like Joseph Rotblat and Alice Stewart. Richard regarded these people as having extreme views. That was part of it, and there was obviously a big personality clash between Richard and Alice, which I was in the middle of in a sense, in that I was a witness to it on the sidelines. Our part of the department was in Keble Road, which was next door to the house Alice occupied, it had connecting doors—so I saw a lot of Alice and some of those interactions in seminars. It was muted, it was never openly aggressive, but you had to read between the lines to see the aggression. I never got to know Richard, it was always a very professional relationship; you always got the impression that you were talking to a brain.[43]

Alice Stewart had a reputation for taking on lame ducks, and in 1962 George Kneale joined her team while still a schoolboy. "Everyone knew he'd been a sort of problem child. He was exceptionally clever, but he could never make friends."[44] Kneale was by any standards an unusual character—a self-taught statistician, who was anti-social, painfully shy, and "very difficult to get along with."[45] Together Stewart and Kneale continued to work on the causes of childhood leukaemia, and by the end of the decade they were propagating a controversial theory about the dangers of low doses of radiation. In 1970 *The Lancet* published their paper in which—in combination with a particular set of estimates of foetal doses—they derived from the OSCC data an excess risk of childhood cancer per unit dose of radiation received by the foetus. It was quickly followed by a reply in *The Lancet* from Seymour Jablon and Hiroo Kato of the ABCC, who concluded that the risk coefficient derived by Stewart and Kneale was way out of line with the bomb survivors' data for those exposed ante-natally.[46]

This led Stewart to question the Japanese findings on the grounds that the experience of the survivors of the explosions was unrepresentative as only the fittest, who might have been less susceptible to the harmful effects of radiation, would have survived. Such a hypothesis might have accounted for a deficiency of effects seen in the first years after the explosions but is unlikely to have generated the dramatic long-term under-estimation that Stewart and Kneale postulated:

> We'd said that if you give one million children one rad of ionising radiation shortly before birth, you can expect in the next one to ten years to get about six hundred cancer deaths. But if we were right, the A-bomb

studies should have turned up 26 cases of childhood cancer—and they found one. Therefore, they said we'd exaggerated the risk by a factor of 26.[47]

The dispute helped shape Stewart's adversarial attitude towards the value of the bomb survivor data for radiation protection purposes. It also marked the beginning of a new field of research for Stewart and Kneale, and became one that saw them lionised by some, and condemned by others. In 1970 Doll was the most experienced and eminent epidemiologist in the field of radiological protection; believing the A-bomb data to be the most accurate indicator of the hazards of radiation, he rejected the Stewart and Kneale theory. Moreover, Alice Stewart was now occupying territory that Doll believed to be incompatible with that of a serious scientist: she was making a political campaign out of the work she was doing. Peter Smith knew Doll found this unacceptable:

> He came off the fence once he formally retired, but with smoking he stepped back from any advocacy role for anti-smoking, and his expressed view for that was: "If I become too obviously anti-smoking then people will question my science." Just as it did with Alice Stewart—she became so associated with anti-radiation, people became unsure as to where her politics stopped and where her science began.[48]

Building on the achievements of the Nuffield Benefaction, Doll set about strategically modernising Oxford medicine. A new chair of social medicine was to be established with money secured from the Nuffield Hospital Trust and at long last Stewart thought she might, approaching the end of her career, receive the professional recognition she and many others believed was truly deserved. "He could have arranged it— at least until I retired. It would have made a difference to my pension, but that was the least of it—there was my pride. It would have said, the only reason I hadn't had it before was because they'd been short of money."[49]

Malcolm Pike was another member of the MRC's statistical unit who had come to Oxford with Doll in 1969; he believed the Richard Doll of the

Oxford era was very different from his London persona.[50] Julian Peto, who joined the epidemiological unit in 1974, saw both the power Doll wielded and his achievements of that early period as staggering.

> When he came to Oxford he was knighted within two years, it went with the job—and to suddenly become Sir Richard Doll, the most powerful person in medical academia, was an extraordinary change. He had real power and he used it, and Alice Stewart was an early victim. She was the reader in social medicine, and it was odd that she wasn't given a chair really because she was quite eminent and was a real founding father of the science. But what happened was Richard created a new chair—social and preventive medicine and gave it to Martin Vessey—and that was a bit peculiar because Alice was only about two years from retirement. It just seemed so natural that she should have it—and it could have gone to someone else two years later. And at that time Martin had assisted Richard with various things, but he didn't have an outstanding reputation, and for him to be given that chair at 37 years old, over her, was the most extraordinary affront, and it really was a bit of power politics. He had crossed Alice off his list because she campaigned over radiation, and in his view exaggerated the risks—I think he was right about that one.[51]

Stewart left Oxford when she reached the mandatory retirement age in 1974, embittered by not having been made a professor—a title which, at the time, was awarded only very rarely except to the holders of established chairs. Richard Doll was the last in a long line of power brokers at Oxford who did not support Stewart in her wish to achieve professorial status; however, by then he believed that she was not a very good or careful scientist. "It was utterly impossible for me to give her a professorship. I tried to persuade John Pemberton to take the chair, but he was reluctant to leave Belfast, and I also approached George Knox, but I didn't push for Martin Vessey—he came in response to an advertisement for the professorship."[52]

Gerald Draper, who joined Stewart's team as a statistician in the 1960s, and owed his career in medical research to the existence of the

OSCC, attended Alice's farewell party. "Alice didn't have much of a sense of humour—she only made one joke during my period in Keble Road. At her retirement, during which Richard Doll gave a moderately gracious speech, Alice then responded, saying that she was preceded by John Ryle, and succeeded by Martin Vessey, and she made this lovely joke, which I'd never heard before: 'Here you have an example of someone who's fallen between two stools—or should I say, two chairs.' I always suspected that came from Molly Newhouse, the other outstanding woman epidemiologist at the time."[53]

In 1974 Stewart was welcomed as an honorary member of the department of social medicine at the University of Birmingham, where she continued to collect data to extend the OSCC. While visiting the United States to discuss the Oxford survey findings, Stewart and Kneale were invited by Professor Thomas F Mancuso to become consultants on a major investigation he was directing for the US government into the health of nuclear workers at Hanford, the weapons complex that had produced plutonium for the Manhattan project. Designed to parallel that of survivors of the Japanese A-bombs, this long-term study became known as the Hanford survey.

At that time it was the largest study of its kind into the long-term health effects of low-level radiation on workers in the nuclear industry. Since the industry was required by law to work within the exposure levels laid down by the International Commission on Radiological Protection (ICRP), the study was seen as a test of these standards. The Stewart-Kneale analysis revealed roughly ten times the cancer incidence predicted from the A-bomb survivor studies. This work became even more controversial than the Oxford Survey. Mancuso, Stewart and Kneale presented the results of their collaborative study in the November 1977 issue of *Health Physics*, results which they claimed showed that the risk of cancer produced by low-level occupational exposure to radiation had been substantially underestimated. The authors came under virulent attack and were severely criticised by distinguished epidemiologists and statisticians for using inappropriate methodology and making unsupported inferences. Over the years Stewart and Kneale tried to answer the scientific criticisms of the 1977 paper in later publications, though by then their work was viewed sceptically by epidemiologists, nuclear physicists and radiologists.

Stewart's passionate and uncompromising promotion of the connection between low-dose radiation and cancer was instrumental in propagating the idea, but brought her into confrontation with other scientists, a confrontation which was in keeping with her personality but which did not serve her science well. She became the representative of less orthodox scientists, and was glorified by non-scientific groups with a definitively anti-nuclear agenda. Ultimately, the controversy about her methods of analysis had to be seen in the context of the very small numbers of cancer cases amongst the Hanford workers.

In the forefront of the opposition to Stewart's alarming findings with regard to the health of the Hanford workforce was Doll who wrote:

> This proved to be the turning point in her career, for she relied on analysis of the findings by a young statistical colleague, George Kneale, who had had no epidemiological experience and who devised a method of analysis that produced grossly biased results. His method has been discredited by every medical statistician who has heard him explain it. In practice its use could lead to such absurd results as that, in some circumstances, there was a greater risk of cancer from background radiation alone than actually from all causes combined.[54]

Greene's biography is a hagiographical work. She is right, however, in advancing the belief that Stewart's early work did not receive the praise it undoubtedly deserved from the scientific community, but she fails to pay sufficient attention to Stewart's own role in this failure to achieve proper recognition. On page 228 of the book, for the first time she reveals part of the problem. An unnamed friend of Stewart is quoted as saying that the papers of Stewart and Kneale are

> convoluted and difficult to read to the point where other specialists in the field have simply not been willing to invest the time it would take to follow them. Alice never took the time to sit down and write a clear review paper of all of her work, to bother explaining why she and

George followed very different methods of analysis... And she has not been her own best friend.[55]

"Alice was her own worst enemy," according to Walter Holland, a former professor of social medicine.[56] On her own admission she was not a good writer, and George Kneale, though highly intelligent, was unclear in his style and isolationist by nature. Collectively they were incapable of becoming persuasive crusaders for their dissenting scientific credo while Doll was the quintessence of the scientific ideal. The two camps were on a methodological collision course. John Bithell, one of Alice Stewart's most celebrated collaborators, recognised the nature of the contradiction:

> There was an emotional response there too, but he genuinely believed that she wasn't a very good or careful scientist, I'm sure. And to be honest that's probably fair comment; Gerald Draper always used to say, "She wouldn't read properly, she didn't absorb the totality of things." She prefers that spark of fire that makes her think there's something different—however crazy—to working systematically through a paper making sure she's got all the facts in place. And how opposite to Richard Doll that is—you couldn't think of two people more opposite, nor can you think of two people that characterise aspects of the scientific mind that you need. I think we need Richards and we need Alices, and she did have that spark of insight and natural thinking, she did have ideas—of that there is no doubt.[57]

The schism between the two became greater after 1974, yet, regardless of what other people believed, their relationship was far from belligerent. As Doll wrote:

> Until the Hanford study we had perfectly good relations when she was in Oxford, but she was embittered when Martin Vessey was appointed a professor; there was nothing I could do about that. I liked Alice—Joan and I went see her, we were fond of her, and were not aware of any bad relations with her until really the last few years before her death. We visited her and Molly Newhouse—they were friends of ours.[58]

And from Stewart:

> Doll is very friendly, he wants to be friendly. He's good. He's a consci-
> entious man as well. But I don't think Joan is like that. I've always main-
> tained—my own little model, no evidence of any sort—that it was Joan
> who said to Doll: "You've got a serious rival in Alice, you'd better be
> careful." Otherwise he would have been prepared to be friendly with
> me—I think she put him off.[59]

Alice Stewart was prone to ideas, but this was not one of her most clearly
thought out.[60]

The early years of her association with Birmingham University marked
an extremely difficult time in Alice's life. In 1977 her only son Hughie,
who had suffered a "very troubling time during which he cut himself off
from everyone", overdosed on lithium, according to Greene,[61] aged forty.
Also within the world of serious science Stewart was increasingly treated
as a heretic, and the problem of a lack of funds for research that she had
faced since Ryle's death in 1950 reappeared. Yet, despite this, the quarter
of a century spent travelling between her home in Fawler in Oxfordshire
and Birmingham she saw as a golden period of her life. Initially her OSCC
records were kept in a caravan, but in time were given a home in a capa-
cious corridor. Their existence also meant that George Kneale—of whom
Alice felt emotionally and scientifically protective—could be given a job.

Though Doll made it quite clear that Stewart would not be welcome
to stay in Oxford after her retirement, ultimately she saw it as a serendip-
itous career move. "I don't bear him any ill will, and I often say it was the
best thing I ever did going to Birmingham. So I owe him something."[62]

Stewart was undoubtedly a creative and persuasive investigator who
had many good ideas and a flair for finding associations in complex sets of
data. But she often found it difficult to explain her ideas to other scientists, not least because they were typically fairly complicated. Her analy-

sis of the data on workers at Hanford and other US nuclear facilities had been criticised by other workers,[63] and there was a widely held belief in the scientific community that Stewart was swimming against the tide of reason. Not only was she campaigning over the work she was doing, which was anathema to Richard Doll, but he also questioned the truth of her suggestion—that if you worked in the nuclear industry you would die of cancer. He was not alone in this view. Not surprisingly, Stewart had been invited to give evidence to public inquiries by activists opposing the expansion of nuclear installations in Britain. On no occasion was her evidence accepted by the various inquiry inspectors. Was this because there was an establishment-inspired conspiracy to hide the truth about the health effects of low-level exposure to radiation, or because all of the many subsequent studies of Hanford and other nuclear workforces carried out by other researchers produce results that do not agree with Stewart's?

The first inquiry at which Alice Stewart and George Kneale appeared was the Windscale inquiry in 1977. The cross-examination was rigorous and tough. "There was a deliberate attempt to trip us up, very nasty indeed. They refused to allow George and me to testify together... they set out to make us look foolish, a very unpleasant business."[64] The inspector, Mr Justice Parker, devoted two pages of his report to Stewart's evidence, in which, inevitably, the Mancuso, Stewart and Kneale paper featured large. Parker stated that Stewart "failed to deal with a number of what appeared to me to be valid criticisms [of the paper]," giving three examples, and he found her interpretation of the analysis of the Hanford data "unconvincing".[65] In this he was in agreement with the bulk of the scientific community. He then went on to declare that her figures are "clearly wrong" and the answer she gave under cross-examination was "untenable".[66]

Alice Stewart worked in a period when medical research was very much an old boys' network, and it is true that after Ryle's death she did not have another male patron. Yet, what was also undeniable was that she had a prickly personality and was allergic to the decision-making process. Fiercely independent, she believed that people should automatically welcome her ideas; and when that response was not immediately forthcoming from her adversarial peers, belligerence was, as often as not, her first emotional response. Ironically, many of the harshest critics of Stewart's work have been women. They (Ethel Gilbert, Sarah Darby, Valerie Beral and Shirley Fry) were, however, relegated by her to the convenient category of "honorary men",[67] and their status as scientists thereby dismissed.

It was deeply unfortunate that Stewart did not share the trust of more conventional scientists. Those who disagreed with her publicly often evoked a level of animosity that made rational discourse impossible. It is simply not realistic to suppose that they were all prejudiced, unimaginative, or guilty of conforming to establishment thinking. Had she been able to discuss her ideas more openly, accepting the criticism that is an inevitable part of the scientific life, she might have been able to change thinking in key areas—especially the risk of obstetric irradiation and the ante-natal origin of childhood tumours—more effectively and sooner than she did.

Progressively she and her later work were subjected in Britain to professional isolation, but grants continued to come from America and elsewhere—whether it was cognitive dissonance or a true belief, as scientific recognition eluded her, the 1990s response was typically Alice Stewart. "Good people are seldom fully recognised during their lifetimes, and here, there are serious problems of corruption. One day it will be realised that my findings should have been acknowledged."[68]

Indisputably, Alice Stewart's standing in the world of science had diminished after the febrile disputes ignited by her Hanford Survey. One measure of her decline as a reliable interpreter of the radiological data was her absence from two high-profile court cases concerning British Nuclear Fuels Limited (BNFL) and radiation exposure due to operations at Sellafield. The Merlin case sought to prove under section 7 of the Nuclear Installations Act 1965 that BNFL would be liable if the radiation emanating from Sellafield had caused damage to the Merlin family's house.[69] Doll was called as an expert witness by BNFL, and seen as a formidable opponent. If Richard Doll was there as the representative of epidemiological research, why did not the Merlin's legal team use Stewart as a scientific counterweight to his assertion that the risk of living in the house was "negligible"?[70] Stephen Sedley (now Lord Justice) was the Merlins' barrister.

> In the Merlin case we took a conscious decision not to use Alice Stewart, simply because of the way in which the establishment had branded her an eccentric. She was not the only woman in science to have suffered this kind of thing. Rosalind Franklin was another, and I think science has a shocking old boy network, probably worse than the bar. Franklin had been written out of history. Stewart was rather differently treated—slightly nutty, loose cannon—because she wouldn't accept the conventional wisdom, and now I gather she has turned out to be more right than wrong.[71]

The second historic court case concerning Sellafield was heard in the High Court during 1992-93. The key issue in this case was the allegation that the occupational irradiation of the father before the conception of his child was the cause of leukaemia in the child. In her biography of Stewart, Gayle Greene finds incomprehensible the absence of Stewart from the plaintiffs' witnesses, but as Richard Wakeford, at the time a BNFL research scientist, pointed out:

> If she had bothered to check Stewart's publications she would have found a paper by Kneale and Stewart, based on analysis of OSCC data and published in the *British Journal of Cancer* in 1980, entitled "Preconception X-rays and childhood cancers". The last sentence of the abstract of this paper concludes, "There is no support for the idea that exposure of parental gonads to diagnostic X-rays is conducive to cancer in the next generation." This paper would hardly endear Stewart to the plaintiffs' lawyers given the nature of the claim![72]

John Bithell was not alone in believing that "the world would have been a poorer place without Alice Stewart."[73] She was a loyal and generous friend and a determined, ingenious, and creative, if not always careful, scientist, and she lived in a world that was male-dominated. The unique position Alice Stewart occupied within British medical science was celebrated in a Channel Four television documentary, *Sex and the Scientists: Our Brilliant Careers*, broadcast in 1996. For some reason the programme makers asked Sir Richard Doll to assess Stewart's scientific method, and his remarks were brutal and honest. "She was a bit slap-dash, but that's all I would say. She was very enthusiastic. She got a great deal of co-operation throughout the country, but she tended to accept results at face value without checking to test their accuracy." Of the Hanford survey he was entirely dismissive. "She used a technique which was not considered appropriate, and I think that analysis was a barmy analysis—yes, it just wasn't a scientific analysis." When Doll saw the pro-gramme, he was angry at how the film-makers had edited the piece and badly misrepresented his beliefs. "They used my remarks about her later work and used them to describe her earlier work, and I wrote a letter of complaint."[74]

Michael Dunnill, one of those involved in bringing Richard Doll to Oxford in 1969, had no doubt about the impact of the Doll interview on Alice Stewart. "He absolutely destroyed Alice Stewart on television. He said that her work was 'slapdash'. Doll can be ruthless. He destroyed her really."[75]

In a programme celebrating the contribution of notable women in science, Richard Doll's remarks seemed incongruous; however, even allowing for the editing mistakes, by the 1990s he had had an unbridgeable scientific disagreement with his one-time Oxford colleague. Upon seeing the programme for the first time, Alice Stewart was shocked. "I knew he didn't approve of me, but that he'd say this! It explains a lot—the cold shoulders, the lack of offers or invitations. I see that I haven't made it up."[76]

Doll was scrupulously honest, believing absolutely that Stewart's earlier work on childhood cancers was important and correct, but that her later work was unscientific and wrong. Tellingly, in the Channel Four doc-umentary, when he was asked about Stewart's analysis of the dangers of low-level radiation, he said without equivocation, "I would be prepared to say that she'll never be proved right." The weight of scientific evidence continues to move against the Stewart hypothesis.

By any standards Alice Stewart's work on the Oxford survey was a valuable contribution by a controversial and single-minded woman, without which the risk of X-raying pregnant women would not be as widely accepted as it is now. "That would stand as an adequate memorial for most of us."[77]

The 26 years of "retirement" at Birmingham University were personally fulfilling for Stewart, but the move marked a divide in how her work as a scientist was viewed. The enthusiasm and determination, ineluctable qualities of her scientific career while at Oxford, were still in evidence, but her isolation from discourse with other scientists led her to pursue research ideas viscerally, unfettered by a scientific detachment.

Richard Doll, in his *Dictionary of National Biography* entry for Alice Stewart, let his voice be heard:

> Subsequent investigations by experienced epidemiologists showed that the Hanford workers had suffered no detectable risk, but the claim that Stewart stuck to, that the low doses that the workers had received had caused substantial risks, made her the champion of the anti-nuclear movement and she was idolised by all who wanted to believe that even very low doses of radiation caused substantial hazard. Her reputation as a serious scientist, was, however, destroyed.[78]

As for the anatomy of a scientific dispute, Alice Stewart was right to say "Doll's is a much more powerful voice, mine is a whisper."[79]

Alice Stewart, who died in 2002, was fond of saying, "Truth is the daughter of time," claiming that her work, like that of other scientists seen as heretical in their own age, would only be fully appreciated in the future. Her earlier work in science was ultimately accepted and lauded; her later work may never be—for Stewart's supporters and detractors, the objective should be to avoid conflating the two.

Chapter 20

"An Investment in Happiness": Green College, Oxford

"Now of the difficulties bound up with the public in which we doctors work, I hesitate to speak in a mixed audience. Common sense in matters medical is rare, and is usually in inverse ratio to the degree of education."

William Osler

Doll's career in Oxford will be remembered for three enduring achievements: developing the Oxford medical school into the most prestigious in Britain, for his own scientific work, and for the founding of Green College. Green College is an architectural and academic success. However, by his own admission, the struggle and emotional pain experienced during the early stages of its development were almost without parallel.

The establishment of Green College on 1 September 1979 followed almost a decade of intense discussion, debate and planning around the need to establish a new graduate society to provide for the academic and social needs of the clinical medical students.[1] Its foundation was the latest of a series of developments that accompanied the recovery of Oxford medicine from its nadir in the middle of the nineteenth century.

By the early 1970s, Richard Doll was at the height of his powers. As the world's leading cancer epidemiologist, he had defined and expanded the subject and established the principles of what could be described as the "Doll philosophy".[2] His intellectual stamina, vision and leadership had designed a blueprint to bring the medical school into the new scientific age.[3] Such were his achievements that Michael Dunnill described him as "the greatest Regius Professor of Medicine of them all."[4]

Yet, it was his indispensable role in founding Green College, from conception to initiation to maturity, of which he was most proud. Of course, Joan had always been his greatest supporter allowing him the freedom to concentrate fully on science, but with Green College it was a

315

collaborative effort: they formed a united front. Uncharacteristically—as his reputation was that of a dispassionate scientist—Doll developed an emotional attachment to Green College. It became a symbol of his view of the better society, a physical representation of his love for Joan, and his genuine wish to improve the "academic and social needs of the clinical medical students". With time the college was a success occupying a dominant position in Oxford medical research. However, this was only achieved at great personal cost to the Dolls because the initial support among the medical students for a new Oxford college began to dissipate on the eve of its realisation.

The proposal to establish a new graduate college to provide for the academic and social needs of the clinical medical students may be regarded as the logical outcome of the decision, taken by the university shortly after the end of the Second World War, to offer a complete course of medical education leading to the degrees of bachelor of medicine and surgery. For the previous seventy years, the university had concentrated, so far as medicine was concerned, on becoming, in Sir Henry Acland's words "a place of the most perfect preparation that can be devised for the best clinical study in the completest manner elsewhere". By so doing, it had enabled its pre-clinical school to achieve its high international reputation.[5] The students, however, had to obtain their clinical teaching in large hospitals attached to other universities. That Oxford could change its policy after the war, and accept responsibility for clinical education, was due to three developments: first, the increased size and efficiency of Oxford hospitals, second, Lord Nuffield's benefaction, which had provided for the establishment of a small school for clinical research workers based on five professorial departments, and lastly the experience gained in teaching clinical students who had been evacuated from London in 1939. These culminated soon after in the establishment of a medical research institute in the old Radcliffe Observatory and a medical school with an annual intake of fifty students.

The idea of establishing a college that would have a special concern for clinical medicine arose from conversations in 1970 between Doll and the Nuffield professor of medicine, Paul Beeson, when plans were made for increasing the size of the medical school so that it could accept as many students as graduated from the pre-clinical school. It is doubtful, however, whether a new college would have been considered had it not been for two other factors: the need to provide fellowships for academic staff and college identities for the NHS consultants, alongside the availability of the old Radcliffe Observatory, which would no longer he needed for research laboratories when the second phase of the new John Radcliffe Hospital was completed.

Even in a city of Gothic wonder, the old Radcliffe Observatory is a stunning building described by Pevsner as "architecturally the finest observatory in Europe". The old Observatory was built at the request of Dr Thomas Hornsby, Savilian professor of astronomy, who was unable to find a room that could accommodate the large instruments that were becoming available in the second half of the eighteenth century. The Duke of Marlborough provided the land and the trustees of the Radcliffe the money. Building work was started in 1772 to a design of Henry Keene, surveyor to Westminster Abbey. However Keene died soon after, and in 1776 was succeeded by James Wyatt, the most celebrated and prolific architect of the time. Wyatt modified the design and modelled the second floor of the building on the "Tower of the Winds" in Athens. The building completed in 1794 rejected observatory precedents, and the use of Greek revival was new for both Wyatt and Oxford. Thus, a canted square tower projects from a two-storey base with one-storey wings attached. The sculptor John Bacon carved the low relief and delicate external decoration. The medallions over the windows at first-floor level depict signs of the zodiac, and each face of the tower has a frieze carved with reliefs of the named winds. Hercules and Atlas support the globe on the apex of the roof.

Early in the nineteenth century, the Radcliffe trustees took exception with the university, which they thought had appointed a professor of astronomy who was not a practical man, and they appointed an independent "observer" and kept the building in their own hands. One hundred years later it had ceased to be much use as an observatory and in 1930 Lord Nuffield bought the building and subsequently divided the estate between the university and the governors of the neighbouring Radcliffe Infirmary. The observatory itself, the Observer's House, and the three acres of garden went to the university on the understanding that the observatory would be used as laboratories for the Nuffield Institute for Medical Research, and it served this function until the Institute was re-housed in new buildings near the new hospital and designed specifically for research. Meanwhile, the Observer's House became the base for social activities for the clinical students and was known as Osler House.[6]

By the time Doll came to Oxford, it was a widely held belief among medical scientists and clinicians that they were disparaged within the university by the greatly more numerous arts faculties. In 1971, Trevor Aston, a historian at Corpus Christi College, felt that the marginalisation of medicine had become so pronounced within the university that only a new institution dedicated to the subject would liberate it from this growing sense of neglect.

Following a conversation with Doll, Dr JM Holt, then secretary of the sub-faculty of clinical medicine, placed on record in June 1971 the need to create a new college "which might be called Radcliffe College, (and) would be primarily but by no means entirely, devoted to medicine".[7] This was reaffirmed by Dr TDR Hockaday, chairman of the sub-faculty of clinical medicine, who suggested that the problem of entitlement would be substantially aided by the foundation of a new college based on the Radcliffe Observatory, Osler House and the adjacent buildings.[8] This would, it was hoped, provide not only some residential accommodation but a "college focus" for clinical students not resident in the college, as well as a source of attachment for postgraduate students primarily but not exclusively medical.

Doll, as the Regius Professor of Medicine, saw himself as the custodian of things medical within the university, and as the fortunate sequence of events began to unfold, he realised that this unique opportunity had to be seized if his wish of establishing a new Oxford college was to be achieved.

In 1971 a working party had reported on the development of the medical school.[9] An increase in the annual intake from 50 to 100 students was suggested. Consequent on this recommendation, which was endorsed by the university grants committee in 1972, it was agreed that the annual intake of clinical students should be increased to 100 in 1977-78 to coincide with the projected opening of the new John Radcliffe Hospital in Headington.

Another crucial factor which stimulated the renewed interest in a postgraduate medical college was that the site of the Radcliffe Observatory as a permanent base for medical students had become even more attractive when it became known that the Radcliffe Infirmary was likely, on economic grounds, to remain as a teaching hospital for the foreseeable future. Also, and again significantly, the university took the decision in 1974 to create a separate faculty of clinical medicine with the general board taking over direct control of the greater part of the Nuffield committee's funds, thereby bringing the administration of clinical medicine directly within the control of the central university bodies.

The Nuffield Committee for the Advancement of Medicine agreed to make a grant of £500 to meet the initial cost of a feasibility study of the Observatory site and a working party on the development of the Osler House site was instituted early in 1972. The grandiose plan for the new college had to be temporarily abandoned due to the economic climate which first discouraged the export of money from the United States and then made it extremely difficult to raise any in England.

Despite the initial failure, Doll was not defeated, merely delayed, in his attempt to attract the finance to ensure the college's independence. Ideally, he wanted to find a modern-day Lord Nuffield, a philanthropist, who possessed a vision of what the future needed, and with an unshakable ability to deliver it.

If money was still a central problem, the location for a new foundation was not, and nor was a rationale to end the discrimination that the clinical students were subjected to. As Doll's clinical lieutenant, Jim Holt was conscious of the injustice and sought to transform the standing of medicine within the university. His view was that "colleges looked upon clinical students as a 'bloody nuisance' that they could collect college fees from.

So, we were advised that we should start thinking about a new foundation, and with Derek Hockaday, we wrote a paper to the Nuffield committee advancing the argument for a separate foundation, we called it Radcliffe College, and it was accepted, there was enthusiasm for it."[10]

In Michaelmas term 1975, the clinical medicine board approved a paper from Richard Doll, the first part of which dealt with the academic and social needs of the clinical students, while the second set out in general terms the proposals to establish a graduate society based on Osler House and the Radcliffe Observatory.[11] The junior members would be mainly but not exclusively clinical students, the senior members would be largely, but again not entirely, drawn from the staff in the department of clinical medicine who were entitled to fellowships.

It appeared that the obstacles that had previously restricted the growth of medical science in Oxford were about to be removed in an elegant and egalitarian manner. The vice chancellor of Oxford University saw Doll's actions as visionary: "There was a crying need for a new college, in that there was the general problem concerning those who were university lecturers and not fellows, but there was the specific problem of doctors who worked in the Radcliffe Infirmary who weren't fellows. So it was a stroke of genius to establish a new college."[12]

Clearly the meticulous planning that was needed to establish the intellectual and physical foundations for the college captured Doll's imagination. As secretary of the medical school, Peter Garnham saw at firsthand the importance of the project to Doll "steering it first of all through the University, which was really very much his forte in diplomacy and charm. I think that Richard feels that Green College is his real big achievement in Oxford."[13]

Yet, as the plans for Green College began to move rapidly through the medieval structure of Oxford University governance, Doll's *modus operandi* and motivation were questioned by some powerful vested interests. In the autumn of 1975, the clinical medicine board approved a paper making the formal suggestion that a new college be established based on the Radcliffe Observatory and its associated buildings, which would have, as its primary concern, the welfare of clinical students and would include among its fellows a majority with clinical interests. It would, however, also include a proportion of students and fellows from other faculties, preferentially those whose work had some bearing on human welfare and the environment. The council of the university, without committing itself on the merits of the proposal, sought the opinion of the conference of colleges (a body on which each college had two representatives) noting only that the needs the proposed college sought to meet were real and that the proposed solution deserved serious consideration.[14] In the event, the conference was in favour of continuing to explore the possibility of establishing the proposed college, and council consequently set up a committee to prepare a detailed scheme.

Fundamental to the proposals for a new college were drastic changes in the whole organisation and the future status of the Osler House Club. It was therefore essential that from the earliest possible moment full and lengthy consultation with the students was undertaken. Accordingly, in April 1976, Doll and Holt consulted the students concerning the provision of accommodation and facilities that the students required.[15] Although the response rate was poor, the results suggested that approximately two-thirds of the students would join the new society. Doll subsequently attended a meeting of the Osler House Club on 26 April. This generated "much heated discussion", but the general opinion of the students attending was "very much in favour of setting up a college if possible".[16]

As the director of clinical studies, Jim Holt was one of Doll's closest emissaries:

> In the run up to all this Richard asked me to sound out opinion as to whether a new foundation would be popular, recognising that it would have to be based around the Tower of the Winds and Osler House. And my advice to Richard was: "Yes, lots of enthusiasm, lots of support from the students, from the recent graduates." As it turned out I gave him bad advice. Because what then happened, one or two people in the clinical school, and Bent Juel-Jensen was one of them, and although he's a great friend of mine, John Ledingham also, they set out quite a powerful movement, antagonistic to Richard and the

idea of a separate foundation, on the grounds that we didn't want a college dedicated to one subject—understandably as that was most un-Oxford."[17]

The students had expressed great concern at the shortage of social facilities in the John Radcliffe Hospital. This was limited to a small single room opening on to a recreational space common to all who worked in the hospital. The students were dissatisfied with this arrangement and sought premises for a social club on or near the John Radcliffe site in Headington. Their disquiet was no chimera. Although the centre of gravity of Oxford medicine was moving from its historic setting at the Radcliffe Infirmary to the new John Radcliffe Hospital in Headington, no analogue of Osler House, with its resplendent social facilities and camaraderie had been thought of, or planned. As Andrew Millar, one of the last alumni of the old celebrated institution, remembered: "Osler House which had been the centre of student activity was a fantastic place to interact with teachers, the people we were going to learn from and work with. And we all felt a great deal of affection for it. We all knew we were going up to the John Radcliffe—at which there were no facilities designated for students, no resources available for students to be up there."[18]

In November 1976, the conference of colleges supported the idea of a new college by the substantial majority of 22 to five. During Doll's speech he mentioned that one of the old buildings near the Observatory known as the "animal house" would be used as "student accommodation". This evoked such laughter that "I realised there wasn't a better way to end my case, so I decided to sit down and end the presentation there."[19]

On 20 January 1977, council promulgated a statue to establish a new college "primarily to meet the social needs of clinical students" and legislation was approved by Congregation on 22 February. But without adequate financial backing the project would again have been doomed. Given that the intention was to make the college financially viable from the outset and independent of university subsidy it was agreed that it would not seek support from the college contributions fund (as Linacre and St Cross colleges had done). By early 1977 the funds raised were already in excess of £250,000, including substantial contributions from the Rhodes trustees, Radcliffe trustees, the EP Abraham Cephalosporin Fund, BH Blackwell Ltd, and GD Searle and Co. All this indicated that sufficient funds were likely to be available to establish the society, but there was little doubt, as Richard Doll succinctly put it, that "any offer of a substantial contribution... would be of enormous value and possibly even decisive."[20]

It was with precisely this in mind that in April 1976 Doll had already contacted Paul Beeson, who was now based in Seattle. He hoped that Beeson might be able to reopen negotiations for raising funds in the United States with one or two of the contacts made in the earlier plans for a Radcliffe College, the original name for Green College. With deft philanthropic timing, Dr Cecil Green "an American Lord Nuffield",[21] director of Texas Instruments of Dallas, Texas, appeared on the scene when Beeson suggested to Doll that Green might be interested in helping the project. In response to Beeson's suggestion that Green might be a possible benefactor, Doll contacted Professor William Gibson of the University of British Columbia, who knew Green well and got him interested. Gibson had, as a Rhodes Scholar in the early 1930s, done a DPhil in neurophysiology in Oxford under Sir Charles Sherrington. Through a combination of intrigue, a love of learning and the beauty of the Observatory captured in an Ackerman print sent to Dallas, Cecil Green and his wife Ida became "at least sufficiently interested" to agree to make a visit to Oxford in April 1977.[22]

Doll thought Green "one of the most remarkable men of his generation in the United States".[23] Born in England in 1900, Green was taken by his parents to Canada at the age of two. After studying at the University of British Columbia he took a higher degree at Massachusetts Institute of Technology and applied his scientific skills to exploring for oil. These led to his becoming president of Geophysical Services Incorporated and, owing to a change of direction during the war, he made a fortune as one of the five founders of Texas Instruments. Possessing riches beyond avarice, the childless Cecil and Ida Green had financed professorships and new academic departments in twenty universities across North America, but never before in Britain; the possibility of financing a new Oxford college was an alluring one.

With the invitation already extended, at Richard Doll's request, Bill Gibson was "glad to ask Cecil for a million pounds in order to get the derelict Radcliffe Observatory building back into use for medical science."[24] The Greens' possible benefaction was advantageous to Doll for two reasons: firstly, it was better to have one large contribution than a lot of small ones, and secondly, he was distant from the university and difficult for others to influence.

The visit in April 1977 was highly significant in the history of Green College and was meticulously planned in every detail by Richard and Joan Doll[25]. The factors that transformed an idea into a happy reality were, according to William Gibson, the enthusiasm of the Greens, the friendliness of the Dolls and the excellent group of fellows, students and staff attracted to the college[26]. If Richard and Joan exuded devotion and love, Cecil and Ida were as close as a pair of shoes, so it was a meeting of minds, a shared vision.

However, the timing of the visit was not propitious[27] as the workers at the Randolph Hotel were on strike* and picketing the entrance to the hotel. Accommodation for the Greens was consequently arranged at Weston Manor Hotel, Weston-on-the-Green, a small hotel based on a historic building with classical four-poster beds in its main bedrooms, and the vice-chancellor lent his car and chauffeur for the use of the Greens during their visit. After three days, during which they had been wined and dined in various colleges, explored the Bodleian and seen the plans for the development of the college, they offered a benefaction of a million pounds to enable the plans to be achieved. To some who met the Greens, Ida gave the impression of "being the power behind the throne"[28]; however, Jack Lankaster, the university surveyor and the pro-

---

* The clinical students who opposed the new college accused Green of being anti-trade unionist and of oppressing his workers. Doll thought that Green may well have been anti-trade unionist but that he looked after his workers well.

posed college's architect, recognised that both Doll and Green shared a single mindedness:

> Originally I thought of a modern type building, a statement, but architectural tastes were changing at that time, and people were prepared to accept, and even like, buildings and traditions in the same style as the originals. Green also had very pronounced ideas about what he wanted. He wanted a stone building, brick was out. His idea was to build something solid that looked like one of the older buildings in Oxford. With the magnificent Tower of the Winds already there, he could see what the college was going to look like. So the choice of style was already made—the building I built was very much in the Wyatt style.[29]

The vice-chancellor, Rex Richards, who had already volunteered the use of his limousine to the Greens and whose job was to be "nice" to them during their visit, described how his position gave him a unique insight into the power of money:

> I can clearly remember the final decision was taken and the college was going ahead, we had a big meeting in my office. Cecil said: "OK, the money's in the bag, vice chancellor, provided you can let the contract by 1 January." Now, this would have been impossible, because of planning permission, and some of the building wouldn't have been vacated by then; when I told him this, he replied: "Well, vice chancellor, I've got lots of other people interested in my money; if you can let the contract by 1st it's OK, if you can't that's just too bad."[30]

This stipulation was impossible to achieve, but what could be done was to let contracts for the work to be done in three stages, by 31 December 1977, 1978 and 1979. This the Greens accepted and they signed the formal contract with the university to help in the creation of a new graduate college on August 22. This happy conclusion was a testimony not only to the Greens' generosity but also to Doll's tenacity, foresight and enthusiasm.[31]

Personally and professionally Cecil and Ida Green were enchanted by the Dolls. Doll had assembled an army of the great and the good to flatter them; he had advanced a compelling case for the new college—his persistence and charm were mesmerising. Yet, even he must have been surprised at how the Greens assessed their three days in Oxford and what they found most memorable. "The warden [Doll] reported that Dr Cecil and Ida Green had been extremely happy with the visit and had indeed referred to dinner with the fellows as the most moving occasion since their wedding."[32]

When Doll was planning the college, he looked around for lodgings for the college's warden, which ideally would be capable of being connected with the site. There were about half a dozen houses that met the conditions: a few houses on the Woodstock Road that belonged to St John's College and 1A Observatory Street, the only large house on the street that had been built at the beginning of the twentieth century. Number 1A, Doll discovered, was owned by the diocese and was let to one of the non-residential canons of Christ Church. He then called on the bishop to see if the church was willing to sell the property, but the answer was an unequivocal "no". But after the Greens' visit, he once again approached the Church authorities. On this occasion he was told that the house was to be sold for £40,000, but had not yet been placed on the books of an agent. Without trying to beat the price down Doll immediately bought it. Within a short time he moved the medical administrative offices into it, and the site was now ready for the building work to begin. What a piece of luck.[33]

The whole project forged ahead with remarkable speed helped greatly by David Piper, director of the Ashmolean Museum. Piper was most interested in the fate of the Observatory and quickly arranged for a site visit of a sub-committee of the Fine Arts Commission of which he was a member. The commission's enthusiastic support of the plans to clean and refurbish the Observatory and make it the architectural centrepiece of the college greatly assisted the quick approval of the officials and committee of the city council. Already, the strict building timetable that Green had insisted upon was expediting the planning process.

The Hebdomadal Council, the chief executive body of Oxford University, agreed in principle at an early stage that Green's generosity should be recognised by naming the new college after him. Accordingly, a statute to this effect was promulgated on 1 November 1977, and enacted a fortnight later on 15 November. By this time it had been unanimously agreed that Doll be appointed first warden of the college from 1 October 1979 (following his resignation as Regius Professor of Medicine) until 30 September 1983.[34] The appointment of the first 22 fellows was finalised in October 1977 and their initial meeting as a governing body elect was held a few weeks later on 8 December. Until the college opening in September 1979, governing body meetings were held in the board room of the Radcliffe Infirmary. Following the meetings, the fellows were guests of St Antony's, and dined in one of that college's private dining rooms.

The Greens' benefaction was sufficient for the physical construction of the college, the construction of the entrance and the buildings around what came to be known as Lankaster Quad, after the project's architect, the internal reconditioning of the Observatory and the associated Observer's House for their new purposes. It also covered the replacement of the "animal house", where university staff at the Radcliffe Infirmary had been able to conduct laboratory experiments, by residential accommodation for thirty students. It did not, however, leave anything over for an endowment that would help to fund the activities of the college.

An appeal for that purpose was consequently organised by Irwin Herrmann, an assistant registrar at the university's headquarters, who had been appointed secretary of the college's provisional governing body and one of its provisional fellows. His campaign was brilliantly conducted and succeeded in raising more than £500,000.[35] It appeared that Oxford University's new approach to medical education was seamlessly under way.

Not everything, however, had proceeded as planned; the attitude of the clinical students had changed radically. Personal ambition, misplaced altruism, vengeful antagonism and sheer bloody-mindedness coalesced into a formidable opposition to the success of Green College. For the students the biggest anomaly was that while the college and its facilities were down at the Radcliffe Infirmary, many of the students would be at the new John Radcliffe Hospital "where the provisions for them are going to be dreadfully inadequate."[36]

According to one student, Andy Millar, "We saw Green College come along and this money being spent down at the place where we were about to leave. The simplicity of the inappropriateness was terribly apparent to almost everybody, and while I am quite loud-mouthed and opinionated I don't think there was anybody amongst the students who thought that Green College was a good thing."[37] Millar together with other medical students had deferential discussions with Richard Doll at Norham Gardens. "We formed a committee and voiced our concerns, it was all very civil and we wore jackets and ties and were very polite. We thought that Green had nothing whatsoever to do with Oxford—the idea of a uni-disciplinary college was nothing to do with the ethos of Oxford. But Doll was very experienced and a master negotiator, but we told him we thought it was wrong."[38]

The students complained bitterly about the "inadequate" nature of the previous consultations and the "indecent haste" with which the plans had been "bulldozed through". They were resigned to the uncomfortable reality that "Green College is now a *fait accompli*"[39]—and lamented the dearth of practical public information on the subject. They claimed that it was essential to ensure that Green College was able "to do as little damage as possible to the character of clinical training" in Oxford. Most significantly, they feared that the relationship between doctors and students was threatened and that the college would recreate a division which Osler House had abolished.

In September 1977 Osler House Club was flourishing. It was an oasis in the Radcliffe Infirmary; it was exciting and vibrant. History emanated from it and this is what made it so addictive to Alastair Buchan:

> You could rub shoulders with George Pickering, Richard Doll, David Weatherall, and Peter Morris—there was a sense that things were changing in the RI, but to be there and walk the corridors with the ghosts of Cairns and Osler was what it was all about. During my first

year we loved the place, we lived there; without making it too nostalgic, it was a very nice arrangement, and there were of course only about 60 of us in a year.[40]

On 30 January 1978, Richard Doll wrote to Julius Weinberg, the president of Osler House: "We were very distressed by your statement that the plans have been presented to us as a *fait accompli* with little attention paid to student opinion, as we do not think this is true." Like all great scientists Doll looked at the evidence, and the findings of the earlier dialogue he and Jim Holt had with the students. In the third paragraph of the letter he wrote: "The principles were described in a memorandum that was sent to all Osler House Club members in April 1976 and were elaborated at an open meeting of the club on 22 April 1976 which I attended; I enclose a copy of the memorandum, which was accompanied by a questionnaire to which 54 students replied. Of these, 38 (70 per cent) said they would join or migrate to the new society."

On 16 March 1978, a memorandum to the university committee on Green College came from the Osler House Club:

> The student body feels that there has been inadequate consultation during the planning of the new college. Furthermore the consultation that did occur was interpreted in an over-enthusiastic manner. A poorly worded questionnaire, responded to by less than 35 per cent of the students, and a meeting of only 30 of the 160 students were accepted as showing student support for the college. We believe that a greater effort should have been made to determine student opinion about a matter which will have such great effects upon them.

The clinical students felt that they were "taken for granted"[41] and certainly it was not an easy time for them. As the building progressed, they found themselves being turned out of Osler House into the less comfortable accommodation in the old medical school hut. The temporary metamorphosis of the "luxury"[42] of Osler House into the misery of the "Osler Hut"[43] proved too much for many within the hierarchy of Oxford medicine. The college and Doll faced determined opposition. George

Pickering, Doll's predecessor as Regius Professor, took the side of the students as did John Ledingham, the director of studies: "I can remember him once saying about our fight to preserve Osler House Club. 'Thank God for our medical students'."[44]

But within the medical establishment there was one totemic figure openly antipathetic toward Richard Doll: the university's medical officer, Bent Juel-Jensen. As the students' doctor he was enormously influential in setting them against the college. He referred to the new institution as the "Kremlin on the Woodstock Road"[45] and was known to be "stirring"[46] behind the scenes. The medical historian Dr Trevor Hughes believed Juel-Jensen's preternatural dislike of Doll was easily explained: "Doll was kind to Juel-Jensen, that's why he disliked him so much. When Richard arrived as Regius in 1969, he supported George Pickering's wish to make Juel-Jensen a consultant."[47]

Oxford University had been extremely generous to Richard Doll and the new college by giving them the Old Observatory and a three-and-a-half-acre site, although this would later lead to accusations that Cecil Green had bought "immortality on the cheap"; in 1978 the tension centred on the issue of transference of power.

The governing body elect of Green College set up a committee for consultation with the students. It was clear that this committee (subsequently known as the warden's committee) had an important function to perform. The committee agreed that it was important to maintain the name and traditions of the Osler House Club, and that it should continue to be run in exactly the same way as it had been in the past, subject to the changes necessitated by the limited space and the fact that the college would be financially responsible for maintaining the premises.

The students, however, remained unhappy about these proposals and "unconvinced" that the college was the "best way to improve medicine, or medical education in Oxford".[48] In March 1978, the Osler House Club committee submitted a memorandum to the university's committee on Green College which included the suggestion that "The status of Osler House Club be protected, such that the club maintains control over those facilities it currently controls. The relationship of Osler House Club to

Green College should be the same as its current relationship to the clinical medicine board."

Richard Doll liked to get his own way. In April, at a meeting of the general committee, he tabled a paper on the relationship of Osler House and Green College. In this consultative document it was stated unequivocally that "Osler House Club shall be a club of Green College". The battle lines were being drawn because the new Osler House Club committee was adamant that their club should continue to be "independent" providing for the needs of the clinical students and preferably sited near to the John Radcliffe Hospital where most of the students would be based in the near future. The objection was not to the establishment of Green College as such, but that its position was comparable with the other colleges in central Oxford, unless it was able to provide satellite facilities in Headington.

This clearly posed considerable problems. The university had agreed by statute to transfer Osler House from the management of the medical school offices to Green College on the understanding that the college would assume responsibility for the continued and expanding academic, social and sporting needs of the medical school. The students, however, were implacably opposed to having what they believed was their club "appropriated" against their wishes. Moreover, after reading through the small print of university regulations, it was found that Osler House Club was an independent club of the university, and its destiny was determined by the wishes of its members. United under the leadership of a new president, the sixty medical students spoke with one voice and it became their "raison d'être to say 'no' we're not going to join Green College."[49]

The divide between the students and their supporters and Doll was, by the autumn of 1978, becoming a threat to the financial wellbeing of Green College. Alastair Buchan, ("an awkward and eloquent bastard, I knew he'd go far"[50]), the students' new president, began to seek a solution to what he saw as the most urgent problem: "We were going to move to the John Radcliffe, and the actual relocation of the medical school had been thought through academically with respect to lectures and libraries, but nobody talked about the social side of it."[51] Buchan sought to reposition the medical students so that they could have some sort of fraternity that could exist in a collegiate way outside of the college in Oxford.

From his position in the Observer's House, Buchan with his colleague Jim Heffer as 'scribe' charted a manifesto to replace their lost club with a replacement at the John Radcliffe. With David Weatherall's help, Lady McCarthy, the chairman of the area health authority, thought she might be able to make some accommodation available. Buchan then went back to his mentors and was put in touch with Sir Edgar Williams, head of the Rhodes House Trust, who offered financial support. Buchan was elated and was now exercising real political power within the medical school. "But Doll was not in the picture at all, he was un-knowing, and not involved and I'd basically pulled off a piece of real estate, not a mortgage, but a down payment to make it happen, and the agreement of the medical school to do it, and all the Nuffield professors lined up behind me 'putting my head on the block'."[52]

To diminish the flow of potential Green College graduates, the disaffected clinical students sent a delegation to Cambridge to try and dissuade them from coming to Oxford. (Historically a large proportion of the Oxford medical students had taken their first degree at Cambridge University.) Letters were also circulated accusing Texas Instruments of being a "warmongering company" the ethos of which was antipathetic to the values of medical care.

Michael Kettlewell, a founding fellow of Green College and a senior member of a medical team with Alastair Buchan, was a sane narrator of the unfolding drama:

> Richard Doll was hurt by the student unrest. The students and Buchan came from the misconception that Richard, through the university, was taking away their domestic facilities. They would not see the bigger picture: that the government was moving up to the JR, the centre of gravity was changing, the medical school was enlarging, it was a different animal and the university did not want to look after a bunch of students. [The university] wanted to get rid of Osler House, it was nothing to do with Richard Doll, but Richard had the parallel vision to go with

that because the site was being vacated. Architecturally it was there and wonderful, and there was an opportunity that could be lost. So, although he had this tremendous vision, somehow, because of his method of working, he never got the students on side.[53]

Richard Doll was genuinely fond of students[54] and had dedicated himself for almost a decade to advancing their cause within the university. However, there was a sense of trenches being dug, a divide between "us and them".[55] Under the onslaught, Doll needed to give a transfusion of reassurance.

Buchan was being advised on tactics by the distinguished lawyer Lord Goodman, his Master at University College, and believed that he had a mandate to carry out the wishes of the medical students:

> There was a stand-off, whereupon the vice chancellor, Rex Richards, called me in and said that "The Proctors have been very helpful, and I was absolutely correct, but they were about to get a million pounds from Green, and the university would take a very dim view if I somehow disrupted that process." I can remember being in his office looking up at two Canalettos and thinking "I'm out of my depth."[56]

It was to this rather undesirable state of affairs that Richard Doll returned in late November from a term's sabbatical leave in Australia. The position had, however, been transformed in one important respect. Lady McCarthy made it clear that the area health authority would be prepared to allow a building on the Manor House site known as the Dower House to be made available for a social annex, but that the authority could not provide any capital or recurrent funds towards its use for social facilities.

The governing body elect agreed to buy the Dower House for the use of the students. "Ultimately, Green College bought it outright and they were very generous."[57] A variety of options was then available. With the greater amount of space for student facilities, it would be possible to provide separate premises for the use of Osler House Club, which could then remain an independent university club linked (or not) to the college as it thought best. For its part, the governing body elect still hoped to see the club form a close relationship with the college, as it could then more effectively take responsibility for the welfare of the clinical students and develop facilities for them as funds allowed.

The clinical students discussed the various possibilities at an extraordinary general meeting of the club on 25 January 1979. The members resolved by 126 to nil that Osler House Club should remain an independent university club and that the club should seek to rehouse itself in new premises as close as possible to the John Radcliffe Hospital. A third solution "that the club representative should negotiate a relationship with Green College" was carried by 125 votes to two. The general principles of such a relationship were that the Dower House should be owned by the college and provide for the use of Osler House Club, that all the members of the club should have access to certain recreational facilities at the Observatory site, and that all members of the college should be members of the club, junior members being full members, and senior members associates.[58]

The relationship between the clinical students and Green College was therefore by no means as straightforward as had been anticipated in the early plans for establishing a college. The feelings of the students were clear. They wished to be allowed to join the college of their choice as in the past, yet to ensure that those who did not elect to join Green College were not discriminated against in the provision of social activities.

Given the alternative of joining Green College or remaining with the older traditional colleges, most opted for the latter. Each clinical student had the choice of joining Green College or staying with their own college while becoming an associate member of Green, or of not joining the new college at all. By the beginning of 1980, four months after the college had accepted its first students, only eleven of the 204 clinical students had become full members, one had become an associate member and the remainder had no direct association with the college.[59]

The poor response of the clinical students to forming an association with the college when it opened its doors on 1 September 1979 was "a bitter blow".[60] In many respects, according to Doll, "what saved the college in its early days" was the suggestion made by Professor AH Halsey, director of the department of social and administrative studies, that it would be a good idea to promote the cohesion between clinical studies and the applied social sciences, thereby enhancing the complementary nature of the two fields.

It could not be denied that there was an element of expediency about the need for Doll to attract students since the vast majority of the clinical students had voted to excommunicate themselves from Green College. Doll, nonetheless, philosophically wanted to make a commitment to the other caring professions who were not medically trained.

As Halsey saw it:

> I can remember when I first met him he called to see me soon after he was elected to the post of Regius. He wanted quite clearly to establish more of a link between medicine and social studies—I distinctly remember him turning up, but I was a bit surprised to find the Regius Professor of Medicine turning up here—but he was a brilliant and concerned social man, wasn't he? Then later he started talking to me about Green College, and he wanted very much to get rid of the monopoly that medicine had over it and to extend it into a set of people who were, as he put it then, "the environment".[61]

Doll was a long-termist. He recognised that once the belligerent generation of clinical students had moved on, he, as warden, would lead Green College into a period of steady growth. The College opened in September 1979 with 30 fellows and 27 students, all unsure about college life.

Richard and Joan Doll's leadership was crucial to the institution's stability. Joan was intimately linked to the Green College experiment and woven into the fabric of the institution. When the immense task of converting the Observatory began, Joan undertook the planning, furnishing and decoration, in conjunction with Jack Lankester, the architect. Joan working with a very limited budget immediately threw herself into the challenge of decorating and furnishing the new college. She had the drive, artistic talent and motivation to bring the finishing touches to the magnificent project. As Dr EWL "Watty" Fletcher, the radiologist, wrote:

> At first she looked in furniture shops but she rapidly decided that factory visits were the only way to get good quality, good-looking furniture, carpets and curtains at budget costs. In the dining room the carpet, tables, chairs, cutlery, glass, china were all chosen by Joan. Even the decoration was chosen by her and she even went to the trouble of varying the decorations in students' rooms so that they were individual.[62]

Joan was a very forceful woman and the relationship between her and Lankester was not always a tranquil meeting of minds:

> She was a very difficult person, I'll tell you that. I sometimes wondered how the hell [Doll] put up with her... She was a very powerful personality and she wanted to be involved. I admired him because, although she seemed more aggressive than he was, it didn't seem to upset him, in the sense that it didn't seem to deter him. But she was a very difficult person, she didn't have an official role in the matter, she was just there and made suggestions, particularly when we got to the finishing stages and the question of furnishings, and she thought she knew best.[63]

The Dolls' dedication to the college in the early years was total. Every evening Doll could be found in the college bar, silver tankard in hand, talking to students and fellows with equanimity. Indeed, in the beginning, Joan and Richard would study pictures of the students over breakfast, memorising names.

The college was officially opened on 13 June 1981 by the then chancellor, Sir Harold Macmillan. It was a memorable occasion on a hot summer afternoon. Macmillan arrived and mounted the platform slowly and unsteadily. With his drooping eyelids and arched eyebrows he resembled an old, lost bloodhound. He peered at his watch. Did he know where he was? Did he know what he was doing? In fact, "He worked the audience like a comic,"[64] said Doll, while, according to the vice-chancellor Rex Richards, "Macmillan's speech was a really sentimental piece which all the Americans loved—it had an electrifying effect."[65] With beguiling aristocratic ease Macmillan portrayed Green College's benefactor as a great figure in the history of Oxford University, and succeeded in endowing the Greens with a sense of destiny. When Green addressed the crowd in the Lankester Quad, his opening sentence captured the moment: "My presence here today, and the involvement that my wife Ida and I have had in Green College, can best be described as 'an investment in happiness'."[66]

By the summer of 1981, the college had seen a slow but steady growth from its small beginnings. It had shown that it was capable of providing a focus for clinical medicine in Oxford and a base for visiting scholars in this and related fields. Moreover, it served the interests of clinical medicine in Oxford on a broader basis by setting an example for other colleges, rather than by attempting to consolidate the subject within the confines of a single college. The change of direction that resulted from the complex negotiations with the clinical students eventually resulted in a solution which was seen as "a happy symbiosis".

Far from being "a Black Hole on the Woodstock Road", Green College had helped make Oxford one of the most desirable centres in the country at which to study medicine. Yet within Oxford medicine there continued to be bitterness towards the college, and Richard Doll's role in creating it. John Ledingham, for example, was one of the pillars of Oxford medicine who took the students' side against Doll. "For the first five years of its life, Green College was commonly known as 'The University of the Doll's House'. I hope he doesn't hold it against me. Doll of course was a great warden, and Green College has succeeded, it's a great tribute to him."[67]

Richard Doll had an irrepressible belief in Green College and through his leadership and force of will the college became established. For the Christmas edition of the *British Medical Journal*, Doll wrote an article entitled "Green College, Oxford: its contribution to clinical medicine". The cover carried an illustration of the Tower of the Winds. For David Millard, one of the college's founding fellows, it was a defining moment. "We knew then, as far as the medical profession nationally was concerned, we were home and dry."[68]

When Doll retired as warden in 1983, he had made Green College into an architectural and academic success, and the status of medicine had been re-established in the forefront of academic life. At a dinner to celebrate his custodianship of the college, Cecil Green announced a scholarship worth over half a million pounds in recognition of Joan and Richard Doll's achievement. At the beginning of the twenty-first century Doll was still a dominant presence in the life of Green College. Other wardens followed him, but no one was under any illusion: it was *his* college.

In 2005 Doll could not help but be amused at one of those classic coincidences that occasionally happen at Oxford University. Dr Alastair Buchan, the student campaigner, was elected to the chair in gerontology at Oxford University. The professorship had a college attachment and Buchan had changed along with the times: "All's well that ends well, and Green College is obviously very successful—I look forward to taking up the chair. But I'm conscious of what David Weatherall called the Homeric irony of it."[69]

Chapter 21
Expanding the Frontiers of
Epidemiology

"My personal desire was to press forward with a giant project similar to
that under which the atomic bomb had been developed in World War
II, or the man placed on the moon in the NASA project, to funnel
money into a massive effort to find a cure for cancer and also be uncovering the cause at the same time."

Senator Ralph Yarborough

The modern war against cancer began in the United States in 1970 with
the publication of the Yarborough report, which advanced a set of recommendations and a strategy for the "means and measures necessary to
facilitate success in the treatment, cure and elimination of cancer—at the
earliest possible date."[1] President Richard Nixon signed the National
Cancer Act into law on 23 December 1971 with a propitious wish: "I hope
in the years ahead we will look back on this action today as the most significant action taken during my administration."

The prescribed ideals of Nixon's war on cancer angered Sir Richard
Doll. How can you make a plan if you do not know the nature of the
human cell or the nature of cancer? In 1970, Sir Harold Himsworth had
published a book on the theory of scientific knowledge[2] in which he
observed how scientists add to it and make it grow. He rejected the
Baconian picture of natural knowledge as a ramifying tree, which scientists explore by climbing like squirrels up and out along the branches. He
substituted the model of a great sphere into which, more like moles, scientists burrow centripetally from multiple starting points on its surface.
At any one point they start with a concrete problem and a practical aim.
Himsworth, who had a profound effect upon both medical science and
Doll's career, set out the Medical Research Council philosophy on
research in his Harveian Oration in 1962:

Research being inquiry into the secrets of nature, the condition for its effective prosecution is an undivided attention to the phenomena of the natural events under study. Human needs or wishes are, in this context, aberrations. It is essentially a voyage of discovery. As such it cannot be charted in advance, and only in the broadest terms can the aim of the individual project be formulated. All that organisations can do is choose the right man as the leader, equip him to the best of its ability with men and materials, and trust to his judgement. In research, policy expresses itself not by prescription but in the informed selection and variety of projects for support so that over the subject as a whole the approach is sufficiently comprehensive to provide, so far as is humanly possible, for any eventuality or opportunity that may arise.

Until about 1980, the task of identifying what makes a cell turn into a cancer cell was formidably difficult. Literature existed about the kinetics of multi-step carcinogenesis but little was known about the order of events or the forces that drive these events. As Doll knew well, the whole weight in prevention depends on identifying the rate-limiting variable in the environment and lifestyle that determine cancer rates. Epidemiology had shown that the incidence of nearly all forms of cancer depends almost entirely upon external factors. At the time of the Yarborough report about one third of all cancer deaths in the US were caused by cigarette smoking. Since the ultimate aim of cancer research had to be prevention (as cures to the big killers did not exist) Doll had directed his work and that of his colleagues into the epidemiological understanding of the causes of cancer.

Doll's arrival at Oxford in 1969 had had an electrifying effect upon epidemiological research there. With Alice Stewart's retirement in 1974, Martin Vessey was appointed to the chair of social and preventive medicine, and Richard Peto was given an independent appointment as Imperial Cancer Research Fund reader in cancer studies with his own research budget. In response to Nixon's war on cancer, Doll and HRL Cohen of the MRC engineered the creation of the cancer and epidemiology unit. Funded by the Department of Health, and under the directorship of Malcolm Pike, the unit attracted intellectually curious explorers of science who expanded the field of epidemiological inquiry by looking for logical sense behind clinical phenomena.

Around this time, a young Australian doctor called Bruce Armstrong joined Doll in a study that has been both a source of optimism and frustration in epidemiology's ability to tell us about the causes of cancer. Doll and Armstrong looked at the correlation between cancer incidence and mortality in different countries with diet.[3] After looking at incidence rates for 27 cancers in 23 countries and mortality rates for 14 cancers in 32 countries, they found the following: "Dietary variables were strongly correlated with several types of cancer, particularly meat consumption with cancer of the colon and fat consumption with cancers of the breast and corpus uteri. The data suggests a possible role for dietary factors in modifying the development of cancer at a number of other sites." This sanguine prediction remained stubbornly intangible, and thirty years later their colleague Leo Kinlen wrote: "Bruce Armstrong and Doll's well known paper in 1975 seemed to point to diet as holding the key [to finding another major cause of cancer], though sadly those hopes were not fulfilled."[4]

From his pre-war concern with the effect of malnutrition, and his 23 years on the wards of the Central Middlesex Hospital, Doll had been fascinated by the impact of diet on disease. The role of tobacco was incontrovertible, but was animal protein nourishment also a contributory factor in cancer induction? The proportion of cancers due to diet was, and still is, elusive of measurement. At the time of the study Armstrong was a Seventh Day Adventist. The church is known for its emphasis on diet and health, recommending vegetarianism and abstinence from pork and shellfish, together with the avoidance of alcohol. Armstrong was indeed a vegetarian in 1975 and his investigation seemed to provide a scientific vindication of his religious beliefs.

Armstrong still believes the intrinsic worth of the study—that the strength of the association with meat and animal protein and colorectal cancer that they found is probably correct but "has not yet been realised".[5] In contemporary Britain people are on average about five per cent heavier than they were a decade before. So the advice that fruit and vegetables have a protective affect on colorectal cancer incidence is good public health advice if it helps prevent people consuming calorie-laden saturated fats. In the conclusion of their paper the researchers stated: "The strongest points to emerge from these analyses are the suggestions of associations between cancers of the colon, rectum and breast and dietary variables—particularly meat (or animal protein) and total fat consumption."[6]

One of the great conundrums for Doll as a cancer researcher was the virtual disappearance of stomach cancer in developed countries during his lifetime. Every twenty or thirty years, stomach cancer mortality halved in many countries while there had been little change in the curability of the disease. What was the explanation? Was it the increased use of refrigeration, the discovery that peptic ulcers were caused by the bacterium helicobacter, or a change in the human diet? Certainly, the stomach is the recipient of all dietary products. Logically it is reasonable to expect that dietary factors will eventually be found to have a major role in the prevention of cancer. It is also, however, still equally reasonable to expect the opposite. Armstrong still believes, as he and Doll did in 1975 "that the subject warrants more attention" and that their scientific method was valuable while having limitations. "There may be something about diet in early life and breast cancer incidence, but it's difficult to carry out a study using conventional epidemiological methods. Many of the hypotheses we investigated have been confirmed—others can't be confirmed by epidemiological techniques."[7]

This is hardly surprising. Eating habits change and it is extremely complicated to obtain dietary histories that are capable of objective validation. Moreover, the precise agents within foods that are beneficial or harmful are not clearly defined. Armstrong and Doll did believe a decrease in the consumption of fat would reduce the risk of ischemic heart disease—but that the only dietary factors to affect the incidence of cancer in Britain were obesity and the consumption of alcohol. In the study of diet and cancer, all we know for certain is that we do not know very much for certain.[8]

Doll disagreed with the views of the philosopher Ivan Illich, as expressed in his book *Medical Nemesis* (1976), that suffering was an

inescapable feature of the human condition.* For Doll severe and prolonged suffering, like severe and prolonged poverty, is for the majority of
people degrading rather than elevating. In the mid-1970s there was a belief
that health care had taken a wrong turning with the idea that the body is
a machine, and that medicine should concern itself with identifying and
correcting faults and defects when it goes wrong. Doll's science emphasised a different philosophy: that what we needed to do was identify and
correct the external events that led to the faults in the human body.

The asymmetrical relationship that initially existed between Hill and Doll
was similarly replicated between Doll and Richard Peto when they began
their twenty-year investigation of doctors' smoking habits. Einstein
showed us that everything is relative, and Peto was in short trousers in
October 1951 when the first questionnaire was sent to all the men and
women on the British medical register. In 1971, when the two began their
investigation, Peto was 28 and Doll was 59; but, just as in the earlier study,
the junior collaborator took on the weight of the analysis. By this time,
especially after Malcolm Pike's departure to California in 1972, Peto had
become Doll's closest colleague, and his principal statistical inquisitor.
Peto, the natural scientist, accepted the reality of the situation. "He knew
so much more about the subject than I did. It was not until the late 1970s
that we were collaborating as equals with different perspectives, although
he remained the senior figure."[9]

The publication in 1976 of "Mortality in Relation to Smoking: 20
years' observations on male British doctors"[10] found that the death rate
in middle age from all causes was twice as great in smokers as in non-

---

*   Illich thought that modern medicine was having a negative effect on society as
well as on individual patients. He argued that modern medicine harmed more
people than it cured. Illich died of cancer at the age of 76 in 2002 after adminis-
tering his own medication against the advice of doctors.

smokers. The revelation led the *British Medical Journal* to call for a fresh offensive to be made against the lethal weed: "A summary of Doll and Peto's report should be made available to every doctor, schoolteacher, and others concerned with advising young people."[11] The distinctive features of this study were the completeness of follow up, the accuracy of death certification, and the fact that the study population as a whole reduced its cigarette consumption substantially during the period of observation. "As a result lung cancer grew relatively less common as the study progressed, but other cancers did not, thus illustrating in an unusual way the causal nature of the association between smoking and lung cancer."[12]

The twenty-year study of British doctors showed that between 1951 and 1971 the average number of cigarettes smoked per day by doctors fell from 9.1 to 3.6 and that this contributed to a steady decrease in the incidence of lung cancer deaths in those aged under and over 65. Meanwhile they found the chief ways in which smoking caused death, especially in middle-aged men, were heart disease, lung cancer, chronic obstructive lung disease, and various vascular diseases. Smoking was confirmed as the nation's most serious health hazard and one that was avoidable. Doctors as a group improved their health expectations, partly by younger ones not taking up the habit, but mostly by older ones giving up smoking or reducing their consumption.

From the smallest of measurements came the biggest of ramifications. The paper itself is a masterpiece of objective narrative and statistical logic; the evidence is weighed, and conclusions drawn. There was no campaigning—yet.* For now that would be left to others. The study itself was "demanding"; they had nothing like the computing capacity of today and with a 99.7 per cent follow up it took five years to bring the evidence

---

* Earlier in Doll's career it had been one of his principal characteristics that he did not enter directly into political lobbying for the changes that his epidemiological work indicated as essential for the improvement of public health. However, he later came to support the campaigns of groups like ASH and was its honorary president at the time of his death.

together. Unlike the 1951 survey the researchers now had a population group that had altered their smoking habits over the previous two decades; consequently it is a more multifaceted review than the 1954 breakthrough paper. Doll and Peto would follow their diminishing army of doctors for another thirty years in what Himsworth might have termed a "voyage of discovery".

Information about the death of doctors was obtained directly from the registrars general of the United Kingdom, who provided particulars of every death identified as referring to a medical practitioner. One of the 10,072 doctors known to have died before 1 November 1971 was Richard Passey, the emeritus professor of experimental pathology in the University of Leeds. Historically, Passey had been sceptical of the causal link between smoking and lung cancer;[13] indeed Doll and Peto referenced the pathologist's work in their paper, and Doll had addressed Passey's criticisms of the correlation between smoking and lung cancer in a paper with Pike in 1965.[14] But Passey was never converted. The underlying causes of death of the doctors were classified according to the seventh revision of the *International List of Causes of Death*. When Doll received Passey's death certificate in his Oxford office and it read "lung cancer" he is reputed to have said: "Do you think he still doubts it now?"[15]

As we have seen, scientifically Doll was a conservative in the sense that the evidence had to be overwhelming. If he could not prove something to be true, then there was uncertainty. In 1976 no uncertainty existed about the dangers of tobacco on the health of the public. Doll and Peto showed that smoking was a most serious health hazard and one that was preventable. The facts had spoken. (Well, not quite. Peto, who had proofread the paper in a London café missed a typing error under "cause of death". "Prostrate" had been entered instead of "Prostate"—it seemed to be one of the few errors they made.)

Scientifically Doll and Peto made a wonderfully catalytic combination.[16] They had what one of their colleagues described as a "father-son relationship".[17] It was a mutual admiration society; they had different styles, but the product was much greater than the sum of its parts. As much as collaboration, theirs was an interaction. Intellectually they were equals, but in personal terms, according to Julian Peto, "they were utterly different in every sense." Richard Peto was seen as the *enfant terrible* of Oxford medical science—uniquely innovative, iconoclastic and unrelenting, he earned that most valued of epithets from Doll: "the nearest thing he had come to genius".* Doll was reassured that his legacy and the future of epidemiology were in the hands and brain of Richard Peto.

While they represented contrasting historical experiences and divergent backgrounds, collectively their endeavours expanded medical knowledge and reduced human suffering. Both were single-minded about science and saving lives. Peto was less judicious than Doll and this brought a campaigning evangelism to their scientific discoveries, seeking to embarrass the tobacco companies for purveying a dangerous and highly addictive drug. Peto thought that it was pernicious that tobacco companies should deliberately try to get new populations in China, Asia and Africa addicted. Peto became a champion of the cause.[18]

In 1976, without the combined efforts of the media, the exchequer and Doll, the moderate reduction in smoking that had taken place could easily have been a moderate increase. The *British Medical Journal* called for a campaign to "make smoking unattractive and socially unacceptable".[19] Stephen Lock, its editor, described the cigarette as "the greatest medical evil of our day."[20] In Britain alone it was responsible for at least 40,000 deaths in adults and 1,500 extra perinatal deaths a year. Lock cited Doll and Peto's work as evidence that the message on cigarette packets should state that smoking "will" damage your health.

When, in 1956, the minister of health was going to make a statement about the implications of Doll and Hill's work, Prime Minister Harold Macmillan had recognised the contribution tobacco revenue made to the NHS when he wrote, "I only hope it won't stop people smoking."[21] However, in 1976 this was no longer the case. By then the *total* care of smoking-related disease cost far more than the revenue that such taxes

---

* This was said by Doll in the presence of David Weatherall. As Weatherall observed, "Coming from Doll that is something."

brought in.

Doll was not a dictatorial abolitionist. It was not for him to tell people to stop smoking. His duty was to bring enlightenment with the power of numbers. "If you smoke, this is what the evidence suggests is most likely to happen." He thought he could best serve public health by informing people about the true nature of risk—by bridging the gulf between what people thought was harmful and what was truly dangerous. Medical science proceeds by the gradual accumulation of evidence; in the 1970s most people had some idea of the dangers of cigarette smoking. Yet clearly, as with other dangers in life, they did not believe that it could hold any risk for them personally. If doctors could be persuaded to quit smoking and avoid chronic ill health and premature death, what would it take to induce the rest of the population to do the same? Doll was a serious person and he wanted to use science to help people live their full biological span of life, free of avoidable morbidity. He wanted to change the world and he had a protégé who was also focusing on a global perspective.

The year 1976 was a defining one in Richard Peto's scientific life. Based on his distinguished work in the MRC's statistical research unit, he published his first book*, and was also the dynamic force behind a research paper** that demonstrated controlled clinical trials could be carried out on a large enough scale (that is, with tens of thousands of patients rather than a few hundred) to enable moderate effects to be established. This is of major importance for conditions that are simultaneously serious and common such as heart attack, stroke and cancers of the breast and bowel. His remarkable methodological achievement— showing the importance of large numbers to finding reliable answers—

---

*   Fletcher CM, Peto R, Tinker CM, Speizer FE, *The Natural History of Chronic Bronchitis and Emphysema* (Oxford University Press, 1976).

**   Peto R, Pike MC, Armitage P, Breslow NE, Cox DR, Howard SV, Mantel N, McPherson K, Peto J, Smith PG, 'Design and analysis of randomised clinical trials requiring prolonged observation of each patient. 1. Introduction and design', *British Journal of Cancer* 1976; volume 34, pp.585-612.

changed medical practice. In doing this he fulfilled the objectives of accuracy that were essential for Hill* and those of co-operation among scientists that Pickering** predicted would come with collaboration.

With the follow up study of British doctors, Peto had secured an international reputation in the field of tobacco and cancer, and the new statistical techniques that he pioneered helped bring epidemiology into the forefront of the fight against preventable diseases.

While nurturing and mentoring a new generation of medical scientists such as Richard Peto, Doll also took a leading part in a wider social discourse. In 1973 he was invited to join Sir (later Lord) Brian Flowers's Royal Commission on environmental pollution which reported in 1976. The august membership considered the same contentious issues that would engage society a generation later: the threat of nuclear terrorism, concern about the spread of nuclear weapons, the disposal of toxic waste and the dangers of radiation exposure for the industry's workforce. The commission delivered its findings three years before the accident at the Three Mile Island nuclear generating station accident in Pennsylvania (where workers were injured). And, according to Lord Flowers, the commission "shook up the [British] nuclear industry about looking after nuclear waste. They never solved it completely. [But] that was one of the commission's great effects."[22]

The industry was alarmed when Flowers, a distinguished nuclear physicist, warned that the dangers of building nuclear power stations had not been properly disclosed and the problems of disposing of spent

---

* "It is not difficult to show that a new drug will reduce the death rate of patients from, say, 30 per cent to 10 per cent. The change is pronounced. We can hardly miss it. But, in the modern world, with one potent drug following another, the problem is to know whether a new one will reduce that 10 per cent to seven per cent. That small difference in mortality is likely to be regarded as important by at least three per cent of the patients. Without a very large scale and meticulously conducted trial it may be impossible to detect it."

** "A controlled clinical trial is the quickest way to get knowledge; it improves enormously the good fellowship amongst doctors, and has to my way of thinking an undoubted educational value."

nuclear fuel remained unresolved. The commission's recommendations covered issues such as discharges of radioactivity to the environment and the disposals of radioactive wastes.

Doll was also concerned that a report* on the mortality of Windscale workers who had been exposed to plutonium included only the numbers of deaths observed and expected among those who were actively employed. This led to the recommendation for a complete national register of radiation workers to be kept by the National Radiological Protection Board, with a section comprising those exposed to plutonium and would include those who had retired or left the industry. Over the following 25 years the National Registry of Radiation Workers would encompass 120,000 men and women, some of whom were first employed in 1955, and were present at the Windscale fire in October 1957**. This cohort, it was hoped, would provide an estimate of risk at very low doses, such as those incurred from natural background radiation, or laboratory experiment.

Doll had established with Court-Brown that radiation caused cancer, but would there be a measurable excess of the disease among workers in the industry? One intriguing health feature of the workers in the nuclear industry was that their lung cancer rates were less than those found in the national population: this may have been because smoking was banned in Britain's nuclear plants.

By the end of the 1970s the epic endeavour of Nixon's billion-dollar war against cancer had not provided the panacea that was envisaged.[23] The great improvements in treatment that had taken place were confined to the rare types of cancer that occurred in children or young adults; while the fatality rate for most of the common cancers remained depressingly high. For Doll, the fact that cancer had become one of the leading causes of death was not so much an indication of an increase in the risk of devel-

---

*   Dolphin GW, 'A Comparison of the Observed and Expected Cancers of the Haematopoietic and Lymphatic Systems among Workers at Windscale', National Radiological Protection Board report, 1976

**   Lorna Arnold, *Windscale 1957: Anatomy of a Nuclear Accident* (Macmillan, 1992).

oping the disease at any given age, but attributable to the elimination or control of so many other diseases.

Continuing in the scientific tradition of Sir Ernest Kennaway, who in the 1930s had identified a chemical that was capable of causing cancer in animals, Doll gave a series of lectures at Oxford that defined the modern programme of cancer detection and prevention.[24] He showed that the risk of developing each of the common cancers varied greatly with place, community, or time, and often all three. For Doll, "By far the greater part of the variation must be due to differences in the environment in which people live or in the way in which they behave."[25] Whether it would be possible to eradicate cancer entirely as had been done with poliomyelitis was impossible for him to say, but he did think that a quarter of all deaths in men in Britain under the age of 75 could be reduced by 80 to 90 per cent. Inspiring devotion in some and scepticism in others, he stated, "The identification of environmental hazards and clarification of the mechanisms through which they cause disease are thus among the highest priorities in cancer research."[26] One epidemiologist looked upon Doll's hypothesis as "an old man's paper", and indeed some slept through his lectures; Peto, on the other hand, found them inspiring. Doll's teaching crystallised in him what he had been thinking for some time,[27] and he gave himself a challenge: to deploy the accumulated knowledge of the causes of the disease and reduce the risk of developing fatal cancer.

Since Rachel Carson's 1962 book *Silent Spring*, which showed chlorine pesticides did in fact damage birds eggshells, there had been a desire in the US to attribute a very high proportion of disease to industry, and especially to the chemical industry which had expanded enormously. Then, in the 1970s, with the failure of Nixon's programme to eradicate cancer, the environmental movement grew strong, and its theories of cancer causation were in disagreement with Doll. One of the most influential of the environmentalist theologians was Professor Samuel Epstein of the University of Illinois. In his book *The Politics of Cancer** he con-

---

*   Sierra Club Books, 1978.

cluded that the majority of US cancer deaths could be prevented by the testing and regulation of environmental contaminants and that the main obstacles against doing this were political rather than scientific. The politics of cancer in the US was becoming increasingly polarised, with environmentalists taking one extreme view and industrialists another. This was at a time in American history when cigarettes caused over 100,000 deaths every year from lung cancer or chronic obstructive lung disease, and while the tobacco industry refused to admit in public that cigarettes caused either disease.[28]

In 1978 Doll was pre-eminent in the epidemiological investigation of industrial carcinogens. He had, after all, been the first post-war investigator to discover the ten-fold increase in asbestos workers at T&N's factory in Rochdale. Asbestos became the world's greatest industrial carcinogen, and most litigated industry. He also recognised that the environment in which we live is complex, changing rapidly, and interacts with our genetic constitution in many ways; but he did not think that occupational and environmental pollutants caused the majority of avoidable cancer deaths. He called for the equivalent of the committee on the safety of medicines to advise on the introduction of new material into industry to detect new hazards quickly, and he could see "no reason to be anxious about the direct effect on health of the further growth of industrialisation".[29]

In 1978 the political and scientific landscape in the United States on the causes of cancer changed dramatically with the publication of the Califarno report. Joseph Califarno was the health, education and welfare secretary in President Jimmy Carter's administration. The report estimated that as many as half of the eight to eleven million workers who had been exposed to asbestos could develop serious diseases such as cancer or asbestosis; and it estimated that six occupational sources were responsible for between "20-38 per cent " of all cancers. This estimation Doll described as "quite ludicrous". Califarno's unpublished typescript was prepared by a working group of nine scientists, including Arthur Upton and David Rall, and directors of the National Cancer Institute and the National Institute of Environmental Health Sciences. Califarno was altruistic and wanted to help: others thought that his actions were sincere but wrong.[30]

The claim that industrial carcinogens were responsible for a great proportion of cancer was readily accepted by a lot of people, but it was contested by industry. Doll looked upon the "environmental movement" as causing a distraction from the real dangers facing humanity: these included ionising and ultraviolet radiations, viral and parasitic infections, hormonal secretions, natural and man-made foods, chemicals met with at work, at home and in the general environment, medicines, and the so-called drugs of solace.

To Doll, humanity's challenge was to learn to control the social environment we make for ourselves by living closer together in large towns, with a high standard of living and with ample leisure. Under these conditions the individual needed self-control of appetites for concentrated food, and for mental stimulus whether by tobacco, marijuana, alcohol or aggressive driving. Doll was not clairvoyant; as an epidemiologist he did what psychiatrists and historians do—he explored the past. This led him to the optimistic belief that cancer could be significantly reduced, but that it would not be easy to prevent the disease. Three decades studying cancer induction led him to a realistic observation: "For if, as I suspect, these hazards are associated with the common diet of developed countries, the problems that we are now having to face in preventing tobacco-induced cancer will seem childishly simple."[31]

By 1978 the view of the "environmentalists" had become more than a hypothesis; it had assumed the status of a climate of opinion and Doll and Peto were looked upon as dinosaurs.[32] A year later, the shifting sands of scientific debate stabilised when Doll was presented with the Mott award, from General Motors' Cancer Research Foundation, for helping to demonstrate the vast hazards of tobacco in developed countries such as the UK and US. He was the first recipient of the prize, and his acceptance speech opened with a joke: "In Oxford, it is widely held that two in one of all the professors have split personalities"—because he wanted to acknowledge the debt he owed to his mentor and long-term collaborator, Austin Bradford Hill.

Could the war on cancer be won? What were the possibilities for its prevention? These were the questions that by the late 1970s exercised the minds of American scientists and politicians. The somewhat acrimonious climate of opinion led the Office of Technology Assessment (OTA) that had been set up to guide Congress to try to resolve the impasse. The OTA was asked by its political masters to provide background material for their assessment of "Technologies for Determining Cancer Risks from the Environment".* However, the OTA was unable to find an independent scientific adjudicator in the US who either did not attract the wrath of industry or the rage of the environmental movement. So they looked outside the US for a reliable assessment, and turned to Oxford epidemiology and Richard Peto, who was mandated by the US Congress to write a report on the causes of cancer. He accepted on the condition that he could co-write it with Doll.[33] In the fight against disease, Doll was still in the vanguard of the scientific army. As epidemiologists, they could no more avoid tackling the causes of cancer in twentieth-century America than Snow could avoid the problem of cholera in nineteenth-century London.

---

*   Office of Technology Assessment, US Congress, 1981.

Chapter 22

"Are We Winning the War against Cancer?"

"Over the past few decades, many of us in Oxford have made a minor epidemiological industry of studying tobacco. Indeed, it seems that epidemiologists need smokers more than smokers need epidemiologists— where else are we ever going to find one thing that causes a third of all cancer deaths, and that kills even more people by other diseases than by cancer?"

Richard Peto

In 1977, the author Susan Sontag in her essay *Illness as Metaphor* attacked the idea that cancer afflicts people of a certain "character type" who are then left feeling that they are to blame for their illness.* She argued that two diseases had been "spectacularly, and similarly, encumbered with the trapping of metaphor"—tuberculosis in the nineteenth century and cancer in the twentieth. Her book was an attempt to make sense of cancer to the individual and to society.

Doll and Peto had the same objective as Sontag but their *scientific* investigation into the causes of cancer came at a time of great controversy in the United States about the extent to which environmental factors, particularly chemicals, were contributing to cancer rates. The authors brought more than arithmetic to the dispute about what might be the best preventable measures for the avoidance of human cancers. The object of the exercise was to publicise the solid facts that medical science had uncovered about the illness.

Using statistical data from 1978, Doll and Peto set out to anatomise cancer. The result was their work *The Causes of Cancer: Quantitative*

---

* Sontag was diagnosed with advanced (stage 4) breast cancer in 1975. She died of leukaemia at the age of 71 in 2004.

*Estimates of Avoidable Risks of Cancer in the United States Today** published in 1981. They found that cancers of three organs (lung, breast and large intestine) accounted for half of all the US cancer deaths and that cigarette smoking was correlated with cancer of the lung, mouth, larynx, bladder, oesophagus, pancreas and kidney. Also, they found that there were sufficient valid data to attribute 30 per cent of the total cancer deaths to tobacco smoking (122,000 men and 27,000 women annually). Another 35 per cent was attributed, albeit with somewhat less certainty, to aspects of diet, seven per cent to reproductive and sexual behaviour, and up to four per cent to occupational exposure.

The authors' magnum opus reflected the interaction of their different interests and academic training: Doll's was in the epidemiology of large-scale determinants in human cancer and medicine and Peto's in mathematics and statistics. Both aimed to reduce premature deaths. Although they argued over every line, Peto believes that it was the best work they ever did together and much better as a collaborative enterprise than it would have been as an individual endeavour.[1] They rejected what they termed "the common belief", held by the "environmental movement", that the majority of cases of cancer could be prevented by the stringent control of chemical pollution of air, food, water and of occupational exposure. Rather their population-based research pointed towards an optimistic trend away from the perception that the US was experiencing an epidemic of cancer due to new factors. "Indeed, were it not for the effects of tobacco, total US death rates would be decreasing substantially more rapidly than they already are, and we are more encouraged by the benefits that are already being demonstrated from the control of known causes of cancer and other diseases than we are dismayed by the appearance of new ones."

The Causes of Cancer had a profound influence on society's knowledge of cancer causation in a number of ways. First, although it contained no original research it told a coherent story with a numerical perspective.

---

* Journal of the National Cancer Institute, June 1981; volume 66, Number 6 Special report, pp. 1191-1308.

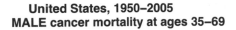

United States, 1950–2005
MALE cancer mortality at ages 35–69

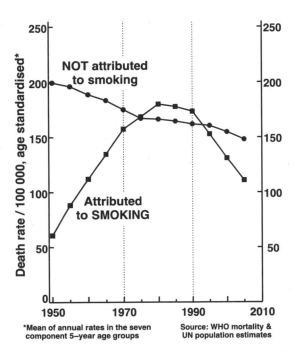

*Mean of annual rates in the seven
component 5–year age groups

Source: WHO mortality &
UN population estimates

The authors were united in their belief that cancers attributed to industrial and occupational exposure had been overestimated and this had distorted the real danger—tobacco—facing American citizens. Second, by showing that smoking was causing more than twice the number of cancer deaths than all the other reliably known causes put together, they believed that the most important public health message was to highlight the hazards of tobacco. Third, Doll and Peto estimated that nearly two-thirds of all cancer cases in the US were preventable, giving hope for the control of the disease.

In 2005 *The Causes of Cancer* was judged to have stood the test of time as a hypothesis of how to avoid some of the risks of the disease when it was given this medical assessment in the US. "Importantly, this document laid out a blueprint for epidemiological research that has guided investigators around the world."[2]

The Causes of Cancer had its origins in Doll's investigations into smoking and occupational cancers in the 1950s, his statistical analysis of *Cancer in Five Continents* in the 1960s and 70s, and his later contributions to diet and disease with Burkitt and Armstrong. Its 116 pages of narrative, stochastic graphs, statistics and six appendices reflected his lifelong thinking on the aetiology and teleology of the disease. It stands as a lucid and irrefutable indictment of the damage being done by tobacco and other carcinogens and it changed people's thinking and helped to clarify how to prevent cancer. The clear message was: make cigarettes less dangerous, and most importantly, promote the health benefits of quitting.

If Doll's role in the co-discovery of the dangers of tobacco is widely acknowledged, his work on the proportion of cancer deaths attributed to diet is viewed tendentiously.[3] In *The Causes of Cancer*, his "best estimate" of the proportion of cancers due to diet in the US was 35 per cent and that "the figure chosen is highly speculative and chiefly refers to dietary factors that are not yet reliably identified." However, he and Peto also suggested that the proportion of cancers due to diet could range between 10 and 70 per cent—a variation that induced incredulity as well as hope. In 1999, James Le Fanu, the physician and science writer, criticised this statistical inexactitude as a form of public health quackery: "Sir Richard Doll subsequently conceded the weaknesses of *The Causes of Cancer* but never publicly retracted his conclusions, and the claim that he had 'proved that food caused more than a third of cancers' was repeatedly cited by all those who had an interest—nutritionists, health educationalists, food fanatics and others—in incriminating the Western diet as a major cause of death and disease."[4]

In their survey Doll and Peto wrote that the natural history and biology of cancers of the gastrointestinal tract pointed towards dietary factors "but that there is as yet little decisive evidence on which firm conclusions can be based." In Doll's investigations of radiologists, asbestos and nickel workers the importance of occupation on the causes of cancer and the ways of preventing it was shown because the exposure to a specific carcinogen could be measured and a dose-response relationship established. However, this biological gradient was not possible for Doll to isolate in his work on diet because "we don't eat individual things, and this raises the potential for confounding, making it difficult to distinguish what is the causal factor."[5]

In 2007, the World Cancer Research Fund assembled a group of experts who wrote an overview of all the data written on diet and cancer.* This weighty volume of the American Institute for Cancer Research offered little to those who sought a way of obviating cancer through dietary means. The only definite causal conclusion of the panel of judges was: "The evidence that red meats and processed meats are a cause of colorectal cancer is convincing." So thirty-two years after their paper first put forward the relationship between red meat and cancer Armstrong and Doll had been vindicated. Similarly, the most learned body ever assembled to analyse the various elements causing cancer quoted the 1981 Doll and Peto definition: "A number of different types of exogenous (environmental) factors are known causes of cancer. These include some aspects of food and nutrition that are established as carcinogenic by the International Agency for Research on Cancer, although it is difficult to estimate the proportion of cancer directly attributable to these."[6] The panel concluded: "Currently, no firm judgements can be made on any possible relationship between dietary patterns and the risk of cancer."

Professor Timothy Key of Oxford University has spent more than twenty years looking for a relationship between diet and cancer. With the notable exceptions of obesity and alcohol, little progress has been made, according to Key, since Doll and Peto. "A quarter of a century of research hasn't been able to categorically find any aspect of our diet that is protective, which is a rather frustrating position."[7] For those looking for salvation in stalagmites of broccoli, garlic or blueberries the evidence, according to Professor Key, is wanting. It has been a source of disappointment that growing levels of obesity and alcohol consumption need acts of willpower to prevent them while the discovery of a miracle ambrosia that could be

---

* World Cancer Research Fund, *Food, Nutrition, Physical Activity and the Prevention of Cancer: a Global Perspective* (American Institute for Cancer Research, 2007).

taken to actively inhibit cancer has not materialised.

The force driving the quest for the dietary Holy Grail is that there must be some thing in the common diet that causes intestinal cancer but it has not been found by epidemiological research. In 2002 *The Lancet* published a review article by Professor Key and his colleagues entitled "The Effect of Diet on Risk of Cancer".[8] Its opening line stated that the likely role of the human diet in the cause of common cancers had not been attenuated by a generation of research. Nonetheless, "Diet-related factors are thought to account for about 30 per cent of cancers in developed countries." Doll had shown that the rates of liver cancer vary more than 20-fold between different parts of the world and that countries with diets high in animal fats had higher rates of cancers of the colorectum, breast, prostate and endometrium than countries with low intakes of animal fats in their diet.[9] The authors of the *Lancet* review concluded their examination of the definitive correlation between diet and cancer and found only scientific uncertainty. The prediction that Doll had made in 1977[10] about the complexity of finding the cancer hazards associated with the common diet were no less insurmountable for other epidemiologists in 2002. As Key put it: "At present, prudent advice is to maintain a healthy weight, restrict alcohol consumption, and select a conventionally balanced diet ensuring an adequate intake of fruit, vegetables, and cereals."[11]

Doll believed that scientists had a responsibility to give early warning of the way hazards could be avoided as they had to warn about the possible existence of new hazards. But if they were to give advice, it was important that they should distinguish between advice based on established fact, and advice based on a personal assessment of the most likely interpretation of the evidence. Unless this was done, subsequent admission that some of the advice was wrong (as some certainly would be) would detract from the confidence that people have in advice that is known to be solidly based. Doll was sometimes thought of as an austere scientist, but his advice to people who were worried by health scares was to ignore the majority of them. "Grilled and smoked foods carry a cancer risk," he said, "but I haven't given up my grilled kipper or smoked salmon." You can choose not to smoke but you cannot choose not to eat.

"Are We Winning the War against Cancer?"

Lung cancer is the most common fatal cancer in the world. Heavy smoking increases the risk of the disease by around thirty-fold, and tobacco causes over eighty per cent of lung cancers in developed countries.[12] This was the big picture that Doll and Peto had wanted to convey about the avoidable risks of cancer in the United States. But could Doll and Peto have been wrong? Could investigators like Professor Samuel Epstein[13] have been correct in arguing that a major cause of human cancers was due to man-made pollutants? Such a leap of faith would, to quote George W Bush, have required a belief in "fuzzy math". In the late 1970s if all the reliably known "environmental" causes of cancer—as opposed to speculated causes—were added together, they would have been equivalent to half of all tobacco cancers.[14] The politics of cancer was heating up.

Peto thought that "environmentalists" like Epstein started from the proposition that there was a generalised increase in cancer rates while he and Doll found that trends were not going up.[15] In 2007, an American epidemiologist, Devra Davis, in her book *The Secret History of the War on Cancer**, made a assault on *The Causes of Cancer*. On page 255 of her book she makes this apparently sentient observation:

> I was confused. Lilienfeld had taught me that the incidence of cancers—the rate of new cases of the disease—was the most important indicator of factors affecting the disease. Incidence also was the best predictor of future demands for medical care. Yet Doll and Peto had not looked at incidence at all, nor had they included the growing rates of cancer in blacks. Instead, they had considered the other end of the process: causes of death and only in whites. We both knew that at the time, four out of every five cancer deaths occurred in people over

---

*   Basic Books, 2007.

65. Why, then, did Doll and Peto restrict their work to deaths that occurred in whites under 65?

Unfortunately for Davis's thesis, in *The Causes of Cancer* on facing pages 1,284-1,285 the book gives "cancer mortality in middle age" (under 65), and "cancer mortality in old age" (aged 65 and over). The data was put on facing pages deliberately so as to enable researchers to contrast and compare them. As for Davis's observation that Doll and Peto only looked at mortality and not incidence, on page 1,286 they describe trends in incidence* both for "whites only" and for "all races"—so the accusation that the data excluded "blacks" or "incidence" is untrue. This was not the first time such an error had been made. Nor may it be the last—because for more than a quarter of a century the same unfounded accusations have followed Doll and Peto through history like a mutagenic meme.

Perhaps the critical response to *The Causes of Cancer* can be explained by the desire of some members of the environmental lobby to disregard anything that contravened their pre-conceived findings. Or it may have reflected an unwillingness to accept that no other industry kills people on anything like the scale of the tobacco industry.[16] Davis in her folksy homily, or as one reviewer described her book "an amalgam of history, speculation and memoir"[17], disingenuously attributes to *The Causes of Cancer* the status of "a bible of cancer epidemiology".

But did the book bring enlightenment to public health medicine? Their emphasis on the hazards of tobacco may have contributed to the halving of US cigarette consumption between the mid 1970s and 2000. This led to an historic counterpoint with the country having as many ex-smokers as current smokers: and a corresponding fall in the rates of male lung cancers. While Doll and Peto found no evidence of the existence of any new risk, "the lack of any apparent overall upward trends in cancers ...

---

* The most precise way of finding incidence rates is to look at mortality rates in middle age because they will have been recorded accurately whereas with older people the artefactual trends are quite substantial.

Proportions of cancer deaths attributed to various different factors

Text section No.	Factor or class of factors	Per cent of all cancer deaths	
		Best Estimate	Range of acceptable Estimates
5.1	Tobacco	30	25–40
5.2	Alcohol	3	2–4
5.3	Diet	35	10–70
5.4	Food Additives	<1	-5ᵃ–2
5.5	Reproductive [b] and sexual behaviour	7	1–13
5.6	Occupation	4	2–8
5.7	Pollution	2	<1–5
5.8	Industrial products	<1	<1–2
5.9	Medicines and medical procedures	1	0.5–3
5.10	Geographical factors [c]	3	2–4
5.11	Infections	10?	1–?
5.12	Unknown	?	?

a Allowing for a possibly protective effect of antioxidants and other preservatives.

b See section 5.5 for intended meaning.

c Only about one per cent, not three per cent could reasonably be described as "avoidable" (see text). Geophysical factors also cause a much greater proportion of non-fatal cancers (up to 30 per cent of all cancers, depending on ethnic mix and latitude) because of the importance of UV light in causing the relatively non-fatal basal cell and squamous cell carcinomas of sunlight-exposed skin.

(Table from *The Causes of Cancer* JNCI, Volume 6, June 1981)

do not of course, guarantee that apart from tobacco all is well." Doll had a serious interest in industrial health and he wanted industry to keep records in such a way that any dangers could be detected sooner rather than later. When writing about the causative role of industrial products in contemporary US cancer rates Doll and Peto noted that while there was no cause for alarm: "There is too much ignorance for complacency to be justified."

Indeed, in their survey Doll and Peto had underestimated radiation as a cause of cancer because they completely missed Radon gas (a naturally occurring radioactive gas that causes lung cancer) in houses. They were more insightful about infections and the possible importance of "the hepatitis B virus... with the development of cancer of the liver". But it was not until 1982 when molecular biologists discovered HPV 16 that it was possible for modern medicine to protect against viruses. In *The Causes of Cancer* Doll and Peto estimated that infections accounted for between one and four per cent of cancers within "a range of acceptable estimation" of about four to ten per cent. Doll and Peto could not predict technological advances in medicine and, as a result, their analysis of the causes and avoidable risks of cancer in the US contained those notable underestimations.

The Causes of Cancer has, however, entered the canon of knowledge on the aetiology of the disease and the evidence is there to be judged on its intrinsic worth. Doll and Peto synthesised their skills to provide the best possible analysis of the chief determinants of cancers in the US. In 1965, Sir Austin Bradford Hill, in his classic paper "The Environment and Disease: Association or Causation?" had explained why the work of investigators like Doll and Peto was an affirmation of the scientific endeavour. "All scientific work is incomplete—whether it be observational or experimental. All scientific work is liable to be upset or modified by advancing knowledge. That does not confer upon us a freedom to ignore the knowledge we already have, or to postpone the action that it appears to demand at a given time."[18]

The US Congress had offered Doll and Peto a nominal fee for writing *The Causes of Cancer*. Peto did not want to accept any payment but Doll told him to take it "and give it to some thing you like".[19] Both of them, as was their custom, gave the money to charity. The destination of Doll's cheque was Green College. Peto's nomination was altogether more of a problem for the United States government. He wanted the cheque to be paid to Amnesty International. However, at the time it was a proscribed organisation in the US, and the Congress initially refused to sanction the payment. Eventually a way out was found. Congress made the payment to Green College and they forwarded the money to Amnesty.

Doll was not protective of his sensibilities. He was sensitive, but the acrimonious attacks on his scientific integrity did not hurt him emotionally. For Doll the point was not whether the perfidious accusations against him were fair or not, nice or not, but whether they were true or not. What seemed wrong to him was the extent to which things that were much less important than tobacco were being taken much more seriously. The quest for knowledge often carries risks. Doll, in the face of the environmentalists' scientifically lightweight but politically heavyweight attacks, could defend *The Causes of Cancer* and his integrity as a scientist by replicating the stance of Martin Luther. In 1517 Luther posted his 95 theses on the door of the chapel of Wittenberg University. Doll too refused to recant his position. Luther said defiantly, "Here I stand. I can do no other."

Tooth decay remains a major public health problem in most industrial countries. Many scientists believed that water fluoridation, first introduced in the US in the 1940s was the best way to eradicate this human avoidable human tragedy, others however, did not.

In January 1976 Doll was one of the authors of the Royal College of Physicians report on the effect of fluoride on teeth and health. The report stated that: "There is no evidence that fluoride increases the incidence or mortality of cancer in any organ"[20] and it recommended the adding of fluoride to water supplies to prevent tooth decay.

Two years later, on 13 September 1978, Strathclyde regional council as the statutory water authority decided to co-operate with health boards in the progressive fluoridation of water. The purpose of fluoridation* was to reduce the excessive incidence of dental caries which were endemic in Strathclyde (the problem was greater in Scotland than in other parts of Britain). The issue had for some time aroused great passions in British medical history and in 1951 Aneurin Bevan, then minister of health, had resigned from the Cabinet in protest at prescription charges being introduced for dental care and spectacles. A quarter of a century later, the UK was still suffering from two great public health failures—smoking and tooth decay—and the *British Medical Journal* while calling for boldness about dental disease also took the opportunity to highlight the political machinations at the heart of the war against cancer:

> First is to have the courage to act on another known benefit to mankind, the artificial fluoridation of drinking water supplies where this is indicted. Dental disease is the commonest preventable abnormality in our population and yet we shrink from applying a proved, safe, and cost-effective method to stop it. Why? We all know the answer: despite the weight of evidence presented by unbiased report after report, not to mention the experience of other advanced countries who have gone ahead with fluoridation, the opposition is noisy and effective. Why does our society still listen to these scrannel pipes, and why do the opponents of fluoridation not turn their energies and enviable abilities to dealing with the cigarette?[21]

Doll's belief in the safety of fluoride was based on his own research work. His investigations had been inspired by claims that cancer mortality in the United States[22] increased more sharply in cities with fluoridated water than in those without. Dr John Yiamouyiannis and Dr Dean Burk had carried out a study in trends in crude mortality rates from cancer between ten fluoridated and ten non-fluoridated cities and suggested that

---

* Fluoride is a mineral occurring naturally as a trace element in almost all waters throughout the world as well as in many common foodstuffs and at high concentrations in tea.

fluoride had been responsible for 35,000 cancer deaths in 93 million persons who regularly used fluoridated water in the United States in 1975. As we have already seen, the death rate calculated for a population covering a wide age range is called a crude death rate. In a comparison of the mortality between ten or twenty populations, the crude rates may be misleading. This is because cancer death rates vary grossly with age and can differ widely between sexes and races of the same age.

That fluoridation may have been responsible for such a catastrophic loss of American life led Dr DS Fredrickson, director of the National Institutes of Health, to examine the demographic changes in the population of the cities selected by Burk and Yiamouyiannis to see if these demographic changes could have contributed to the findings. Fredrickson reported that "the differences in the trend in the crude rates of cancer mortality between the two groups of cities can all be attributed to differences in the racial and age composition of the populations involved."[23] This judgment was reinforced in 1977 by Doll, in collaboration with Leo Kinlen, who found that when account was taken of age, sex and ethnic group "the ratio between observed cancer mortality and expected cancer mortality fell slightly in the cities with fluoridated water and did not change in the non-fluoridated cities."[24] This conclusion should have ended the controversy, but it did not, and in 1981 those "energies and enviable abilities of the opponents of fluoride" that the BMJ had noted were exercised.

This happened when Catherine McColl, a 69-year-old woman from Hutchesontown in Glasgow, complained that her rights had been infringed by the decision of Strathclyde regional council to put fluoride in the water supply. She did not want her grandchildren[25] exposed to a "horrible poison"—and with the assistance of an unusually large legal aid award, she sued the water authority. The hearing commenced on 23 September 1980 in the court of session in Edinburgh, in front of Lord Jauncey. Described as a "courteous and patient judge",[26] he particularly needed the latter quality as the trial continued until 26 July 1982, making it, at the time, the longest and costliest civil case in Scottish legal history.

Ironically, Mrs McColl, who was toothless (Juancey described her as "edentulous"), only appeared in court on the first day, and then briefly on one other occasion, but the munificent legal aid award enabled her legal team to call witnesses from around the world. As the judge noted in his opinion:

> There can be no doubt that the petitioner, through the granting of legal aid, has been enabled to pursue a litigation of unprecedented length and expense which only an individual with unlimited means at his disposal could have afforded to pursue. Whether such an individual would have considered that expenditure on this action was the most cost-effective way of avoiding the effects of fluoridation must be open to question.[27]

The debate over whether there was any reliable evidence that fluoridation of water caused cancer moved from the pages of medical journals to the altogether more combative arena of the court room. Doll's mantra of "only write a sentence if you know that you can defend it in a court of law" was about to be put to the test. If there were any shortcomings in either side's methodology it would be demolished under the accumulated weight of expert witness testimony and coruscating legal cross-examination.

In support of her proposition that the addition of fluoride to a water supply at a concentration of one part per million would increase the cancer death rate, Mrs McColl's lawyers relied not only on epidemiological evidence but also on biochemical evidence as showing that fluoride was an agent capable of interfering with the mechanism of the body in such a way that it acted either as a carcinogen, or as an agent which stimulated tumour growth. These two sources of evidence were, the petitioner maintained, mutually supportive although each was capable of standing on its own if the other were held to fall. The biochemical evidence upon which Mrs McColl's case relied upon came largely from John Yiamouyannis, who had received his PhD in biochemistry from the University of Rhode Island in 1967. He then worked at the Western Reserve University medical school until December 1968 when he became an editor in the biochemical section of the chemical abstract service of the American Chemical Society. In April 1972 he lost that job because of his stand against the fluoridation of drinking water. From 1980 Yiamouyannis had been president of the Safer Water Foundation, which was concerned primarily with opposing fluoridation of water.

Yiamouyannis had given evidence on behalf of organisations opposing fluoridation in several cases in the United States Courts. About one-third of Lord Jauncey's 292-page "opinion" was devoted to arguments derived from cancer deaths in the 20 American cities that Yiamouyannis and Doll had metaphorically locked horns over. The written record of evidence ran to 21,000 pages and nearly a quarter of it was contributed by expert statistical witness for the defence. Of these the greatest amount was contributed by Doll. In his crystalline testimony he explained to the court that after many years of research he had come to the conclusion that the rapidly increasing incidence with age of the great majority of the so-called epithelial cancers was due not to age as such, but to the greater length of time an older person is likely to have been exposed to a carcinogenic agent.

Some forty individual agents were known to be capable of causing cancer in humans and the characteristic of all these agents was that the risk of their producing cancer increases progressively with the duration of exposure. It was, Doll stated, very seldom that any effect is seen within the first five years of exposure but thereafter the risk of cancer incidence increases rapidly. He outlined to the judge that there are several stages in the conversion of a normal cell into a recognisably cancerous one. The chemical agent exposure which causes the first change in the cell leading ultimately to cancer, he described as an *initiator*. If exposure to that agent ceases after the first change a further chemical may act on the change already formed by the initiator to produce a cancerous cell. This second chemical Doll described as a *promoter*: and that it was proper to describe both initiators and promoters as carcinogens. A substance which merely increased the growth of an existing tumour was not a carcinogen but an *accelerator*. Doll told the court he was unaware of any chemical taken by the mouth which acted as an accelerator. Lord Jauncey, "quiet and thoughtful by nature",[28] wrote that "Sir Richard's evidence on the foregoing general matters was neither controverted nor seriously challenged and I have no hesitation in accepting it."[29]

On the American side of the scientific argument, confusion reigned. Yiamouyannis thought that there was no reason why fluoride should affect one tissue type more than another. In expressing this view, he was not only departing from the earlier view attributed to him in 1975 but he was, according to Jauncey, "demonstrating his lack of sound scientific knowledge on the subject of cancer".[30] Doll explained to the court that there was only one known factor, namely ionising radiation, which appeared to be capable of causing cancer in every organ whereas the vast majority of agents caused cancer in only one or a few sites because they or their metabolic products only came in contact with certain sites. On page 77 of his opinion, Jauncey determined the scientific foundation of his judgement when he wrote: "I have no hesitation in preferring the evidence of Sir Richard on these matters to that of Dr Yiamouyannis whose practical experience thereanent was virtually nil."

If fluoride is an accelerator, as the lawyers for Mrs McColl suggested would be the most attractive explanation for the way in which it was working, it would be unique as the only known chemical which, if taken orally, can accelerate tumour growth. Dr Dean Burk accepted that fluoride would be unique in that it produced the greatest increase in cancer death rates so soon after fluoridation but he did not say whether it would be unique as a carcinogen or as an accelerator or as both. Indeed Dr Burk's evidence on the subject of cancer did not impress the judge. This was in marked contrast to Doll's testimony[31] whose account of how certain chemicals can cause cancer Jauncey found of "considerable assistance". The epistemological uncertainty upon which the Burk and Yiamouyannis supposition was built was exposed under legal examination during which Burk appeared to dismiss the distinction between fluoride acting as an initiator or as an accelerator while Yiamouyannis recognised the distinction but was unable to say which of the two roles fluoride was fulfilling.[32]

Lord Jauncey retreated to his beloved Perthshire home with his "patient temper"[33] and volumes of legal evidence for almost twelve months before emerging with his 392-page opinion, delivered at 10am on 29 June

1983. Although Mrs McColl was not in court to hear the decision, Jauncey ruled that Strathclyde Regional Council had exceeded their statutory power by adding fluoride to the water, and found in her favour. However, he emphasised the safety of fluoride at a concentration of one part per million and made it clear that although he had found against Strathclyde regional council this did not reflect on the efficacy of the chemical for the health of the Scottish public. "Since I have concluded that fluoridation would not have an adverse effect upon health it follows that fluoridation of water which was already wholesome would not render that water unwholesome rather would it render it more beneficial or more whole-some in the wider sense to some of the consumers."[34]

Michael Ashley Miller, a senior medical officer at the MRC, was working in Scotland at the time of the court case and viewed the judge-ment as a vindication of fluoridation's safety. Scottish medicine took the case seriously and wanted "to bury the issue conclusively and forever."[35] He was also convinced that the anti-fluoridation lobby was behind Mrs McColl's litigation. Before the court case, Doll's academic papers had been criticised by Yiamouyannis for being "so replete with errors that space does not allow a full discussion of each point here"[36] but when their different explanations of medical data were rigorously analysed under the micro-scope of expert opinion, it was Yiamouyannis's science that was found to be erroneous. No biochemical mechanism had been demonstrated that fluoride at a concentration of one part per million was likely to cause cancer, or accelerate existing cancer growth. Jauncey made his decision based on science. None the less, fluoride was taken out of the water supply. As a result, Catherine McColl's grandchildren who were after all the *raison d'être* for her litigation, may well, in the light of the region's history, have followed her edentulous journey into adulthood. In March 2006 while recovering from a stroke, Lord Jauncey of Tullichettle could still recall the case clearly and that Doll's evidence was "very impressive".[37]

Doll's *Causes of Cancer* and his support of water fluoridation put him in the telescopic sights of critics who may not have possessed his scien-tific skills but their political influence, was, to quote George Orwell's *1984*, about to make "the clocks strike 13."

One of the people who wished to emphasise the importance of occupational and environmental pollutants, and that there *was* an increase in US cancer onset rates over and above that attributed to tobacco, was Samuel S Epstein. Professor Epstein, a self-confessed "non-epidemiologist"[38] in 1998 devoted an appendix of his book* to Doll. In the opening paragraph the reader is told of Doll's pioneering investigations warning that smoking, and exposure to nickel, asbestos and radioactivity were all causes of cancer. The admiring paragraph concluded, "In the late sixties, Doll could even have been considered a radical."[39] Thereafter Doll's scientific biography is critically reassessed. Professor Epstein portrays Doll as "a major defender of corporate industry interests". He cites eleven examples of Doll's supposed volte-face that include: "In 1976, in spite of well-documented concerns on the risks of fluoridation of drinking water with industrial wastes, Doll declared it was 'unethical' not to do so." And:

> In his 1981 report on causes of cancer mortality in the US in the absence of any scientific evidence, Doll trivialised the role of environmental and occupation causes of cancer. He claimed that occupation was responsible for four per cent of mortality rather than at least twenty per cent, as previously admitted by consultants to the American industrial health council of the Chemical Manufacturers' Association.

The claim that twenty per cent of cancers were a result of the actions of a rapacious chemical industry created an apologia for Big Tobacco. It was a fissure in the edifice of the causes of cancer that they readily exploited. In 1980-81 the American cigarette industry had a record year with the largest increase (two per cent) in cigarette sales for some time. Commenting on this, the chairman of the largest American cigarette manufacturer was reported as saying that he thought the "cancer problem" was no longer hitting sales as hard as before because "so many things have been linked to cancer" that people might be getting sceptical.[40] Tobacco companies defended by the greatest legal minds that money could buy

---

* Epstein, SS *The Politics of Cancer, Revisited* (East Ridge Press, 1998).

would try to cast doubt on tobacco's role in causing cancer. It would be left to scientists like Doll, who felt a moral responsibility not to run away from their scientific discoveries, to face the tobacco lawyers in the American courts.

Doll did not retire early as Hill had done. In fact, he never retired. However, in 1983 his tenure as warden of Green College came to an end. It marked a transition in his life and he was now free to take up a new occupation: full-time cancer research. With emeritus status, he was recruited into the cancer epidemiology unit and Richard Peto's clinical trials studies unit where he embarked on a remarkable Indian summer of epidemiological research spanning 22 years. In 1997 under cross-examination in a Florida tobacco trial, Doll was asked by a lawyer if he knew Richard Peto. Doll replied, "Yes. He was once my protégé, but I'm his now."

Part Four 1984-2005
The Revolution in Public Health
The Doll Legacy

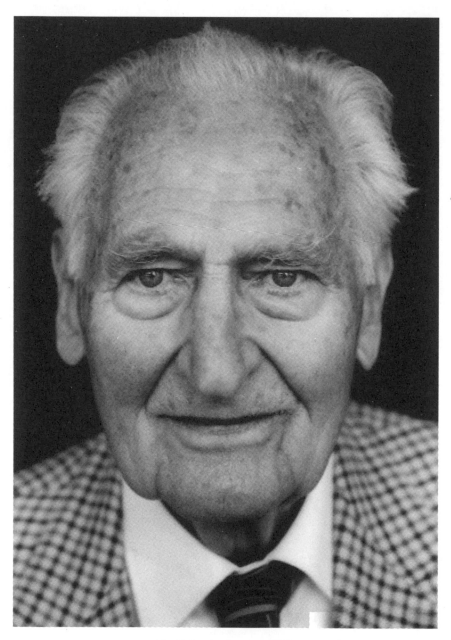

Prodigious retirement, 1998

Chapter 23
Waiting for the Barbarians

"The judiciary mechanism of independent and searching inquiry through the cross-examination and direct confrontation of the ways and methods used by scientists can be of outstanding importance for the quest for truth."

GM Reggiani

When Richard Doll first "retired" in 1979, he was simultaneously the director of the cancer and epidemiology unit at Oxford, the Regius Professor of Medicine at Oxford and the warden of Green College, Oxford. It took three people of international standing to replace him. Malcolm Pike returned from the United States to run the cancer and epidemiology unit, Henry Harris became Regius Professor of Medicine and John (later Lord) Walton became warden of Green College. Doll's second "retirement" in 1983 as warden of Green College neither diminished his energy for work nor his scientific influence. Liberated from medical and academic administration, he now sought to extend the comfortable symbiosis he had with science into his domestic life.

For their retirement Richard and Joan bought 12 Rawlinson Road, a double-fronted Victorian house with a large enclosed garden in leafy liberal-minded North Oxford. Doll wanted the move to represent a break with the past, to mark a new beginning. In 1961 Steve had been employed as their housekeeper but with time she had become a great deal more. With her Calvinist work ethic she had been a housekeeper, child-minder, chauffeur, companion and, during the Green College years, head porter. Steve had been a loyal workhorse. Both Richard and Joan had their vanities and it may, once Joan had retired from the MRC, have been convenient to have Steve drive her around Oxford and "admire her".[1] If the relationship between Joan and Steve was relaxed, that between Doll and Steve, at least from his standpoint, was functional and increasingly unnecessary. The children had long gone: Nicholas to become a GP and Cathy a social worker; the entertaining of visiting dignitaries had now eased, life was going to be altogether more tranquil and Doll wanted Rawlinson Road to be a home for just him and Joan.

So in 1983 Doll tried to end Steve's employment. But the house was large and Steve had nowhere to go so ultimately he relented.[2] That was his last stand. Twenty years later when he became physically frail there was a growing recognition of her worth, and he admitted that he "was probably pleased to have her".[3] The Richard-Joan-Steve relationship was emotionally complex and it transcended the decades, changing function, purpose and obligations. From 1961 until 2001 Richard Doll, Joan Doll and Steve had lived under one roof. Perhaps the one thing that can be said is that throughout those four decades Doll and Steve shared one thing in common: they both loved Joan.

By the time of his formal retirement Doll had become a respected medical statesman trusted as a dispassionate scientist. In this role he was called upon to adjudicate on national and international scientific controversies, and, as with smoking, radiation, and asbestos, these would lead him into political minefields.

All wars cause health problems. The troops who served in Vietnam were no exception and soon after returning home they began to display higher rates of psychiatric disorder, heart disease, alcoholism and alcohol-related disease than the rest of the population. Among them were 46,000 Australian troops of whom 31,000 were wounded and 500 killed. But there had been an extra ingredient in the Vietnam war: in their fight against the elusive Vietcong, the Americans had deployed a new tactic, spraying unthinkable amounts of Agent Orange,* a defoliate herbicide (a 50:50 mixture of butyl esters of 2,4-D and 2,4,5-T) on the forests of Vietnam. The Australian Vietnam Veterans' Association believed that

---

* The name derived from the orange colour of its storage tanks. The chemical was produced by Monsanto, the US chemical giant.

Agent Orange had caused and was causing cancer in the Vietnam veterans, but for more than a decade after the end of the war in 1973, no formal investigation was undertaken.

The situation was changed dramatically on 5 March 1983, when Bob Hawke (who had opposed the war in Vietnam) was elected prime minister of Australia. His political opponents had sent the Australian forces into the war, and he saw it as his administration's duty to appoint a Royal Commission to carry out a judicial inquiry into the use and effects of chemical agents on Australian personnel in Vietnam. There is some difference of opinion over whether the Labour Party government had an open mind on the matter, but no one could doubt the intellectual calibre of the commission's composition and the dramatis personae that appeared before it. The Honourable Mr Justice Phillip Evatt was the commissioner, a decorated submariner, who came from a Labour background. John Coombs* QC assisted the commissioner.** Barry O'Keefe and Graham Ellis represented Monsanto Australia Ltd, whose American parent company manufactured the Agent Orange used in Vietnam.

Doll was not called to testify before the commission but his views permeated its philosophy, and his adjudication of the work of one of the epidemiologists who did give evidence had important and long-lasting repercussions. Epidemiology is the science dealing with the environmental causes of diseases of humans as inferred from observations of human beings. The subject involves the mathematical testing of a possible relationship between a health association and a postulated source of that phenomenon. In this instance, the evidence of a correlation between herbicide use and cancer centred on the work of two Swedish scientists, Dr Olav Axelson and Dr Lennart Hardell. Their epidemiological research was

---

* He was the son of Dr HC Coombs, the economist and public servant. Always know as "Nugget" Coombs, he was a distinguished Keynesian economist and government advisor. In retirement he became chairman of the Australian Council for Aboriginal Affairs.

** His younger brother was Johnny O'Keefe, aka "The Wild One" (1935-78), the pop singer and star of the classic rock'n'roll era of Australian music.

crucial to the Vietnam Veterans' Association of Australia to support their claim that the incidence of lymphomas, or soft tissue sarcomas, or of cancers generally is increased as a consequence of exposure to Agent Orange or other phenoxy herbicides.[4]

From the start, the atmosphere was uncompromising and bruising, with O'Keefe having Hardell's working notes subpoenaed for the commission. Hardell did not want to appear before Justice Evatt, and, according to Ellis, asked for "some outrageous amount of money (in the region of $1,500—about $10,000 in today's money) so Monsanto called his bluff."[5] The commission went to San Francisco where Hardell was cross-examined by O'Keefe.

In any case-control study great care has to be used if the play of chance, bias or confounding are not going to distort the accuracy of the investigation and the relationship between dose and response. Under rigorous cross-examination, Axelson admitted that his study of cancer mortality among railway workers exposed to 2,4,-D, 2,4,5-T could have been the subject of observational bias.[6] This led the commission to conclude "that because of the number of faults, together with the extent of uncertainty or error in the data, Professor Axelson's doubtful positive conclusions should be given little or no weight."[7]

At the time, the only epidemiological evidence to support an association between exposure of humans to phenoxy acids and an increased incidence of soft tissue sarcoma and malignant lymphoma was the work of Hardell. This led the commission to examine his work with forensic diligence. It noted that a ban on the use of 2,4,5-T had been imposed in Sweden in 1979. In August 1977 Hardell published the findings of his research in northern Sweden, where he reported having found seven patients with soft tissue sarcoma and some exposure to phenoxy acids and other herbicides in the ten to twenty years preceding diagnosis. The commission noted in its conclusions that these observations received widespread publicity and that Hardell gave a number of newspaper and radio interviews and appeared on television. This campaigning earned him a reputation for being a "battering ram" against phenoxy herbicides.[8]

Hardell's eminence on the subject was based on three epidemiological investigations among Swedish workers: the north Sweden study concerning the incidence of soft tissue sarcoma; the south Sweden study, also concerning soft tissue sarcoma: and the malignant lymphoma study. During what one lawyer described as "probably the best performance of Barry O'Keefe's career",[9] O'Keefe pointed out that no one had been able to replicate the findings in Hardell's studies relating to soft tissue sarcoma and malignant lymphoma, and the results of his three studies were contrary to the finding of Professor Allan Smith in New Zealand. Under claustrophobic cross-examination Hardell's over-statement of exposure (dose) and shortcomings in methodology were revealed and admitted. In relation to the former, O'Keefe was damning. "The description of the exposure of the cases in the series as 'massive' and 'quite massive' is not only inaccurate, it is emotive. It is not the language of a detached scientist."[10]

The possible danger of bias and its distorting effect on any epidemiological study was also examined in front of Justice Evatt. Hardell was asked by O'Keefe about information bias:

O'Keefe: "And in the case of cancer I put it to you that the existence of controversy and of publicity was one factor that could operate in that regard."
Hardell: "Yes."
O'Keefe: "You may also have information bias?"
Hardell: "Yes."
O'Keefe: "As a result of which there is a differential treatment by the interviewer between cases and controls?"
Hardell: "Yes."[11]

Doll had been following the commission's investigation and felt that Hardell's studies had transgressed the accepted rules of an epidemiological study. On 4 December 1985, after "weighing the evidence", he wrote to Justice Evatt with his independent judgement. He stated that, having examined the documents submitted to him, he was of the opinion that:

your review of Hardell's work with the additional evidence obtained directly from him at interview shows that many of the published statements were exaggerated or non-supportable and that there were many opportunities for bias to have been introduced in the collection of his data. His conclusions cannot be sustained, and, in my opinion, his work should no longer be cited as scientific evidence.[12]

Doll saw it as his professional duty to advise governments, industries and legal investigations on controversial scientific issues. He voluntarily wrote to the Royal Commission with his judgement that methodological errors had engulfed Lennart Hardell's work. Doll's answer to the question of whether exposure to Agent Orange and other herbicides used in the Vietnam war was likely to have caused cancer: on the evidence he had seen was "no".

When the commission delivered its conclusions on Hardell's studies, it judged them as "widely recognised as flawed … unacceptable as proof of the results claimed" and such "that they cannot be taken at face value … Accordingly the commission does not accept the Hardell studies as proving, on the balance of probabilities, any causal association, between Soft Tissue Sarcoma, and Lymphoma and exposure to 2,4,-D. 2,4,5-T, and DDT."[13]

John Mathews was the chief scientific advisor* to the commission and he was not convinced by its "not guilty" verdict on Agent Orange. Mathews had been one of Doll's post-doctoral students in Oxford and would have been happier with the Scottish law verdict of not proven. However, he understood Doll's scientific philosophy and how his scientific mind worked. If Doll could not prove something to be true, then there was uncertainty. This synthesised with his professional conservatism, which Mathews summarised thus: "Effectively Doll puts a minimum estimate and others a maximum estimate and the truth lies somewhere in the middle."[14]

---

*   Mathews together with Coombs and Ellis went to Saigon in 1985 and the communists had kept the Australian embassy exactly as it was in 1975 when the city fell to the Vietcong. They were the first Australians back into the building since the fall of the regime.

The commission's findings and treatment of Axelson and Hardell sent them into a vengeful rage. The unprecedented interaction between medical science and Australian politics led the two Swedish physicians to write to the governor-general of Australia to protest against the handling of their data and evidence by the Royal Commission. Axelson's final paragraph summaries the intensity of their feelings:

> To the extent that the report of this commission achieves appreciation and its viewpoints become the "truth" in Australia, I am afraid that also the mid-80s in Australia might go to the history of science as the time when a Royal Commission's report became a sort of modern substitute for the stake as scientific counter argument. Its flaming lies may cast shades on Royal Commissions.[15]

The volatile dispute then found its way on to the pages of the *Medical Journal of Australia* when Bruce Armstrong, in an idiomatically titled article "Storm in a cup of 2,4,5-T", attempted to bring some balance to an increasingly unbalanced standoff. He recognised the difficulties of the task which the Swedish investigators had set themselves. Trying to provide statistical evidence that a chemical agent causes cancer is fraught with several difficult problems. For example, the long-time interval between exposure to the chemical agent and the onset of the disease, often decades later, is not easy to correlate biologically. Showing compassion to his fellow scientists, Armstrong tried to evaluate how the commission's conclusion regarding Hardell's studies stood up. While acknowledging Hardell's failure to adequately rebut the commission's claims that his methodology* was biased, Armstrong also recognised the

---

* Hardell L and Sandstrom A, 'Case-control Study: soft-tissue sarcomas and exposure to phenoxyacetic acids or chlorophenois', *British Journal of Cancer*, 1979; volume 39, p711-717, and Hardell, L, 'Epidemiological studies on soft-tissue sarcoma and malignant lymphoma and their relationship to phenoxy acid of chlorophenol exposure' (Umea University Press, 1981).

argument that the bias was not sufficient to have undermined Hardell's findings.

One observer thought that there were no derogatory intentions of Hardell as a scientist or any misgivings about his professional skill and eligibility, least of all a falsification of what he submitted as testimony during the "courteous and searching questioning".[16] Mr Justice Phillip Evatt, chairing the proceedings, is on the record requesting repeatedly the examiners to let Hardell answer in his own way. He said, "He (Dr Hardell) is an expert, a scientist and one has to give him the possibility to qualify his answer in his own way."

Armstrong was of the impression that all had not been equal before the law; and that there was a lesson to be learned—for the Royal Commission at least: that sometimes unnecessary personal comments can undermine the acceptance of otherwise sound conclusions. In 1986 Armstrong was way ahead of the game when he wrote this prophetic summation of the destiny of the debate. "Axelson and Hardell are certainly receiving a sympathetic hearing for their grievances among scientists in Europe. In the emotion-filled atmosphere that still surrounds the question of exposure to herbicides in Vietnam, the reactions of Axelson and Hardell could have a significant effect on public acceptance of the commission's findings."[17] Certainly, the findings of the Australian Royal Commission on the use and effects of chemical agents on Australian personnel in Vietnam was a warning for scientists who enter the public arena—the rules and methods of combat are very different; only the fortunate can expect to emerge unscathed.

But what of the real casualties in this story—the Australian Vietnam veterans? They had fought an unpopular war because of a quarrel in a far away country between people of whom they knew little. At least the Royal Commission was successful in persuading the government to provide access to health care for the veterans who were suffering from high levels of alcoholism and post-traumatic stress. However, Bob Hawke's government refused to undertake an investigation into purported birth defects in their children.

While the Australian Vietnam veterans received no compensation, it was a different story for US troops. In 1978 Maude de Victor, a Chicago veterans' caseworker, reported a pattern of cancers and other illnesses suffered by Vietnam veterans and linked those illnesses to exposure to herbicides like Agent Orange and its dioxin counterparts. Studies were carried out on the crews of the UC-123s, the fixed-wing aircraft that carried out the spraying, and the results were negative, except for an excess of adult onset diabetes. Epidemiological studies, too, have found no excess of cancers in the Vietnam veterans, and not one case of chloracne* has been diagnosed among American veterans.

Fearing, however, being swamped in litigation, the administration acted expediently, and in 1991, despite the lack of scientific evidence, untruth prevailed.** The decision to provide financial compensation to Vietnam veterans was a political decision by the Congress of the United States although they knew full well that the science could not establish a cause and effect relationship. It has now entered American folklore that Agent Orange kills people although there is an absence of any epidemiological evidence. The US is paying as presumptive compensation almost $5bn per year to Vietnam veterans who claimed exposure to Agent Orange.

Even such an august body as the International Agency for Research on Cancer (IARC) stated in 1986 that there was "limited evidence"[18] for the carcinogenicity of chlorophenoxy acids as a class. IARC disregarded both the alternative possibilities of "sufficient evidence" that is, a proved case of causal association in humans, as well as, at the other end, the "inadequate evidence" category, that is, that the causal association was not credible.

Doll had always thought it was important for academics to work openly and honestly with industry so that industry could identify occu-

---

* The Ukrainian politician Viktor Yushchenko was diagnosed with chloracne from dioxin poisoning in 2004.
** On 6 February 1991 President George Bush signed the bill. "I am pleased to sign into law H.R. 556, the 'Agent Orange Act of 1991'. The legislation relies on science to settle the troubling questions concerning the effect of veterans' exposure to herbicides—such as Agent Orange—used during the Vietnam war."

pational hazards at an early stage. His objective was to make sense of, or ignore, the cacophony of sound coming from interested parties. The world of occupational exposure and environmental claims was chaotic and there were always going to be periodic alarms coming from vested interests.

This happened in 1984 when Doll was approached by a London-based medical adviser of ICI chemicals called Brian Bennett, who wanted to know whether Doll would carry out a review of the safety of vinyl chloride (which is used in the manufacture of plastics). Bennett told Doll that the Chemical Manufacturers Association, ICI and Dow Chemicals would pay for the investigation. Doll agreed, on the condition that his report would be published whatever it said. The fee was set at £15,000 plus expenses—which Doll asked to be paid to his nominated charity, Green College, Oxford. Doll's 1988 review of the evidence concluded that vinyl chloride was associated with liver cancer but that there was no significant extra carcinogenicity associated with the manufacture of the chemical.[19]

In the final quarter of his life, Doll had given hundreds of thousands of pounds to Green College, which he founded, to enhance academic research in medical sciences. He also gave money to the Medical Foundation for the Victims of Torture. It was a prophetic charitable bene-faction—and while Doll was too formidable to take on in any serious way while alive, he would become a victim of persecution after his death.

In December 2006, more than one year after Doll's death, an article enti-tled "Secret Ties to Industry and Conflicting Interests in Cancer Research" that was later published in the *American Journal of Industrial Medicine* was leaked to the *Guardian* newspaper.[20] The journal article's principal author was Lennart Hardell, and in it Hardell *et al* "revealed" that Doll had "failed to disclose" fees that he received from chemical com-panies. They suggested that these payments undermined Doll's work on the environmental cause of cancer. Hardell's accusations were based on letters found in Doll's archive deposited for public scrutiny at the

Wellcome Trust Library.* Doll did not hide his relationship with industry and the fact that he had documented his ties to industrial epidemiology negated the idea that there was anything "secret" about the association. Doll's 1988 review of the effects of exposure to vinyl chloride,[21] according to Hardell *et al*, "made no declaration of vested interests or payments in relation to chemical companies," and the "article remained the gold standard for more than a decade."

Other scientists who were also accused of a conflict of interest by Hardell *et al* said they were "honoured to be included in the company of the late Sir Richard Doll, even in such a baseless attack."[22] Doll's reputation was based on integrity. Nowadays medical publications have to include disclosure statements about sources of funding but this was not standard practice in the 1970s and 1980s. Doll approved wholeheartedly of its introduction. If Doll did not treat his association with Brian Bennett as a secret, and if he received no direct financial reward for his investigation of vinyl chloride, how does the accusation that his role as a consultant "influenced his statements" stand up?

Vinyl chloride was under scrutiny again in June 2007, when 25 scientists from eight countries met at the International Agency for Research on Cancer to reassess its carcinogenicity. They found that vinyl chloride increases the risk of liver cirrhosis,[23] that it is a risk factor for hepatocellular carcinoma, and that the results provided evidence in humans that vinyl chloride "causes angiosarcoma of the liver and hepatocellular carcinoma."[24] Almost twenty years after Doll's investigation, the only cancer for which there was "sufficient evidence" linking exposure to vinyl chloride was liver cancer. Doll, on the basis of the evidence, and as an independent cancer researcher, had called it right.

Inevitably, the other subjunctive charge of venality made against Doll concerned Agent Orange. In his Wellcome Trust archive, Doll had deposited a letter from George Roush Jr, the director of Monsanto's medicine and environmental health, dated 29 April 1986:

---

*   In 2002 Sir Richard Doll deposited articles, letters and papers from his life in medical research at the Wellcome Institute

Dear Sir Richard

This letter is for the purpose of extending your Consulting Agreement with Monsanto Company dated May 10, 1979. The Consulting Agreement is hereby extended for an additional one year period beginning June 1, 1986 and ending May 31, 1987.

During the one-year period of this extension your consulting fee shall be $1,500.00 per day. All other terms and conditions of the Consulting Agreement of May 10, 1979 shall remain in effect during this extension period.

If the foregoing meets with your understanding and approval, please so indicate by executing this letter in duplicate and returning one of the signed duplicates to us.

On 11 July 1986 Doll wrote to Dr W Gaffey, Monsanto's director of epidemiology: "I greatly appreciate the offer to extend my consulting agreement and for the increased fee, and I have signed and am returning one contract note. I enjoy the meetings with your company and will look forward to another one."

The deliberately misguided impression given by Hardell *et al* was that the $1,500 was paid in perpetuity. The monies only went to Doll's nominated charity on the days that Doll acted as a consultant to Monsanto. Terry Leet was a Monsanto epidemiologist at the time and can remember meeting Doll on at least two occasions in the US. He remembered Doll providing insightful information about how to improve the quality of their research and to communicate it more clearly. "I never got the impression that his work with any organisation prejudiced his scientific independence. On the contrary he was a brilliant epidemiologist who was able to compile evidence from around the world to support or negate the role of occupational or environmental risk factors for specific diseases."[25]

Doll recognised that a direct financial relationship with a company could have suggested accusations that the role of an independent researcher could be called into question. While an MRC employee, all of the investigations he undertook, whether in the gas industry, asbestos industry or nickel industry, were done without payment. Also, in retirement Doll would appear in court cases (sometimes for an expert witness fee and sometimes not) mostly against tobacco companies which were trying to undermine the causal link between smoking and lung cancer. In one such case, in 1997, Doll was questioned by Theodore Grossman* who sought to determine whether Doll was a truly independent scientist, free of the contaminants of secret financial ties. Doll was on oath during the cross-examination.

> Q. "And you have done some consulting work with drug and chemical companies; is that correct?"
>
> A. "I have not been paid for it. I have advised them."
>
> Q. "You have advised them. You have provided advice to pharmaceutical companies?"
>
> A. "Not to my knowledge. Monsanto, I wrote them a very long report on the carcinogenesis of chemicals, on condition they gave something to charity. I have never taken any money from chemical or pharmaceutical companies for giving them advice."
>
> Q. "But you have been, you have happily provided them with advice on epidemiological work on their behalf; is that correct?"
>
> A. "No. I have never done any epidemiological work other than what I wanted to do myself."
>
> Q. "But you have worked with them?
>
> A. "On controlled trials, pharmaceutical companies, yes."
>
> Q. "That is, you have conducted controlled trials on behalf of pharmaceutical companies?"
>
> A. "No, I don't think I ever have. I have done on behalf of the Medical Research Council, and that has had some support, possibly, from the companies."

---

* Sir Richard Doll Defence Discovery Deposition, 15-16 January 1997, Florida. In the United States, the defence (the tobacco lawyers) get the chance to cross-examine the expert witnesses first.

Doll looked upon it as a travesty if the most reputable scientists were not available to advise companies or governments on controversial issues. The ideal for Doll was that quality science should and must be the foundation for public policy and legal discussions. However, he had seen how science could be corrupted by financial dependency on industry and he was not inhibited about revealing it.

On 28 October 2003, his 91st birthday, Doll appeared in the outer house court of session in Edinburgh as an expert witness in the case of McTear v Imperial Tobacco Ltd. Doll was brought to the court to explain the intellectual journey of the acceptance of the idea that smoking was the main cause of lung cancer. When Doll was confronted with the name of Professor Hans Eysenck he was transported back to an altogether unhappier time in the 1960s. Eysenck, like Ronald Fisher before him, promoted the notion that the association between smoking tobacco and lung cancer is not causal, but reflects a predisposition in people with certain genetic or psychological characteristics. Doll and other researchers knew that Eysenck received money directly from the tobacco industry to promulgate theories to undermine the epidemiological evidence. The barrister for Imperial Tobacco Ltd asked Doll about Eysenck's work on introversion and extroversion and the relationship between personality types and the development of lung cancer.

Mr Jones. "I have not heard of a death bed conversion. Did he have one?"
Doll. "No, it was not a death bed conversion, but there was a death bed recognition of where he received his funding."
Mr Jones. "I see. Is the suggestion that you are implying here, Sir Richard, that he was in some way compromised in his integrity because of his funding?
RD "Yes I am saying that. He was a liar"*

---

* On 31 May 2005, Lord Nimmo Smith wrote in his judgement in the case of McTear v Imperial Tobacco Ltd: "Eysenck was on Sir Richard's list of eccentrics; indeed he would go further and come straight out, he was a liar." Interestingly,

Doll knew the rules of the game, and it would have been a departure from his scientific philosophy to transgress in such an uncharacteristic way. He dismissed the validity of Eysenck's work as unscientific and tainted by the source of its funding: clearly if Doll had been receiving secret payments then to deposit evidence of them for public examination in his academic archive would have been grossly inept.

Another scientist, Dr Alvin Young, also served as a consultant on the Australian Royal Commission. An American government scientist, he was there to provide background on the use of herbicides in Vietnam. He too acted as a consultant to both Dow and Monsanto on issues related to Vietnam and Agent Orange, and also advised the Department of Defence on the same issue. "I see it appropriate to provide the best scientific advice that I can to my government. I suspect that Sir Richard viewed this in a similar way."[26]

The malicious attack on Doll by his detractors again revealed his status as epidemiology's custodian and his uncompromising attitude towards inferior research and the partisan reporting of results. As with the Eysenck episode, he spoke out if he felt this had occurred. "Naturally," as Richard Wakeford wrote, "this did not go down well with those on the receiving end of his criticism, and perhaps an element of this can be detected in the article of Hardell *et al*".[27]

Hardell had developed a reputation for finding stronger associations between agents studied and the diseases of interest than other environmental epidemiologists in the field, and by the 1980s he had become "the Swedish champion of cancer scares".[28] He had implicated everything from tampons to breast milk, and used television sets as causing increased cancer risks.

Nimmo Smith in his ruling rejected the evidence of Doll and other medical experts on *causality* mainly because of their association with ASH and because they waived their expert witness fee. Bizarrely, those experts who appeared for Imperial Tobacco Ltd and accepted a fee for appearing in court were given more credence by the judge.

These alarms, according to Inger Atterstam, a Swedish journalist, were prominently featured in the Swedish daily newspaper *Dagens Nyheter*. In 2002 Atterstam decided to investigate Hardell's career and the story took her to the north of Sweden and the University of Umea. While there, Atterstam found that Hardell's superior, Professor Lars-Gunnar Larsson, had discovered gross methodological shortcomings in Hardell's study of the association between herbicides and soft-tissue sarcoma. According to Atterstam's article,* Larsson decided to conduct an entirely new study to check the research and eliminate all suspicions of wrongdoing. This is not how it turned out. Lars-Gunnar Larsson is quoted by Atterstam as saying: "What happened was extremely traumatic. One of the worst things I have experienced."

Doll and Hill in their innovatory epidemiological studies had emphasised the need to check for bias at every opportunity. To prevent any bias entering into Hardell's study, the questionnaire responses from the participants who had developed cancer (the cases) and the healthy controls would be sent unopened to another department at the University of Umea and not to Hardell personally. The responses would then have their identity removed and no one knew which were the cases and which were the control group; then an unbiased assessment could be made of dose (exposure to herbicide) and response.

No such probity, however, was discovered by Professor Larsson. Instead, Inger Atterstam's article reported that it was discovered that questionnaire responses from several cases, posted in groups in separate envelopes from a few post offices in Borrbotten province and from Sundsvall, did not correspond to the respondents' home addresses: "In a report that remains confidential to this day, it was established that Lennart Hardell had collected the questionnaires himself, put them into new envelopes and, either by himself or with the help of someone else, posted them in groups from various post stations." Perhaps now, as Barry O'Keefe wrote in 1988: "The Hardell studies should now be laid to rest."**

---

*   *Svenska Dagbladet*, 19 September 2002.

**   In Young AL, Reggiani GM (editors), *Agent Orange and its Associated Dioxin:*

Richard Doll, probably remembering his days on the retreat to Dunkirk, was heard to say once: "Everything I need I could get in one rucksack."[29] He was interested in money but he was not for sale. For Steve Sutherland, Doll was "a man of the highest integrity—you could trust him to the end of the earth. To me that is his greatest virtue."[30] As a scientist he was called upon to adjudicate in some of the most emotive medical issues of our times, and the more responsibility people take on, the more enemies they can make. Doll's relationship to industry and government was transparent and documented in his archive for all to see. The danger, however, was obvious. If incorrect statements* are repeated frequently, they might finally come to represent the truth. In December 2006 some of Doll's scientific colleagues sought to right the wrong in the letters column of the *Guardian*, the newspaper that first published the allegations. They wrote: "To this day and in the years to come, many tens of millions of people in the developed world will owe their lives and health to his skills. He should be remembered with fondness, respect, and gratitude."**

Assessment of a Controversy (Elsevier, 1988).

*   *The Weekend Australian*, 9-10 December 2006 under the headline "Scientist was on Agent Orange payroll" by Clara Pirani. "Ron Coxon, national president of Vietnam Veterans' Association in Australia said Sir Richard's connection to Monsanto should have been revealed. 'At the time, we suspected that some of the experts giving evidence might have had links to companies, but we didn't know,' Mr Coxon said, 'I think it's disgusting but I'm not surprised. At the time, there was medical evidence of the damage that herbicides caused, but the problem was there were experts like Richard Doll who had come out and said there was no link.'"

**   *The Guardian*, 9 December 2006. Letter from Professor Colin Blakemore, chief executive of the MRC; Dr Mark Walport, director of the Wellcome Trust; Martin Rees, president of the Royal Society; Professor John Bell, president of the Academy of Medical Science; Professor Alex Markham, chief executive of Cancer Research UK.

Chapter 24

Nature, Nurture and Luck

"Harm of a new sort or of an unfamiliar origin is considered worse than harm that is familiar. Risks that are endured by choice are of less concern than those that are suffered involuntarily."

Richard Doll

In the 1980s the nation and public health agencies were anxious. With the advent of the acquired immune deficiency syndrome (HIV/Aids) the fear grew that a human catastrophe was unfolding. Humans are not the only biological organisms that change. Micro-organisms continue to evolve and when changes occur in those that infect humans, new epidemics result. From the days of leprosy and bubonic plague onwards,[1] governments had fought epidemics with legislation as well as information, and laws had been on the statute books since the Public Health Act of 1875.[2] Predicting the path of epidemics is notoriously difficult and while Doll and the science of epidemiology had succeeded in plotting the lung cancer epidemic, the ethical questions surrounding HIV/Aids were execrable. With both a vaccine and a cure many years away, the immediate task was to find out if the epidemic was growing. People felt they were living on the frontier between life and death.

Historically, unlike other casually contagious diseases, sexually transmitted diseases had inflamed the sensibilities of mid-Victorian legislators and prophylactic laws had been passed, found to fail, and subsequently abandoned. The decisive experiment was the Contagious Diseases acts, passed in the 1860s in the hope of preventing the British armed forces being defeated by syphilis. Desperate diseases may require desperate remedies. The acts specified that in named ports and garrison towns the police should be empowered to detain any woman suspected of being a prostitute, compel her to undergo medical examination, and, if she were found to be infected, enforce treatment.

The acts aroused great hostility from feminists incandescent at the use of the double standard, while Sir John Simon, one of the nation's leading doctors, thought the legislation a perversion of medicine and sure to threaten professional integrity. Pressure from all sides brought their repeal in 1886. Since then public policy for combating sexually transmitted disease has been voluntary. It is a misfortune not a crime to contract a disease but by December 1986 it was already a criminal offence knowingly to infect someone with the human immuno-defi-ciency virus (HIV) in New South Wales. Various Canadian provinces had made Aids a notifiable disease, and had proposition 64* been approved in California drastic powers would have been available to police the lives of sufferers.

Doll's epidemiological involvement with Aids dated from a visit in the 1980s made by Sir James Gowans, secretary of the MRC, to Donald Fredrickson, the director of the National Institutes of Health (NIH) in the US. The infection was known to have been present in the US in 1978 and several years earlier in tropical Africa.[3] At the time the vast majority of cases in the developed world had been in male homosexuals, drug addicts who injected drugs intravenously and patients who had received intra-venous injections of whole blood or blood products. The spread of the infection was not, however, limited to the two principal modes of recep-tive anal intercourse and intravenous injection. The experiences of spouses of infected haemophiliacs showed that infection could be trans-mitted from male to female by vaginal intercourse, and the results of studies in Haitian men in New York and Miami showed that it could be transmitted in the opposite direction.

Gowans, a former student of Howard Florey, was an immunologist, and he went to Fredrickson with a simple inquiry. "We don't have many cases of HIV/Aids in the UK, what is your advice about how to contain

---

*   Proposition 64 was a proposition in the state of California in the November 4 1986 ballot. It was a statute that would have added Acquired Immune Deficiency Syndrome (Aids) to the list of communicable diseases. It was defeated by 71 per cent to 29 per cent. Opponents characterised it as an effort to force HIV-positive individuals out of their jobs and into quarantine.

it?"[4] Unfortunately the NIH did not have an answer. In 1986, 19,000 cases had been reported in the US; this suggested a reservoir of infection some 50 to 80 times greater than the number of reported cases. Gowans returned to the UK and in the British tradition "cobbled together" an Aids directorate which brought a scientific armoury to bear on all aspects of the disease. Max Perutz ran the chemotherapy programme, Robin Weiss oversaw the serology and the search for antibodies, and Doll was appointed chairman of the epidemiological subcommittee of the Medical Research Council's working party on Aids. In the mid-1980s in the UK a central question facing medical scientists was how prevalent was the disease.

Doll, calling on his knowledge as a founder of the National Blood Service, came up with an ingenious idea for Gowans. One way of measuring the spread of HIV/Aids in the heterosexual community was to use the blood samples from women in obstetric departments. Obviously all the women were sexually active and as the blood was going to be disposed of it would be a simple procedure to analyse the samples and monitor the spread of the infection through society. Gowans was keen on the idea and sought approval from Sir Donald Acheson, the chief medical officer of health. Acheson told Gowans that he was "vehemently against the idea and even said it was 'unethical and bad epidemiology'."[4] His reasoning for describing it as unethical was that if a "positive" was found it was not possible to do anything about it.

Gowans then took the idea to the full council of the MRC* but they rejected it as being "too political". For a sexually transmitted disease, society needed to know the degree of heterogeneity in sexual activity that prevails in the population, for as Julian Peto pointed out: "The behaviour

---

*   The MRC, according to James Gowans, had been criticised for not doing enough to determine a scientific understanding of the disease, and Lord Jellicoe, chairman of the Medical Research Council and a subsequent trustee of the National Aids Council, had been reported as saying "Why don't we leave it to the clever Americans to [to find the answers]." This exasperated many within the British scientific community.

of the most promiscuous one or two per cent may be more influential than the average number of partners in determining the rate of spread of venereal disease. This neglected part of disease epidemiology may be important to limit the Aids epidemic."[6]

Doll and Gowans knew that the only firm conclusion, however, was that without better epidemiological data on transmission, contact and seropositivity rates they could not predict the eventual scale of the epidemic or plan effective action to limit it.

Fearing the possible loss of hundreds of thousands of lives, they decided to act. They wrote an article, which they hoped would be published in *The Lancet*, stating: "The idea that the disease would be self-limiting, because it was restricted to promiscuous male homosexuals and drug addicts and others who shared needles for injection is clearly untrue." The evident spreading of the disease outside its original spheres of containment* (in truth little was known about the evolution of the disease) and the social stigma that it carried presented great difficulties. Medical science can cause volatility and public or ethical disquiet. This had been true of the implications of Snow's finding in the middle of the nineteenth century and of Doll and Hill's investigations a century later.

---

*   Doll carried out three investigations into the spread of the disease within haemophiliacs. With Sarah Darby doing the statistical analysis they measured the incubation of the virus in haemophiliacs. It was a complete population many of whom had been given transfusions from imported, bought blood, from the US— some from infected drug-users. This blood proved to be a motorway for infection. Working closely with Dr Charles Rizza at the Oxford Haemophilia Centre, a collection of national data on HIV infection in haemophiliac patients was undertaken. In April 1987 Doll wrote to Dr Rizza: "I enclose a graph showing the survival time of haemophiliac patients following seroconversion. As only two of your 131 patients were classed as dying of Aids compared with that of haemophiliacs who do not convert—partly because it makes a more interesting graph and partly because some of the deaths could perhaps have been due to Aids though not described as such. The numbers are small and the graph is consequently not smooth, but it suggests that after three years some 17 per cent have died."

Public health involves a subtle balance between the rights of the individual and the collective well-being of the wider society: and Doll's campaign for the anonymous testing of Aids set him on a collision course with the law.

Gowans obtained the Treasury solicitor's views on their initiative and wrote to Doll that the legal advice was unambiguous: "Testing blood without consent is regarded as unlawful and that the taker of the sample and those authorising him would be guilty of assault and battery."[7] Both Gowans and Doll wanted to let the public know the obstacles they were up against and to this end they sought the advocacy of Sir Donald Acheson. Gowans asked Lord Jellicoe "to make a last ditch attempt to discover why Donald was still unhappy with our paper. He failed."[8] Acheson then visited Doll at 12 Rawlinson Road but the meeting was not a success. In a letter to Gowans dated 8 December 1986 Doll wrote, "He still doesn't like the idea of anonymous testing, though I couldn't make out the reason for his objection."

On the same date Acheson wrote to Doll about their Saturday afternoon meeting.

> Dear Richard
> I'm glad I came to see you. I will write from the office about the points you raised re Haemophiliacs etc. Perhaps I could come again sometime in the New Year.
>   As far as any future press coverage of your article of course my remarks about free condoms are non-attributable—too 'deeply held!'
>   I hope it will go into *BMJ* /*Lancet* and I hope to avoid any implication of it being an official view—it will be on a personal basis.
> As ever
> Donald

However, even after much letter "bombardment" it was still not enough to persuade the editor of *The Lancet* to accept the article advocating anonymous testing. Nor indeed was Stephen Lock, the editor of the *British Medical Journal*, convinced by their thinking; he told Doll over the phone that the article was "too anodyne". Undefeated and standing up for what he believed in, Doll wrote a letter to the *BMJ*, which Lock published on 24 January 1987:

Sir, - For the past six months I have been seeking to obtain the support of doctors for the conduct of surveys to determine the prevalence of infection with the acquired immune deficiency syndrome (Aids) in the general population. I have sought this as chairman of the epidemiological subcommittee of the Medical Research Council's working party on Aids. So far I have failed to obtain it. This causes my colleagues on the subcommittee and me serious concern as the public health authorities and the general public need to have reliable information about the prevalence of infection and the rate at which that prevalence is changing. For this purpose we need information about the prevalence of infection and the rate at which that prevalence is changing. For this purpose we need information relating to more representative sections of the population than those currently being studied (blood donors, patients attending sexually transmitted disease clinics, etc). We agreed that at present it is unacceptable to test an individual's blood and to tell him or her the result if consent for the test to be done has not been given. We are asking therefore only that random samples of blood taken for other purposes should be tested in such a way that the individual is unidentified, except for sex, age, and residential district. Such samples might, for example be obtained from antenatal clinics or casualty departments.

Three objections to this proposal have been raised: that it is unethical, illegal, and imperfect. How it can be unethical is incomprehensible, as it can do no possible harm to anyone and could do much good. If it is illegal the medical profession has been acting illegally for many years and the sooner the law is changed the better. That the proposal is imperfect, because we cannot relate positive samples to specified individuals whose liability to risk cannot be determined, is a more serious objection; but if we cannot inform people of the result without having had their consent for the test to be done we have no alternative. We have a better opportunity for checking the epidemic in Britain at an early stage than many other European countries and we need to take every practicable step that will help us to do so. The testing of unidentified blood samples in the way we propose is, in our opinion, one such step.

Gaining a biological and epidemiological understanding of Aids was the most pressing issue facing British medical scientists. Doll did not toe the establishment line; instead he took on the role of the rebel. He campaigned to shift the balance away from the risks of doing something, and take into account the risks of not doing the research, which might kill thousands—if not tens of thousands—of people every year.

Doll's crusade for the protection of society by the application of science was again thwarted in 1987 by a fusion of politics and ethics. In a letter to Dr M Whissen, deputy director of the blood transfusion service* in Perth, Australia, he described the changing parameters within which medical research was going to have to operate:

> I have had support from nearly everyone concerned with the problem in England except unfortunately from those in the Department of Health who advise them, and the parliamentary committee which considered the question rejected expert medical opinion in favour of a quite irrational statement by a lawyer who has set himself up as a medical ethicist.
>
> It is odd why there has been such a change in attitude over the last 20 to 30 years... My advice has been to carry on making use of laboratory material in the way we have in the past without referring to ethical committees on the grounds that no ethical question is in reality raised!... I suspect moreover that the majority of the population would support

---

* In 1989, Doll was in a team led by Sarah Darby, which carried out three investigations into HIV/Aids in haemophiliacs. They reported "a substantial burden of fatal disease among patients positive for HIV who have not been formally diagnosed having Aids." 'Incidence of Aids and excess in the United Kingdom: report on behalf of the directors of haemophilia centres in the United Kingdom', *British Medical Journal*, 1989; Volume 298, pp. 1064-1068.

us, but unfortunately the only voices that are ever heard are those of the enthusiastic minorities as, for example, in the case of the anti-fluoridisers.

The custodian of moral law that Doll referred to was Professor Ian Kennedy, professor of law and ethics at University College London. When Doll's suggestion of the anonymous testing of pregnant women for HIV seropositivity was discussed by a House of Commons select committee it was fiercely opposed by Kennedy, who, despite assurances that no positive result could be traced back to the particular woman, said that it was a violation of her rights.* The committee accepted this, and the introduction of such testing was delayed by a number of years.

The worrying misunderstanding of unsupported ethical assertions— that led the committee to conclude that "we are therefore unable to recommend the general use of anonymised screening at this time"—created a sense of incredulity among some leading scientists. Doll together with like-minded colleagues made his views known in *The Lancet*, objecting to the logic upon which the decision had been arrived at, and calling for it to be reversed.[9] For Doll the alarming feature was the seemingly irresistible ascendancy of certain ethical considerations over all others. The incremental advance of ethicists into the work of medical researchers had become so pervasive that by the end of the century it would have been impossible for Doll to undertake either his 1950s studies linking smoking to cancer, or his pioneering work on the cause of leukaemia in patients with ankylosing spondylitis.

So what had changed? Why had the Hippocratic oath, which had sustained its pre-eminence since the time of Galen, been diluted in the final decades of the twentieth century? As with so much in Richard Doll's life the explanation may be found in the Second World War. The experiments

---

* 'Problems associated with Aids. Third report from the social services committee, session 1986-87'. Volume 1: Report together with proceedings of the Committee. (HMSO, 1987).

carried out on concentration camp victims by doctors like Josef Mengele who intertwined his roles as an SS officer and physician in Auschwitz-Birkenau were revealed at the Nuremberg trials in 1947. In Nazi concentration camps, the doctors' duty to care for their patients became debased, and the international community in the post-war era sought to restrict medical research with a new ethical code. This was the pre-history to the establishment of the World Medical Association's Declaration of Helsinki of 1964. In its forty-year lifetime, the declaration has been revised five times, rising to a position of prominence as a guiding statement of ethical principles for doctors involved in medical research. The Declaration of Helsinki was designed to prevent a Mengele from conducting eugenic experiments, not to stop benevolent research into the mysteries of virulent epidemics. In 2004, in the Witts lecture theatre of the Radcliffe Infirmary where researchers discussed the increasing restrictions to patient records, Doll in his 92nd year said. "If it was thought to serve a useful purpose I would be quite willing to go to prison over this"—and he meant it.[10] His colleague Sir Richard Peto countered, "You're too saintly. No judge would send you down."

Doll *et al* had stated in *The Lancet* that the testing of pregnant women ought to raise no ethical difficulties provided they are asked whether or not they wished to know if they are infected. On 24 November 1989 the Government announced that unlinked anonymous HIV surveys would begin in January 1990 in order to monitor the prevalence of HIV infection in England and Wales. The populations were selected either because of or regardless of their risks of HIV infection. The surveys included a survey of antenatal serology specimens from 120,000 women.* Today all pregnant women are asked to undergo an HIV test, but they can opt out if they want to. Nearly all mothers have them now as part of routine screening.

---

* Public Health Laboratory Service, Communicable Disease Report Weekly Edition 98/48. 1 December 1989. p. 1.

Doll received the Royal Society's Royal Medal in 1986 in recognition of his "pioneering use of statistics and epidemiological techniques to evaluate environmental factors of disease". A non-conformist at heart, Doll was a member of that most British of species—the scientific intellectual. Influenced by those such as HG Wells, JBS Haldane and John Desmond Bernal, he formed a link with the past, believing in the social function of science and "getting the facts absolutely right."[11] The ability to put into perspective the major and minor causes of disease was not a theoretical exercise; he was conscious that his conclusions must not be wrong as people's lives and livelihoods were at stake. More than a generation after he had begun his investigations into the hazards of radiation in 1954, the public unease at the questions of morality and safety raised by thermonuclear science brought Doll back into the centre of a number of highly emotive epidemiological investigations.

On 14 August 1945 the dean of St Albans had showed his disapproval of the use of the atomic bomb by prohibiting the use of St Albans abbey for a civic service of thanksgiving for peace. "I did not hold a service," he said, "because I cannot honestly give thanks to God for an event brought about by a wrong use of force by an act of wholesale, indiscriminate massacre which is different in kind from all the acts of open warfare hitherto, however brutal and hideous." From its inception, the nuclear age was set against a background of public unease about whether Britain was right to have an atom bomb and H-bomb national defence policy. Certainly the idealism of using nuclear energy for civil purposes—of creating good out of evil for the benefit of the human race—came a distant second to the first priority of producing bombs during the Cold War. In 1956 the Queen opened Calder Hall, the first civil nuclear power station in the world—an event that perfectly reflected the concept of the "white heat of technology" that Prime Minister Harold Wilson would allude to in his speech at the Scarborough Labour Party conference of 1963. Conversely in 1961 the left-wing newspaper, *Tribune*, had attached to its masthead the slogan "The paper that leads the anti H-bomb campaign." As the world's third thermonuclear power, Britain entered a new anthropological period; and Doll—both alone and in collaboration with others—became one of the world's leading experts on the effects of ionising radiation.

Britain's H-bombs were conceived and made at Aldermaston, and tested in four weapons trials, code-named *Grapple*, in the Pacific in 1957 and 1958.[12] The plutonium for the weapons came from the Windscale plant in Cumbria, and, remarkably, Britain developed its H-bomb programme with only 21 weapons tests, while the Soviet Union and the US carried out hundreds of detonations. The experiences of the thousands of test participants, many of them young National Servicemen most of whom had never been abroad, or flown in an aircraft, before their long flight to Christmas Island, became a matter of great public concern. The island left indelible memories in the minds of the British military personnel. It was the largest coral atoll in the world with an area of 248 square miles, half of it land and half lagoons. It had been named by Captain Cook, who had landed there at Christmas 1777; he and the crew of HMS *Resolution* had stayed there for several days. He found no inhabitants, and no trace of previous inhabitation. Despite its sunshine, beaches, and plantations of coconut palms, it was hardly an island paradise—there was no fresh water and it was infested with evil-smelling land-crabs. The Polynesians called Christmas Island Abakiro: "the far away island". It is 1,450 miles from Tahiti and 1,335 from Honolulu; San Francisco is 3,250 miles away and Sydney 4,000.

On 28 April 1958, Ken McGinley, a Royal Engineer from Renfrewshire, was nineteen years old when, along with hundreds of other British servicemen, he was lined up on a beach while eleven miles away a three-megaton hydrogen bomb was detonated 2,500 metres above the sea.* "At the moment of detonation there was a flash. At that instant I was

---

*   Local radioactivity contamination at Christmas and Malden Islands was minimal because there were no ground or tower bursts—which drew up large quantities of soil and rock, much of which returns to earth as heavy particles of local fall-out. All seven big explosions were high airbursts, and the debris was mostly carried very high into the upper atmosphere, to be slowly diffused over great distances. The Christmas Island hospital had no cases of radiation sickness caused by high radiation exposures, and the medical staff's chief worries had been dysentery and sunburn.

able to see straight through my hands—I could see all the veins, I could see the blood, I could see the skin tissue, I could see all the bones, and worst of all, I could see the flesh itself. It was like looking into a white-hot diamond, a second sun."[13] McGinley's health suffered in the years after his experiences in the Pacific and in 1967 he was diagnosed as being sterile. He blamed his disabilities on atomic radiation.

It was not, however, until 1983 that Ken McGinley founded the British Nuclear Test Veterans Association. A sincere man, McGinley became a symbol of the perceived injustice, which he termed a "war crime", conferred on the veterans.[14] Many of the veterans were by then approaching the ages when cancers became more frequent, and anecdotally the feeling grew that their exposure to radiation in the Pacific was responsible for cases of the disease. In the same year, their concern and publicity in the media led the Ministry of Defence to commission the National Radiological Protection Board to carry out a study by Doll and others to find out if the veterans' exposure to radiation had caused an excess of cancer.[15] In 1988, about ninety per cent of the test participants were still alive and they presented a unique opportunity to evaluate how their experiences in Australia and the Pacific between 1952 and 1968 imprinted itself on their life expectancy or not.

Total mortality, cancer deaths and cancer incidence were studied in 22,347 men who took part in the test programme in Australia and the Pacific Ocean and 22,326 controls who had served in the tropics from the same archives but had not witnessed any thermonuclear explosions. *The Lancet* described the undertaking as "one of the most formidable epidemiological studies ever".[16] The results of the study published in January 1988 showed that the total mortality of the participants, and also their mortality from cancer were lower than expected from the experience of the whole population of England and Wales—something that was anticipated because of the selection that required the participants to be fit for service overseas—but that both were similar to that of the control group of servicemen.[17]

There were, however, two notable differences: namely, excesses of leukaemia and multiple myeloma (MM) in the participants in comparison with the service controls. Doll's attention was drawn to these two diseases because if there had been exposure to ionising radiation the logical cancers to expect would include leukaemia and MM. The large difference between the two groups in the mortality from leukaemia and MM (22 deaths from leukaemia and six from MM in the participants against six from leukaemia and none from MM in the controls) was mainly due, according to Doll's colleague Sarah Darby, professor of medical statistics at Oxford University, "to the deficit in the controls rather than an excess in the participants".[18] At the time Doll was unable to come up with a satisfactory explanation for the unusually low incidence among the control group. The authors believed that in "mortality among participants, some of the differences between the values were due to the chance occurrence of very low mortality in the controls."

The painstaking examination of the complex records did not provide the mitigating evidence that the British Nuclear Test Veterans Association hoped for if their claims for compensation from the Ministry of Defence were to be persuasive. But their quest for compensation and moral exoneration was not entirely ruled out by Doll *et al* in 1988 when they wrote, "The evidence related to multiple myeloma and leukaemia (other than chromic lymphatic leukaemia) is confusing, and on balance it is concluded that there may well have been small hazards of both diseases associated with participation in the programme, but their existence is certainly not proven, and further research is desirable."

Commenting on the study in a leading article in January 1988 in the *British Medical Journal*, Martin Gardner, professor of medical statistics at the MRC's environmental epidemiology unit, wrote, "The preferred conclusion so far must surely be that some leukaemias, and probably multiple myelomas, have resulted from radiation exposure during the tests. This is a stronger conclusion than the authors are prepared to reach because of the lack of certainty in the findings." Leukaemia had, however, been the first cancer to show an excess among survivors of the Japanese bombs and rates of multiple myeloma rose among them after a latent period of some fifteen years, according to the Atomic Bomb Casualty Commission and the Radiation Effects Research Foundation.

The Ministry of Defence, which commissioned the study, regarded the 1988 results* "as fully vindicating its view that the radiological protection measures adopted were effective and that the chance of anyone suffering harm to health as a consequence of participation is extremely small."[19]

For Doll, however, the investigation had raised too many questions not to be extended, and he was "adamant" that a further analysis was required to remove unexplained anomalies and establish scientifically authoritative findings. After all, some 17 per cent of participants, mainly those serving in the Royal Air Force or Army, were not on the original lists and hence were excluded from the study. Some of the army personnel were missed because their service records had been removed as disability claims had been made. There was also the discovery that the cancer experience of the controls had been surprisingly low, which contrasted with accusations of the test veterans that many of their members who had contracted cancer were absent from the study. Accordingly, the Ministry of Defence agreed to a recommendation from the study's authors to continue to observe mortality and cancer rates for a further seven years' follow-up. In the second study, a group of participants who had been omitted from the records initially provided by the MOD and identified independently by other bodies, including the British Nuclear Test Veterans Association, were included. This was published in 1993.[20]

The second study found that between January 1984 and December 1990 the number of cases of multiple myeloma in the participants was

---

* "The lower mortality in the participants to the controls from both chronic bronchitis and lung cancer suggested to the authors that the participants may have smoked less, perhaps as a result of a greater response to health education." At a meeting of the British Nuclear Test Veterans Association in London, Doll congratulated the assembled men for quitting smoking. However, Colin Muirhead, an NRPB statistician also in attendance, recalled: "As the meeting ended, *en masse* the audience lit up and a blue haze enveloped the hall ... "

three while in the controls it was six. For leukaemia the cases in the participants numbered six while in the controls the cases numbered eleven. So between the first and second studies there had been almost a complete reversal between participants and controls in the occurrence of cancers that were known to have an association with ionising radiation. The authors concluded

> that participation in the nuclear weapons programme has not had a detectable effect on the participants' expectation of life, or on their risk of developing cancer or other fatal diseases. The suggestion from a previous study that participants may have experienced small hazards of leukaemia and multiple myeloma is not supported by the additional data, and the excesses observed previously now appear likely to have been a chance finding, although the possibility that test participation may have caused a small risk of leukaemia in the early years after the tests cannot be completely ruled out.

Doll had decided to undertake these complicated studies to investigate the claims that the test veterans were dying because of their exposure to radiation in Australia and the Pacific Ocean. He had great respect for the armed forces forged on the beaches at Dunkirk and sacrifices at Salerno. The fact that the data gathered did not show an excess of deaths from all causes among the test veterans compared to the control population—and was lower than the national population*—should have been a cause for celebration. Instead, some criticised the authors for the findings and Doll was labelled a "government stooge" because the report's conclusions exonerated the government from claims for compensation made by the British Nuclear Test Veterans Association. On 13 June 1998 the British soldiers and civilians who witnessed the weapons tests had their

---

* The mortality from all causes and from all neoplasms was similar in both groups and less than expected from national rates; the only notable excess of deaths when compared with national rates was from accidents and violence, which occurred equally in both groups.

claim for compensation rejected by the European Court of Human Rights in Strasbourg.

It was true that the authors of the reports had very limited information on radiation exposure levels, but by excavating every available data source their investigation was, according to Darby, "quite a challenge—but we were successful."[21] She described the report's conclusions as "very good news" for the test veterans and claimed to be baffled by the veterans' insistence that they were still suffering. "The veterans have vested interests I haven't," she said, "I'm only interested in what the data points to."[22]

Over the decades that Doll studied radiation he had politically and professionally metamorphosed from being an active communist in a nascent discipline to becoming a liberal democrat who was the most influential medical scientist in Britain. He had, after all, helped found the Medical Association for the Prevention of War, which had pre-dated the Campaign for Nuclear Disarmament. By the 1970s, however, he had come to the view that nuclear power was far less polluting than any other existing form of power generation. He recognised the contribution that wind and solar power could make in conjunction with energy conservation, but he believed the nuclear industry was arguably essential to the economic survival of western civilisation, and in terms of avoiding dangerous pollution.

While working on the first study into the test veterans, Doll had come out of retirement and was acting director of the cancer and epidemiology unit. In 1989 Professor Valerie Beral succeeded him as director. "Before I came to Oxford I would have said that 'Doll the establishment man' was the prevalent view, but when I got to know him that wasn't true."[23] Doll's work was recognised throughout the world and his integrity and contribution to the health of humanity won him many awards and honorary doctorates. Perhaps the one he was most proud of was the Ettore Majorana – Erice - Science for Peace Prize, which was presented to him in the beautiful Sicilian town of Erice in 1990. Peace and science were as close to Doll's heart when he wrote his paper on the *Bravo* detonation in 1954 as they were when he studied the mortality and the incidence of cancer in the men who took part in the atmospheric nuclear weapons tests in Australia and the Pacific Ocean. *

By now Doll was eighty years old and many of the political causes that had directed his life were extinct or so corrupted that they left him cold. But one element in his political past that continued to be a bright shining light involved the bonds of friendship made in the time when left-wing politics was synonymous with equality, decency and the fight against fascist injustice. WH Auden's description of the 1930s as "a mean and despicable decade" captured the spirit of the times, and the appalling social conditions, malnutrition and poverty had instilled in Doll an unshakable belief that society had been sleep-walking into a cataclysm and that something had to be done to end people's suffering. In 1992 his friend Alex Tudor Hart, a communist who served with distinction in a field-operating theatre in the Spanish Civil War, was dying in the Radcliffe Infirmary where Doll often visited him. Doll had supported the Spanish Republic in the 1930s raising money for the Medical Aid Committee and he had a deep admiration for Tudor Hart's sacrifice because his involvement in Spain had been to the detriment of his medical career. Tudor Hart was a strong-willed individual and he was unafraid of death. On his final visit Doll showed a side of his character that was rarely seen. "He wanted to die and had refused food. He wasn't able to speak so I kissed him on the cheek. I could see from his eyes that he appreciated the comradeship."

---

* In July 2006 Roy Prescott, an ex-service man who was exposed to radiation in weapons tests, was awarded $75,000 compensation by the United States, which considered that his lung cancer was caused by radiation released in tests. Prescott was a member of the Royal Engineers who was seconded to the US military when it was testing its nuclear bombs off Christmas Island in the Pacific. He told the *Guardian* newspaper on 26 July 2006: "I am a casualty of the Cold War and, whilst I am pleased that I am receiving compensation and recognition from the US government, it really galls me lying here, a critically ill man, that the British government continue to fail in their duty of care towards me and thousands of other nuclear test veterans by denying that we were exposed to radiation during service."

By the early 1990s Doll had given evidence in numerous legal cases. It was an activity that he found exciting, and his sharp mind and precise use of language made him a formidable expert witness. He felt it to be his duty to disseminate knowledge beyond the scientific community, and he agreed with the mathematician AFM Smith that the discipline of statistics is "vital to the honest and decent conduct of public affairs".[24] Yet seldom in contemporary British history did statistics arouse greater public concern than over the discovery of an unexpectedly large number of cases of leukaemia in young people living near the Sellafield nuclear reprocessing plant in north-west England.

Between October 26 1992 and June 29 1993, the civil law cases of Reay versus British Nuclear Fuels (BNF) plc and Hope versus BNF plc were heard simultaneously in the High Court of Justice, London. These two personal injury actions were among the longest, most expensive and most complex to come before the English courts.[25] Doll's testimony was crucial to the outcome of what in effect became a public inquiry into the putative hazards of the nuclear industry. It was a bruising encounter for all involved and the nation's attention was trained on the unfolding drama.

Leukaemia is a rare disease. The incidence of childhood leukaemia in the United Kingdom is around one in 2,000. Clusters of childhood leukaemia were noted before nuclear installations existed,[26] but with the advent of the Windscale fire in October 1957*, the world's first major reactor accident, the phrase radioactive contamination came to the fore. The fire did not give rise to any seriously high radiation doses and no

---

* In November 1957 seventeen miners were killed and eleven injured in a mining disaster at Kames colliery, in Ayrshire. Most people soon forgot the Kames tragedy, but the Windscale accident where there were no deaths and no known injuries captured the headlines and preoccupied politicians. This was because atomic energy was a special case, involving international relations, the defence of the realm and national prestige.

immediate medical response was required. A committee of inquiry appointed by the government was satisfied that it was in the "highest degree unlikely" that any harm was done to the health of people in the area, the workers at the Windscale plant, or members of the general public. Few people in the country understood much about nuclear power, knowing only that it was a futuristic technology in which Britain proudly led the world. But the accident at Windscale undermined Churchill's description of nuclear power as "a perennial fountain of world prosperity" and Windscale itself began its process of transmutation in the public consciousness.

Questions about the incidence of childhood leukaemia near nuclear power stations were not first raised in the scientific literature but by a Yorkshire Television First Tuesday documentary, *Windscale: the Nuclear Laundry*, broadcast on 1 November 1983. James Cutler, a television producer, had gone to west Cumbria to gather information for a programme on the health of employees at the British Nuclear Fuels reprocessing plant at Sellafield (formerly known as Windscale). With the help of a local GP, Cutler's research team discovered that seven children and young adults had leukaemia diagnosed between 1956 and 1983, whereas less than one case of leukaemia would normally be expected among residents at those ages.

Public interest was intense and it was widely believed that discharges from the Sellafield site had caused the cancers.[27] Fears were compounded by the discovery of deposits of nuclear waste in the estuary near the reprocessing plant by Greenpeace activists. Tellingly, the information about the environmental pollution had not come from British Nuclear Fuels, which was increasingly viewed with distrust as the public began to wonder what the levels of undisclosed radioactive pollution could have been in previous decades. In response to the Greenpeace findings, beaches in west Cumbria were closed for the first time in their history.

The Conservative government's response was swift. Sir Donald Acheson, the chief medical officer, asked Sir Douglas Black* to head an

---

* This was the same Sir Douglas Black who in 1980 published the Black Report, much to the political distaste of the newly-elected Tory government led by

independent inquiry. Black's independent advisory group confirmed the tenfold excess of leukaemia among young people living in the coastal village of Seascale about two miles south of Sellafield. It also found that the amount of radiation in the environment and estimated doses of radiation received by the local community were, according to conventional knowledge, insufficient to account for the excess. This led to the conclusion that it remained a possibility that the "cluster" had arisen by chance.

On the recommendation of Black, the Committee on the Medical Aspects of Radiation in the Environment (COMARE) was established in 1985. The occurrence of a cluster of cancers that are among the most easily produced by ionising radiation in a village two miles from Sellafield led many people to suspect that it was a direct effect of environmental pollution from radioactive waste, and this was the first explanation considered by the Black committee and COMARE. This idea was, however, soon shown to be unsustainable, as the discharges from the plant that people were likely to have received were far too small to have caused such a large excess of leukaemia and non-Hodgkin's lymphoma (NHL). Alternative explanations had to be considered and there followed an unparalleled amount of epidemiological activity into the possible causes of the cases of leukaemia and NHL in young people under 25 years of age who lived in Seascale during the period from 1955 to 1983.

Then, in 1986, a smaller excess of leukaemia was discovered among young people living near the Dounreay nuclear establishment in northern Scotland, the only other nuclear reprocessing plant in Britain. Again, the cause of the excess could not be found, but COMARE concluded that "some feature" of the two sites was leading to the increased risk of childhood leukaemia in their vicinity.[28]

Margaret Thatcher. The report found that although there had been some improvement in the health of the nation since the inception of the NHS much inequality still remained—the main cause of which was poverty. The government published the report over a Bank Holiday weekend in the hope of limiting the impact of its uncomfortable findings.

This observation coincided with a change in mood and *modus operandi* as scientific investigation was displaced by restitutive litigation. It was after the publication of COMARE's second report in June 1988 that legal action on behalf of those who had developed leukaemia and NHL while living near Sellafield came to be seriously considered. In July 1988, the London firm of solicitors Leigh Day, who specialised in personal injury cases and David and Goliath legal battles for justice, placed an advertisement in the local newspaper the *Whitehaven News*, inviting those interested in making a claim to contact the firm. Lorna Arnold, who has chronicled Britain's atomic history referred to this prospecting for claims as "very misjudged".[29]

The mystery took a dramatic turn in February 1990 when Martin Gardner, a member of COMARE, and his colleagues published a case-control study which suggested that it was not environmental pollution but the fathers' employment in the nuclear industry which was responsible for the excess in Seascale.[30] The fathers of children with leukaemia had received, the study claimed, relatively high doses of external radiation before their children were conceived. This complex study, which became known as the Gardner report, took six years to complete and sent shockwaves through the workforce of the nuclear industry. One curious finding of Gardner's study was that the association with the fathers' exposure at work was far stronger for children born in Seascale than for children born elsewhere in west Cumbria.

Even so, the implication of the Gardner hypothesis was terrifyingly clear: paternal preconceptional irradiation (PPI) at Sellafield increased the risk of childhood leukaemias through changes induced in the father's sperm. The possibility of the existence of such a genetic pathway understandably caused alarm among radiation workers and their families. Childhood cancer is a rare disease and its causes are, in the main, unknown. However, the Gardner report was given added authenticity when a press conference called by British Nuclear Fuels at their Sellafield plant was addressed by Martin Gardner and his colleague Hazel Inskip from the medical school at Southampton University.

Gardner's hypothesis exposed him to the full spotlight of the media, although, according to Michael Snee, a co-author of the 1990 paper, this attention was not totally unwelcome as Gardner was an "environmentalist campaigner".[31] The story was national news, and its repercussions were immense for the state-owned industry and its workforce. Dr RJ Berry, director of health and safety at Sellafield, unintentionally added to the growing sense of disquiet* when he was reported as saying, "Perhaps it would be best if the workforce didn't have babies at this time." It appeared that the canons of radiation safety were going to have to be rethought.

Unsurprisingly, such a departure from long-established scientific knowledge was not intellectually attractive to Doll. From his visit to Hiroshima in 1957 he knew that no such effect as Gardner *et al* postulated had been observed in the children of the survivors of the Japan atomic bomb explosions. Moreover, the total number of Seascale leukaemia cases found by Gardner *et al* was four and this instinctively triggered in Doll's mind the possibility of the law of chance. Indeed, he had written in 1967 in his landmark publication *Prevention of Cancer: Pointers from Epidemiology* about such an occurrence:

> When a disease is endemic and extremely rare, the appearance of three or four cases in a small area within a short time attracts attention and creates the appearance of a small epidemic. Such "epidemics" are, however, bound to occur from time to time by chance alone and, in these circumstances, it may be extremely difficult to decide whether the amount of clustering that has been observed is more than can reasonably be attributed to chance, or whether it provides *a priori* evidence of the temporary appearance of a causative agent.

---

*   This doom-laden attitude was very different to the public relations exercise that followed the 1957 fire. There had been much more excitement about the accident in London than there was locally, which was probably due to the standing within the area of Gethyn Davey, the Windscale works general manager. A well-known man who, after the fire, went around local pubs and clubs talking to people and explaining how the fire occurred and what he thought the effects would be, the local people trusted him. None the less, according to Lorna Arnold, the 1957 accident was definitely a "fasten your seatbelts" moment in nuclear history.

Battle lines were being drawn. Science and scientists were about to interact with the law and lawyers in a dramatic way. It was to be a juggernaut case bristling with personal and scientific atmospherics. The stakes were high, as children had died and the whole future of a British industrial megalith would be decided in a high court trial. For all involved, scientists and lawyers, it was to be a defining episode. Doll was to play a vital role in the litigation, appearing as an expert witness for British Nuclear Fuels.

But this, of course, was not the first time Doll had appeared as an expert witness for BNF in a legal action concerning their Sellafield nuclear reprocessing plant. In the spring of 1973 Christopher and Christine Merlin had bought a "very desirable property" called Mountain Ash in the village of Ravenglass, six miles south of Sellafield.[32] Their dream was to get out of the rat race, live a quieter life and start a family in bucolic Cumbria. After the birth of two sons their rural tranquillity evaporated when a local pressure group, Network for Nuclear Concern, told the family of their disquiet about levels of radioactivity in the immediate vicinity of Mountain Ash. A local biology teacher suggested that the house be vacuum-cleaned and the contents of the Hoover bag sent for analysis. In 1979 even their cat, a heavy consumer of local fish, was tested with a Geiger counter by a visiting German scientist. Geographically, Mountain Ash was situated on the estuary of the River Esk, directly downstream from the nuclear plant, and this, combined with the findings of the Greenpeace campaigners, troubled the family to such an extent that they decided to sell their dream property.

When Yorkshire Television made the documentary, *Windscale: the Nuclear Laundry*, they persuaded Christopher and Christine Merlin and their children to take part in the film. Mountain Ash featured prominently. It could no longer be thought of as a rural sanctuary and, as Mr Merlin observed, the family began to realise that "to some extent we were living in the outskirts of a sort of open laboratory."[33] According to Martyn Day, the family's solicitor, Mountain Ash "was described, I think without any disagreement, as 'the most radioactive house in the western world'."[34] A year later the Merlin family succeeded in selling Mountain Ash for

£35,000 to a Sellafield employee who was unconcerned at the then much-publicised radioactive contamination of the house, and expressed the view that he had got a bargain.

In 1989 Mr and Mrs Merlin brought a claim for compensation against BNF plc in respect of damage to their property alleged to have been caused by radioactive contamination emanating from Sellafield. The family had lost about £50,000 from selling at a discounted price, and that was the amount of damages they sought from BNF. The case centred on the plaintiffs' ability to prove that the radiation emanating from Sellafield was sufficient to prevent people from buying the house at its market value. The BNF defence was that while the radiation was high in relative terms, it was still low when compared to living in Cornwall where the natural geology created elevated levels of radiation. The Merlin family were represented by Leigh Day Solicitors and Steven Sedley QC, while BNF had Freshfields Solicitors, a big London firm, and Ken Rokison QC.

No money had been spared by the defence. The case lasted three weeks and hinged on the scientific evidence put forward by Professor Edward Radford for the plaintiffs and Doll for British Nuclear Fuels. Radford, who had worked with Doll briefly in Oxford, was an able man but he was giving evidence beyond his area of expertise. He was also confronted by the adversarial intensity of Rokison, whose mastery of the court room went beyond the cross-examination technique. The memory stayed long with Radford: "Rokison was brilliant, and talk about a dramatist ... ! When other witnesses were talking in support of the Merlins he was constantly using distraction tactics, whispering to his colleagues, or shuffling his papers. He was a real pro—if he's on the other side you've had it."[35]

The case came down to assessing the exposure of the respiratory system to minute particles of dust. In 1988 Doll had written an article on

---

* 'The contribution of epidemiology to risk assessment'. In *Risk Assessment of Chemicals in the Environment*. Ed. ML Richardson, pp. 192-194. The Royal Society of Chemistry, London.

risk assessment for the Royal Society, * and when he was asked the question in court, "What do you consider to be the risk of living in this property?" his answer was devastating. "It would be trivial, my Lord, somewhat less than the risk of smoking two cigarettes a year." For Paul Bowden, the Freshfields solicitor, Doll's evidence won the Merlin litigation.

> It was an extraordinary performance. End of case. Richard Doll knew his trade and as an expert witness he knew how to bring things to a climax. His testimony was like a moment from [the television drama] *LA Law*—where the best possible question is asked and the most inconceivably best answer is given. The files are folded and the counsel sits down with the smug smile.[36]

Mr Justice Gatehouse's verdict reflected the evidence put before the court and also Doll's scientific interpretation of risk. On Monday 2 April Gatehouse found for BNF plc, stating: "I am wholly un-persuaded that the actual increased risk in Mountain Ash resulting from the level of radionuclides found there and emanating from Sellafield, was anything other than trivial."[37]

For Doll, the Reay and Hope case would be an altogether more harrowing experience. The trial was highly political,[38] and the lawyers for Reay and Hope offered BNF an early settlement, but the nuclear industry was determined not to give an inch. Financially it would have made sense, as settling the claims would have cost a few hundred thousand pounds, while it had to be expected that the defence of the claims would cost millions. Even so, there were grave issues to be evaluated in the Reay and Hope cases that transcended money, including the adequacy of the scientific basis of radiological protection.[39]

Historically the nuclear industry had been taken very much on trust. The state-run monopoly unambiguously declared that for nearly half a century its workings had been absolutely safe and that it had cost no loss of life—a high claim indeed. The whole future of the nuclear industry was in the balance and the dynamics that were leading to a moratorium on the building of new nuclear power stations were beginning to take shape. There was a sense in the nation and in the court room that this was the industry's one big moment to justify itself. There is no more searching an inquiry than a high court trial, and it was into that arena that Richard Doll went.

Dating from the press conference at Sellafield up until the autumn of 1992, media coverage around the case rose to such an intensity that objectivity was all but discarded. The underlying human search for solutions and the need to seek connections made it difficult to resist the cause and effect hypothesis of the plaintiffs' case. There evolved a tangible "will to believe"[40] that the most significant cluster of childhood leukaemia during a particular temporal period so close to the Sellafield site was too much of a coincidence. Even Ken Rokison's daughter admonished him over the breakfast table for defending such a heinous and obviously guilty client.[41]

In the Merlin case Martyn Day felt on his own admission that his team had "been really mashed from day one" as a result of being underfunded.[42] For the Reay and Hope litigation, he had assembled an impressive team of expert witnesses, geneticists and epidemiologists from around the world to give evidence in support of his case. Awarded a generous legal aid settlement, Day engaged the formidable Ben Hytner QC, leader of the north-west circuit, a man of the people and personal injury barrister, to lead the case in the high court.

Hytner began the trial with a scintillating opening statement outlining the moral and scientific righteousness of the case. He was so persuasive that some on the BNF team believed that speech "won the judge over".[43] The court was told that parental exposure to radioactivity at the Sellafield plant had been implanted as the leading scientific theory responsible for leukaemia and non-Hodgkin lymphoma (NHL).

One of the subjects of the trial was Dorothy Reay, born in 1961 in Whitehaven, west Cumbria, eight miles from Sellafield. She died in Whitehaven at the age of ten months of acute leukaemia, and the litigation was brought on her behalf by her mother, Elizabeth Reay. The other plaintiff, Vivien Hope, was born in 1965 in Drigg, a village four miles south of Sellafield. At the age of six years, she moved with her family to Seascale, about a mile or so from Sellafield. In 1988, at the age of 23 and while still resident at Seascale, she was diagnosed as having NHL. At the time of the trial she was in remission. Both Mr Reay and Mr Hope, the fathers of Dorothy and Vivien, had recorded doses of ionising radiation received while employed at Sellafield by the United Kingdom Atomic Energy Authority (UKAEA) before the conception of the affected children. (Dorothy Reay had been included in the Gardner study, but Vivien Hope was not, having been diagnosed after 1985, the last year of the study period.)

Richard Doll was "a scientist's scientist" but he was good on the witness stand and he had the ability to speak the language of the judge and jury.[44] The Merlin trial had been Martyn Day's first encounter with Doll and he realised what a formidable player he was. "He's the most impressive expert witness I've ever seen—you know that if you're up against him that you are in serious trouble."[45] The thought of again facing such an intimidating scientific brain as Doll's concentrated the efforts of Day and Hytner's team.

If an expert witness can not be shaken, then for Hytner the tactic must be different: "Perhaps one looks to see if they are vain, or arrogant, or some other weakness—then one goes for that." Cross-examination is a stimulating but sometimes disturbing experience. Richard Wakeford, a BNF scientist advising the defence's legal team, has written that the court room was not a place for an expert witness to show arrogance or ignorance. "Top lawyers are extremely clever people and those involved in the Reay and Hope versus BNF litigation had some of the sharpest intellects I have ever encountered."[46]

The day Doll was cross-examined he was not feeling well. On the way to the high court he went to a pharmacy and bought some linctus.[47] He was asked by Ken Rokison QC for the defence: "I think it has been suggested by the plaintiffs that this study lends support to what we all call the Gardner hypothesis of paternal preconception irradiation (PPI) having causal association with childhood leukaemia and NHL. Do you consider

that it does support that hypothesis?" Doll answered "No, I do not."
At this point Ben Hytner QC began his cross-examination of Doll.

Q. "We then have to turn to Professor Gardner. The first thing clearly
that has to be determined is whether his findings are the result of a properly conducted study?"
A. "Yes. I have said earlier that there is an element of what we call subgroup analysis in his examination of the results, and I must retain that
as a possible criticism, about the inclusion of one case which most
people seem to agree now probably ought not to have been included in
the series—the so-called Bristol case.* Otherwise the study was conducted well. The interpretation put on it I think was taken a bit too far,
and I do not think that they recognised the element of subgroup analysis there probably was in the presentation of the results."
Q. "Can I then explore that, because that is your concern? Without that
concern you would be happy with the interpretation that Professor
Gardner puts upon his findings?"
A. "No, I think he has gone too far. I think leaving aside my concerns
about focusing on the subgroup there is material there to formulate a
hypothesis for testing by other means. There is nothing else."
Q. "I do hope that you are not misunderstanding my question and
going too far."
A. "I hope not."

The argument, then, came to be centred on the scientific interpretation of the association. Doll then, much to the consternation of some, suggested the possibility that Gardner had committed what Martyn Day

---

* One of the high-dose cases, and there were only four of them, should not have
been included in Gardner's study. The rules of the study were sacrosanct. Each
case had to be diagnosed born and resident in west Cumbria. However, one young
man was diagnosed in Bristol where he was a student. He was registered with a
Bristol GP and therefore his diagnosis transgressed the original guidelines of the
study. He died in Seascale. But the controls were defined on their GP registration.
If there was ambiguity the defence said, "This Bristol case ought not to be
included."

termed "a cardinal sin in terms of epidemiology."[48] Doll raised the possibility that Gardner's team had begun by collecting data for a wider study of cases in area, and then, as the data started to come in, they saw that they could make a big story if they focused on the small subgroup born and diagnosed in Seascale.

Hytner moved immediately onto the attack because in a subtle way Doll had accused Gardner *et al* of manipulating data.

Q. "Sir Richard, that… is a pretty serious allegation against an epidemiologist, is it not?"

A. "No, I don't think so. It is the sort of thing that happens. Unfortunately I cannot discuss it with Martin [Gardner]. As you know, he has died, but one has to say what you think is right and I would have said that to him in friendship."

Q. "Again, so that there can be absolutely no doubt and to avoid misunderstanding, this is not a suggestion really, but an allegation of fact. Your allegation or suggestion or imputation is not that they exercised judgement in some way which you disagree with, but that factually they made this decision to focus on births in West Cumbria after they knew the details of the dose?"

A. "No, I never said anything of the sort… What I am suggesting is that they focused on cases born and diagnosed as they claimed in Seascale when they saw the way the dose was pointing, the distribution of the doses was pointing."

Q. "Is your doubt about the finding of the Gardner study based upon your belief that the case-control study, as it finally was conducted, was restricted to children born and diagnosed in Seascale?"

A. "Yes. I am sorry, I am confused. I will have to look back."

Q. "Please take your time, because I am not going to hurry you on this, Sir Richard, as it is rather important."

A. "It is indeed."

Q. "If there has been a misunderstanding on your part it is better that it should be clarified and your position amended?"

A. "Or alternatively confirmed."

Q. "Or alternatively I can peruse it."

After looking at the Gardner paper Doll was asked by Hytner if he would withdraw his criticism.

A. "No, it causes me to change the words of Seascale to West Cumbria. The criticism remains."

A sense of theatre gripped the court room. Professor Martin Gardner had died of lung cancer in 1993. Much loved and much respected by statisticians and epidemiologists around the world, he was now having his professional character besmirched. Hytner had studied Doll intently and he was trying to get him to vilify Gardner and put the message across to Mr Justice French that Doll was a pompous, dismissive slightly vindictive old man. Some on the BNF side felt that Hytner went a long way towards succeeding in his objective.[49] For Martyn Day it was "the most dramatic scene" he had ever seen in a trial. So grave was Doll's allegation that a twenty-minute adjournment was called so that he could reflect on what he had said.

Doll held his ground. He had a talent for being able to concentrate even under the most pressurised of conditions and when there was a palpable undercurrent of hostility.

Q. "Professor Doll, if Professor Gardner did that which he says he did at the stage that he did it, do you maintain or withdraw your criticism? A. "I maintain it. The question was when do you publish results? The question to me is when do you publish results? As one reads this paragraph, one reads Professor Gardner's statement: 'It has always been the intention to present findings for the six cases of leukaemia and eight cases of lymphoma born elsewhere. These cases, however, are more relevant to the assessment of such factors as X-rays or mother's age than the Sellafield geographical and occupational environment before birth or at a young age.'*

---

* Doll was reading from the statement of Professor Gardner that was put in evidence because he was unable to give evidence orally.

They are equally relevant to the question of paternal irradiation, and I suggest they were influenced in publishing the data relating to the particular ones born and diagnosed in the area because of the results, rather than continuing with their original intention, which is described here to present findings for the six cases of leukaemia and eight cases of lymphoma born elsewhere. Having said that, I must say I would have probably reacted in the same way as Professor Gardner did. This is a very natural and understandable thing to do, but I think scientifically incorrect."

This answer led Mr Justice French to interject:

"Natural and understandable but scientifically incorrect. Would it be fair or unfair to add, 'I might well have done the same?'"
A. "Perfectly fair, my Lord. The temptation would have been very strong when you have got such a striking result."

Scene by scene, hour by hour, the exchanges between Hytner and Doll were becoming increasingly personal in tone.

Q. "I think it right that you know the relevance in case you should want to add anything to the points that I was going to make. As I say, we want to be absolutely sure that when your back is turned you are not going to have a knife in it. You may get a knife in it, but at least you ought to have the chance of having some armoured plating in advance!"
A. "Thank you."

Beforehand, Ken Rokison's expectation was that Doll would baffle Hytner and that Mr Justice French would be able to do nothing other than admire and believe every word of the expert witness for the defence. But it did not work out that way. Hytner certainly felt he got the better of the exchanges with Doll,[50] and just as importantly, so did Paul Bowden, the BNF solicitor.

I remember sitting back, having watched his evidence, and immediately drawing the comparison with the man who had given evidence in front of Gatehouse, in different circumstances, four years before; and over that period of time, at least in the context of being an expert witness, Sir Richard's powers were waning. I think age had caught up with him. He was 81 years old and I felt pity and guilt that we'd brought him too far.[51]

Martyn Day's interpretation of Doll's performance was very different. "It was quite remarkable. It took a strong character to say what he did [about Gardner]; at the time we hated him—but in terms of standing up under pressure, he was very strong."[52]

Doll was "pleased" that he had cast doubt on the Gardner hypothesis. It did not make biological sense to him nor did it satisfactorily explain the original seven cases exposed in the 1983 film documentary. It might be, however, that Gardner avoided counting the other three in the cluster because one had been born in Oxford and another one was born before 1950, and their inclusion would have contradicted his theory of mutation in the sperm of the father.

In the court room Doll presented evidence from Leo Kinlen* that the excess of leukaemia in Seascale was not limited to children born there, but extended to children born elsewhere but living in the village. Unfortunately Martyn Gardner did not have the opportunity to defend his study. Strangely none of Gardner's six co-authors was called by the plaintiffs' lawyers to validate the contested protocols of the study. Even Dr Michael Snee, who was awarded his DM on the basis of his involvement in the study, was not called to the witness stand.[53]

Clearly the idea that the Seascale cluster could be a chance effect now had to be scientifically abandoned, and Gardner's hypothesis was reduced to three valid cases. Gardner *et al* had failed to explain why there was such a concentration of cases in Seascale when there was no similar excess of cases associated with PPI in West Cumbria outside Seascale, given that the high doses were so prevalent well away from the village. In 1993 a sci-

---

*   LJ Kinlen, 'Can paternal preconceptional radiation account for the increase of leukaemia and non-Hodgkin's lymphoma in Seascale?' *British Medical Journal*, 26 June 1993, volume 306, pp. 1718-1721.

entific paper by Parker and Wakeford *et al* demonstrated that if the Seascale cluster were to be explained by reference to PPI, one would have expected some fifty extra cases of leukaemia in the remainder of west Cumbria over the relevant period, which did not appear.[54] Indeed, Gardner himself asserted that statistics alone could not support a judicial case:[55] evidently another explanation needed to be found.

As long ago as 1988, Kinlen had noted that Seascale had rare demographic and geographic characteristics. It possessed an unusually high level of social class one and two (highly-educated nuclear scientists) and it was very close to the country's largest rural industrial site where most Seascale residents worked and where an atypically large number of mobile construction workers could be found. Kinlen suggested therefore "that childhood leukaemia represents a rare response to some unidentified common infection(s) epidemics of which would be encouraged by mixing of populations* with plausibly different previous experiences of infective agents."[56] Doll's introduction of Kinlen's hypothesis to the trial had an impact that one of the lawyers likened to the Prussians arriving on the fields of Waterloo.[57]

At this point, in terms of judicial psychology, the balance in the scales of justice began to tilt away from the plaintiffs. After re-examination by Ken Rokison, the establishment figure of Doll was rehabilitated in the eyes of Mr Justice French. The wobble was forgotten, and the logic of his thinking—culminating in Occam's razor,** or the law of scientific parsimony—began to make sense to French. The plaintiffs' case was based on using

---

* Kinlen showed that excess risks occurred in many other situations without a source of man-made radiation in which mixing of urban and rural populations had occurred: in rural areas with a high concentration of servicemen, in local authority growth areas, in rural parts of Scotland with high proportions of oil workers, in towns with the greatest increase in commuting to work, and in rural districts that had received most evacuees from large centres during the Second World War.

** Originating from William of Occam, the English philosopher, the principle was that in explaining an event no more assumptions should be made than are necessary.

epidemiological and genetic evidence to persuade French that there was an association between paternal irradiation and Dorothy Reay's death and Vivien Hope's disease.

By Easter 1993, even after Doll had demolished their science, the plaintiffs' legal team still somehow felt they were winning the epidemiological argument. The difficulties arose when they tried to bring the genetic evidence into play. They had relied heavily on the mouse experiments carried out in Japan by Professor Tatsuji Nomura, a distinguished Japanese biologist, who had found high levels of cancers and leukaemias in the offspring of irradiated mice in his laboratory. Unfortunately Professor Nomura was not able to attend the high court hearing, and in his absence the defence were able to demonstrate the unreliability of his experiments. This, in the words of Martyn Day, "opened the lid of doubt,"[58] and when French looked back on the undulating terrain of evidence it was Doll's scientific assessment of probability, chance and bias and Hill's criteria that remained untainted. At the end of the trial even Ben Hytner QC was convinced that "their case was correct and we were wrong."[59]

Mr Justice French, it would be fair to say, was intellectually stretched by the complexity of the scientific evidence whirling around his courtroom.[60] But who would not have been?

The purpose of epidemiological studies is to make an assessment of the probability, first, that there is an association between the exposure in question and the disease of interest and, second, that the association, if any, is causal. On page 74 of his judgement on 8 October, Mr Justice French quoted from Doll's report:

> I have previously concluded that the observation of an excess number of cases of leukaemia and NHL in Seascale was not the result of PPI, but could most reasonably be explained by a combination of chance and the effect of the sort of socio-demographic factors described by Kinlen, and that the statistical association with paternal preconception irradiation found by Gardner was probably due to a combination of chance and the *post hoc* selection of an atypical subgroup of the

young people who developed leukaemia in West Cumbria for concentrated study. The new evidence that has become available supports this conclusion.

"This," Mr Justice French wrote, "is a conclusion which, on the evidence as a whole, seems to me no less plausible than the Gardner hypothesis."

Doll was not in court to be popular; he wanted to find the truth and to get the science right. In retrospect the "Gardner hypothesis" has not stood the test of time or of scientific examination,[61] but this does not diminish his standing in the annals of British epidemiology. For, within that history stretching back to John Snow it would be fair to say that seldom, if ever, has a hypothesis been scrutinised with such intellectual rigour. His obituary noted that:

> Martin made no enemies, because his concern was to get the correct answer rather than to prove himself right or to put someone else down... This [the Sellafield report] landed him in a new world of reporters, television cameras, litigation, and the powers of an industrial/military/political lobby. There could be no greater tribute than that, despite the scrutiny, no one accused him of unfairness or of bad workmanship. [62]

In 1993 the cloud of suspicion that hung over Sellafield was lifted. Doll, the opponent of on-coming bandwagons, held on to his scientific independence under corrosive scrutiny. It may not have been an *LA Law* performance but the verdict was against the claimants, and Doll's evidence was seminal in determining Mr Justice French's judgement: "... On the evidence before me the scales tilt decisively in favour of the defendants and the plaintiffs, therefore, have failed to satisfy me on the balance of probabilities that PPI was a material contributory cause of the Seascale excess or, it must follow of (a) the leukaemia of Dorothy Reay or (b) the NHL of Vivien Hope."

Even in defeat Martyn Day retained his legal objectivity, and saw it as a testament to Doll that he stood up under pressure and showed no weakness. "He was absolutely rock solid, and as a result of that it helped to persuade the judge to go against us."

Doll's work on radiation had transcended the decades and in his 82nd year he approached another landmark publication on the defining subject of his career: smoking. His twenty-year observation of smoking among British doctors had been looked upon as highlighting previously unknown hazards of tobacco, but in his forty-year follow-up even worse was to come.

Chapter 25

One for the Heart

"How the people of England live is one of the most important questions that can be considered; and how—of what causes, and at what ages—they die is scarcely of less account; for it is the complement of the primary question teaching men how to live a longer, healthier, and happier life."

Dr William Farr

Richard Doll was a rationalist, and his scientific training led him to fear the known more than the unknown.[1] He also believed that people should be treated as adults and told the facts. One of the reasons for his continued research into the long-term use of tobacco among British doctors was to make society aware of the devastating effects of the smoking epidemic. When Doll and Hill initiated the British doctors' study in 1951 there was doubt about the role of tobacco in lung cancer causation. Some forty years later, there was also no doubt—and more than 25 other causes of death had been added to lung cancer by Doll and Peto as being "associated with cigarette smoking".[2]

When the twenty-year follow-up of the British doctors had been published in 1976 the death rate in middle-aged men (35-69) from all causes was twice as great in smokers as in non-smokers, but graver hazards were about to be revealed. During the second half of the forty-year follow-up (1976-94), the death rate from all causes in middle-aged smokers was three times that of the non-smoker. There had been a maturing of the epidemic, and at last the true dangers of prolonged smoking had been reliably assessed.

Doll and Peto's main finding was that their earlier work had underestimated the hazards of long-term use of tobacco: and that about half of all regular cigarette smokers would eventually be killed by their habit. Tragically, about a quarter would die in middle age and would lose, on average, twenty to 25 years of the non-smoker life expectancy. Nationally, tobacco was the greatest cause of death while for non-smokers cancer mortality was decreasing slowly and total mortality was decreasing rapidly. One heartening finding of Doll and Peto's meticulous calculations was that quitting really worked. From the 10,807 replies, they found that stopping smoking even in middle age substantially increased the expectation of life—and the benefits of stopping at earlier ages were even greater.

While much of the evidence on the health benefits of quitting came from the British doctors' study, the 1994 findings enabled smokers to avoid the consulting rooms and prognostications of doctors entirely and become active participants in their own destiny. To stop smoking is difficult, but the work of Doll was empowering and the rewards of a life free of premature morbidity and death by changing personal behaviour was being embraced by growing numbers of smokers. His research had the ability to penetrate the mind of the non-scientist even if his identity had not. Coincidentally, the chilling finding that half of all smokers would be killed by their habit was counterbalanced by the same percentage of smokers who agreed with the statement that "Smoking can't be all that dangerous, or the government would ban advertising."[3]

While the report, "Mortality in relation to smoking: 40 years' observation on male British doctors", showed how bad things were for life-long cigarette smokers, its political impact was diluted by a Tory administration reluctant to act on what had become "a great failure of public health".* After 1993 John Major, the prime minister, declined to consider the British Medical Association's plea for a ban on tobacco advertising. The BMA's 1993 annual meeting deplored the decision "not to ban tobacco advertising at places other than the place of sale," and Dr Sandy Macara, the chairman, told Major that the BMA believed that in the light of the British doctors' study the government was undermining its targets and policies set out in *The Health of the Nation*.** The chairman reminded the

---

*   Peto R, 'Smoking and Death: the past 40 years and the next 40', *British Medical Journal*, 1994; volume 309, pp. 937-939.

**   Between 1992 and 1997, *The Health of the Nation* set the context for the planning of services by the NHS. It was a genuine attempt by government to improve the overall health of the population.

prime minister that there was widespread support for a ban from the House of Commons health committee, and the health secretary admitted that the government faced a dilemma over how to persuade young people to stop smoking. An advertising ban and a substantial increase in taxation would, the BMA believed, address this concern.[4]

In a rare combination of ignorance and incompetence John Major saw the answer not in regulation but in the voluntary agreements on tobacco advertising with the tobacco industry. The protectiveness that successive Conservative administrations showed the tobacco conglomerates was matched by the willingness of the industry to employ former government ministers on large salaries in recognition of their political inertia. While there had been a moderate reduction in tobacco consumption in Britain, cigarettes in 1994 were still responsible for thirty per cent of deaths in middle age, and worldwide sales were still increasing. Perhaps without Doll's intellectual leadership, integrity and composed but firm insistence that actions must follow discoveries, the moderate reduction could have been a moderate increase given the power and stealth of the tobacco marketing methods.

In neighbouring France where there had been no equivalent of the Royal College of Physicians reports, or quantitative epidemiological studies, there was a steep increase in tobacco consumption and tobacco induced cancers. In the mid-1990s, more than $5bn a year was spent on global advertising and promotion of tobacco, a sum, as Richard Peto noted ironically, "which, according to the tobacco manufacturers, has no effect on the proportion of children who choose to smoke."[5] The swing in the pendulum of perception of the dangers of smoking that began with Doll and Hill had moved in an arc of reasoned persuasion through the medical profession, politicians and finally to the wider society. In 1950 when Tony Hill had the brainwave of asking British doctors about their smoking habits he would have doubted that the experiment would still be continuing over forty years later. He had died in 1991, but had he lived, he would have applauded Doll and Peto's interpretation of the epidemiological evidence.

In 1990 Sir Richard Doll attracted the bemused attention of the anti-smoking lobby when he told the *Journal of Addiction*: "I don't mind if someone lights up in front of me, it's his life and not mine." This was a comment which some interpreted as a denial of the impact of passive smoking. Four years previously, the *Times*, under the headline "Passive smoking: no significant danger", sparked a medical controversy. The Tobacco Advisory Council, which was funded by the tobacco industry, lost little time in exploiting the *Times'* misleading report and wrote to all members of parliament. On 16 July 1986 an early day motion was tabled in parliament to urge the health minister to stop funding the Health Education Council's campaign on passive smoking.

In 1986 Doll's own research had confirmed that exposure to ambient smoke caused some lung cancers in non-smokers "consistent with a risk of the order of 20-50 per cent".[6] He also thought that the risks of passive smoking "are certainly trivial compared with the risks to smokers themselves." Environmental tobacco smoke contains many carcinogens but the primary message Doll wanted to put across was that smokers kill themselves; some are probably killing other people, but half of all smokers will be killed by their own cigarettes.

Because he found it difficult to access accurately the hazards of passive smoking, Doll took some persuading before putting his authoritative weight behind restrictions on smoking in public places. Once the evidence was there,[7] he felt justified in writing, "the suggestion that the possibility of a cancer hazard should be added to the certainty of unpleasant pollution in the movement against unrestricted smoking in public places seems entirely reasonable."[8]

Undeniably Doll was no Stanton Glantz, the legendary San Francisco-based researcher and outspoken activist against the tobacco industry who tirelessly campaigned on the dangers of second-hand smoke. Glantz's direct-action techniques led to California being the first state in the United States to have smoke-free bars and restaurants. Doll's approach was, as always, more detached but he did campaign for a ban on tobacco advertising and thought it a necessary step in a democratic society in preparing the ground for a restriction of smoking in public places. Perhaps he was not evangelical enough, but it was not his way. He would take on

Big Tobacco in court cases—which other cancer researchers were reluctant to do—if they were making untrue public statements. But even within the corps of his admirers,[9] there was a feeling that his public voice was more circumspect than it needed to have been.

In 1996 his assimilation into the status quo and his contribution to science was given national recognition when he was awarded the medal of the Order of the Companion of Honour. A CH was not awarded just to the standard-bearers of the establishment—Harold Pinter and Eric Hobsbawm were in its ranks too—but it was an unconditional celebration of established eminence. His rehabilitation was complete. Even in the senior common rooms of Oxford colleges the epithet "red" was reduced to a barely audible murmur. His political extremism was now firmly placed in the past. He may not have been the first ex-proselytising communist to be awarded a CH but he was the first practising epidemiologist.

The qualities that made Doll the great scientist he was will have become apparent in the preceding chapters of this book, but predominant among them, perhaps, was that most essential factor—luck. The early papers upon which his career was built were published under "Doll and Hill" although he was undeniably Hill's assistant. In July 2005 Doll acknowledged how this alphabetical good fortune supercharged his scientific career while Hill's contribution has been eroded by time. "I think my whole life could well have been different. Because the 1950 study has been attributed to me—I did a lot of the work, but Hill inspired it, and had these papers been published Hill and Doll, I think my reputation would be very different to how it is now."

Yet his career was not built on tobacco alone. Over a period of sixty years his publications show that nothing he did was far removed from some major human disease. He followed the maxim of the Oxford physiologist, Sir Charles Sherrington: "The more intelligent the question you ask of Mother Nature the more intelligent will be her reply." The most important factor in Doll's later success as a scientist was his sense of direction in research. His work on the contraceptive pill, asbestos and ionising radiation and the molecular mechanisms of cancer expanded our knowledge of disease causation. By identifying and quantifying cancers that occurred in specific occupations, he helped establish the idea that much of the disease derived from environmental risks, and consequently was avoidable.

2 May 1997 was a bright scintillating spring day that heralded a new political dawn and marked the end of eighteen years of continuous Tory rule in Britain. Tony Blair led the Labour Party to victory, securing a greater majority in the House of Commons than even Clement Attlee had achieved in the landslide election of July 1945. As part of their election campaign the Labour Party pledged to ban all advertising of tobacco products. This marked the culmination of a moral and medical struggle stretching back almost half a century.

Alas, the euphoria of the election victory was short-lived. The Labour Party announced that it was going to exempt Formula One motor racing from the advertising ban and that a donation of £1m received from Bernie Ecclestone, the sport's power broker to the party's coffers, was completely unrelated to the stay of execution. Doll was not a supporter of New Labour, but he did encourage every effort to reduce the hazards of tobacco. It was hoped by some that Doll, arguably the most powerful doctor in Britain,[10] would make protestations to the prime minister for the renunciation—he did not. The government's justification for motor racing's immunity was that British jobs would be lost, as the ban would force the teams and their so-called "flying fag packets" abroad. When the legislation was eventually implemented, it contributed to a 25 per cent reduction in smoking in Britain and is seen as part of a trenchant public health policy.

The year 1997 was so productive for Doll that it prompted a congratulatory editorial in the *British Medical Journal*. Aptly, one of the articles he had written for the *BMJ* was entitled "There is no such thing as ageing."[11] In the week of his 85th birthday, the editor described Doll as "perhaps Britain's most eminent doctor"[12] and commended him on his output: in that year he wrote 18 scientific papers. Honouring his work on smoking and health, the editorial put his research into context:

> The reduction in tobacco deaths in middle age has been greater in Britain than any other country. About half of those who smoke are killed by the habit, while among those who have never smoked or who have stopped 80 per cent survive to 70 and 33 per cent to 85. Two thirds of the ex-smokers who have survived to 85 would have died if they'd carried on smoking. They owe their lives to Sir Richard.

Earlier in the decade Doll had cheered the nation's drinkers by recommending far higher levels of alcohol consumption than people had previously thought healthy. Since 1978 he had asked his long-suffering doctors not only about their smoking history, but also their drinking habits.[13] For the 1997 Christmas edition of the *British Medical Journal*, Doll wrote the article "One for the heart"[14] and for the hedonists among the readership it was just what the doctor ordered. Doll enjoyed drinking but was aware of the dangers that alcohol had for doctors * and society. George Bernard Shaw had noted the poisonous relationship that existed between doctors and alcohol, when he wrote "They save others: them-

---

* "The harmful effects of alcohol are much more extensive than the production of disease in the drinker himself, as they include injuries inflicted under its influence intentionally or otherwise on others: but even ignoring these secondary effects of intoxication, the current trends in mortality directly due to alcohol-induced disease must cause serious concern. These trends have accumulated an increase in average consumption of nearly 100 per cent a head since 1950, which threatens to herald an epidemic of alcoholism such as those that afflicted Britain in 1750 and 1870."

British doctors appeared to be particularly prone to alcoholism. First admission rates for alcoholism in Scotland were 2.7 times higher among doctors than among other men in social class 1 and the death rate from cirrhosis among doctors in England and Wales was 350 per cent that of the general population. Alcoholism was also the mental disorder most likely to bring a doctor before his professional disciplinary organisation. Robin Murray. *British Medical Journal*, 1976; volume 2, pp.1537-39.

selves they cannot save."[15] Doll's review of the evidence led him to deliver a clear message. "In middle and old age some small amount of alcohol within the range of one to four drinks each day reduces the risk of premature death." He advised that this daily consumption in people aged 45 and above had a protective effect against vascular disease and death, and it did not matter whether they drank wine, beer or spirits since the benefit was derived from ethanol. At medical conferences around the world, Doll, elegantly dressed as was his custom, could be found at the head of the queue for a glass of lunch-time wine, and his answer to any puritan inquiry was "I'm looking after my health."

Physiologically Doll had chosen his parents well and by his own estimation only spent "on average one day a year in bed because of illness". The only precautionary therapy he took was a vitamin D supplement. His collaborative research* had shown its benefits in preventing fractures—and he also did not like the debilitating impact that osteoporosis had on Joan. But he had already surpassed his biological span of life, and the "enviable stamina"[16] that even regular long-haul flights did not diminish could no longer be relied upon. After his mid-80s, he was suffering from cardiac arrhythmia and the gradual decline in his life force was explained by a diagnosis of heart fatigue.

Some of the immediate dangers were averted when he had a pacemaker fitted, which helped to regulate the rhythm of his heart beat. Doll believed in living dangerously and the only life-style concessions he made were taking more time over breakfast with Joan while they listened to classical music, and getting into the office an hour later, at 10.00am.

He and Joan depended on each other and had always shared similar professional and political ideas. Joan, according to Professor Valerie Beral, was "Richard's sub-conscious". His position at the centre of British

---

*   Trivedi DP, Doll R and Khaw KT, 'Effect of four monthly vitamin D (cholecalciferol) supplementation on fractures and mortality in men and women living in the community: randomised double-blind controlled trial.' *British Medical Journal*, 2003; volume 326, pp. 469-472.

epidemiology, achieved through careful, rigorous investigation, was underwritten by Joan's unwavering commitment: professionally and psychologically he had no greater supporter. In 1946 she had been instrumental in securing his first epidemiological appointment, and, given her status as the most powerful woman at the MRC, rarely had a post-war physician a more influential patron within the nation's leading medical institution.

In retirement, second only to epidemiological research Doll's great pleasure was in travel. He toured the world with Joan, lecturing, visiting medical schools and taking part in collaborative studies. Whereas earlier in his career Doll dressed in bohemian style, in later life his notoriously elegant dress sense was primarily overseen by Joan. When he went on lecture tours, she packed his case with such care that each garment was folded in delicate tissue paper. Compared to Richard's apparent outward severity, Joan was loud and possessed an unfortunate but widely felt tendency to "size people up"—a characteristic that some people found terrifying.[17] Colleen McDonald, their cleaner, however, held an altogether different view: "Even if I won the lottery I'd still clean their home, they were such lovely people."

After more than fifty years of happily married life and three cancer operations, Joan's health began to fail. Physically strong, Joan merely buckled when many would have broken. Her determination was so great that rather than miss a celebration at their beloved Green College due to incapacitating osteoporosis, she made the journey up to the dining room in the drinks lift.

On one occasion, in 2001, the symmetry of their collective decline found them both in hospital at the same time: Joan for an unsuccessful operation to reinforce her vertebrae, and Richard for a successful operation for cancer of the large bowel. The night before the operation he called me to his house and delivered a biographical testament. "There's a risk I won't survive the operation and if that is the case there are things I'd like you to know." He admitted that there had never been a time in his life when he was not frightened of something. He told of the trauma they felt when they were accused of being racists during their expansion of the

Agnostic Adoption Society; of how deeply hurt they were by the revolt against Green College; and the struggle to free Joan from an unhappy marriage.

Their life together had witnessed one of the most turbulent periods in British social history and the most exciting in the entire history of medical science. A friendship formed in the political ferment of the 1930s had survived the Second World War to be transformed into a lifelong love affair. Doll had had to fight for Joan, and he said that she was the best part of his life. A man of deep reserve, he did not talk about his feelings much, but the three great emotional upheavals in his life all involved Joan. The "callow youth" she had known in the 1930s had become the doyen of epidemiology as the world entered a new millennium.

When Joan died in September 2001 nothing could cushion his despair. He knew that he should be more pleased that she had lived than sad that she had died. Oppressed by grief, he was unable to sleep in their bedroom. He missed those enduring decencies—what Wordsworth called "the little, nameless, unremembered acts of kindness and love." At Joan's memorial service, held in a packed Holywell Music Room on a misty medieval Oxford night, Doll somehow controlled his grief and addressed the guests. He told them that Joan had a rare quality: "She was one of those people genuinely interested in the lives of others." This may have been true, but what was more remarkable about the comment was that Richard Doll chose to say it because it was not a characteristic he shared.

From his schooldays onwards his work had a thoroughness about it and even before coming under Hill's spell there was an obsessive feature to his character. Doll's science had humane consequences, and it may even have had humane intentions, but from the early 1950s he did not have— nor did he make—much time for the lives of others. He was not one for small talk—it would have distracted him from medical research. Later that evening at Green College he gave an amusing and sometimes moving account of their life together. He said, "It won't surprise you to learn that Joan and I first met at a committee meeting," which met with a gentle ripple of laughter. Afterwards, as Harry Keen, one of his left-wing medical friends, was leaving, Doll grabbed him by the arm and said, "The committee meeting where we met was the executive of our local Communist Party—but I didn't think they would want to know that."[18]

On 23 July 2002, in reply to a letter of condolence from Chris Birch, a comrade from the Communist Party in the 1950s, Doll opened his heart and reached back to a fateful event in his life.

> Many thanks for your kind letter about Joan. She was a wonderful companion and life without her has (I have to say) lost its meaning—but we did have 56 years together, which, seeing as they didn't start until we were both in our thirties, is a lot to be grateful for. She had a great deal of pain in her last few years which she bore stoically, at first from a poorly repaired fractured femur and then from osteoporotic fractures of her spine. Eventually she died peacefully in her own bed without, I think, any appreciation of what was happening, which is something to be grateful for.
>
> I do, of course, remember you—though I can't say I should recognize you if we met in the street. What a difficult time politically those mid 50s were. I foolishly (in retrospect) continued to believe in the possibility of our movement being genuinely democratic and it was the realization that it never would be that caused us to give up shortly after your report.*

With the death of Joan, 12 Rawlinson Road was now the home of the most incongruous possible pairing. Steve and Doll's relationship, not easy at the best of times, was strained further by the unanimity of their grief. In the wake of this personal misery Doll could only work superficially, and yet, before sitting down at his desk, he and Steve played Bezique together every night. Doll had an iron integrity both in science and in ordinary life, but in his treatment of Steve his fairness wavered. Her friends were aston-

---

* The 25th Special Congress of the Communist Party took place on 19-22 April 1957, and a report on the congress was given by Chris Birch to the Norland branch of the Communist Party, to which Richard and Joan belonged, on 2 May 1957 at Flat 3, 49 Ladbroke Grove, the home of Richard and Eileen Turner.

ished to learn that he had told Steve to put her name down on Oxford City Council's housing list, indicating that he did not see her welfare as his responsibility.[19] Both of them knew this was a violation of Joan's sense of duty to her friend.

Doll did mellow as he grew frailer and as his dependency on Steve increased. But a nadir was reached in December 2003 when he suffered such a virulent and long-lasting bout of flu that his friends feared for his life. At the same time the irreducible Steve was suffering from a bronchial infection so devastating that she thought she too would die. His illness also brought about one of the few truly eureka moments in Doll's life. Weak from days of fever and incapacitation, he felt that a good long soak would lift his spirits. Alas, when he tried to get out after his full-immersion in the bath, his strength had deserted him and he was left floundering in the water. He knew his life depended upon getting vertical and out of the bath. At that moment science came to his rescue. He turned the hot tap on full and gently the water raised him to the rim of the bath where he was able to roll himself out to safety. Eureka! He returned quietly to his bedroom and slept the sleep of the saved.

Through a combination of nurture, nature and luck both of them survived but it was a warning that their days of total independence, collectively or alone, were unsustainable. Doll decided it was time to sell up and begin a new and final chapter in his life. Whether it was his conscience or the deliberations of his children that changed his mind it is difficult to know, but Doll set up a trust fund to pay towards the costs of Steve's sheltered accommodation in a delightful complex in Jericho in Oxford. Over the winter months he decanted the treasures he and Joan had collected during half a century until only those things he knew to be useful or believed to be beautiful remained. After 42 years of selfless devotion, Mrs Isabelle Sutherland entered Dr Richard Doll's study for the last time: "Thank you for letting me share your children and for all the years with you and Joan." His private grief was still predominating, and not looking up from his work, he said "Thank you."[20]

Early in 2004 Doll moved into 9 Observatory Street, one of Green College's Victorian terraced houses. During the previous 25 years he had donated over £750,000 to Green College, and without him it would not have existed. For the first time in his life, at the age of 91, Richard Doll was going to live alone. If Rawlinson Road had been Joan's creation, Observatory Street was entirely Doll's. He had sold or given away the contents of a vast North Oxford house, and into his modest new home he brought his personal artefacts. He chose the art, the music and the friends that crossed its threshold. At last he began to find some inner peace, and his grief began finally to evanesce. He joined the Green College book club, and started to shop and cook for himself. He was constantly visited by a dedicated group of women friends who brought care and companionship. Among them were Rani Lall, Jenny Turner and Lalla Ward, the actor and author married to Richard Dawkins, in whose company he began to shine. Doll was renascent.

The house unified his world. At 9.45 each morning he trundled with ever increasing slowness from his home, down the path that opened onto the resplendent gardens of Green College, past the magnificent Tower of the Winds, and into his office beside the Radcliffe Infirmary. He had come to Oxford in July 1969 at the age of 56; now, 35 years later he was still able to traverse his own universe.

Chapter 26

The Final Frontier

"One owes consideration to the living; to the dead one owes only the truth."

Voltaire

Richard Doll's moral integrity could not be bought. For more than half a century he had shown that lung cancer rates could be reduced by almost ninety per cent if people stopped smoking. In 2001, while being interviewed on BBC Radio 4's *Desert Island Discs*, he gave the audience some candid advice. "Find out what the tobacco industry supports and don't do it, and find out what they object to and do it." His stance against Big Tobacco became less judicious as the industry expanded its operations into the developing world, and deployed subtle blandishments to retain a presence in its traditional markets—this he viewed as thoroughly immoral.

On 15 April 1994, under the headline "Tobacco chiefs say cigarettes aren't addictive", the *New York Times* had reported on one of the most bizarre incidents in the medical history of tobacco. A day earlier, the chief executive officers of the seven largest American tobacco companies testified under oath to Congress that they did not believe cigarettes were addictive. They told the house energy and commerce subcommittee on health and the environment that "cigarettes may cause lung cancer, heart disease and other health problems, but that the evidence was not conclusive." In a phrase redolent of Alexandre Dumas's musketeers, the inseparable corporate collaborators embraced the maxim "one for all and all for one". Their infamous declaration may have been partly explained by the 1988 report of the surgeon general that smoking was addictive but it also marked a sea change in the perception of Big Tobacco in the eyes of the American public.

On 14 May 1994, Michael Moore, attorney general for the state of Mississippi, filed the first Medicaid lawsuit against thirteen tobacco companies, claiming that they should reimburse the state for the costs of treating those with smoking-related diseases. Attorney generals from other states joined the suit, and the great Chinese wall of legal protection behind which Big Tobacco had operated was about to be breached in a dramatic way.* In Florida, Stanley and Susan Rosenblatt, a husband and wife team, brought a historic class action suit in Miami. They claimed that the US tobacco companies withheld critical information from the public on the health hazards of passive smoking. Litigation had become a major battleground in the war between public health and Big Tobacco.

With gathering pace, irresistible forces began to unite, culminating in the tobacco Master Settlement Agreement (MSA) in 1998. This agreement, between the four largest tobacco companies and the attorney generals of 46 states, provided restrictions on practices by the companies and payments by them to the states to compensate for the cost of providing health care for people with smoking related diseases. The MSA was the largest civil settlement in US history.

Both Doll and Big Tobacco knew that a scientific discovery scarcely exists until it is communicated and brought to life in the minds of others. As the world's leading expert on the causes of cancer, Doll continued to be a relentless opponent of the tobacco industry's false claims. His constant research into the effects of smoking kept him both at the frontiers of epidemiology and embedded in the legal process.[1] In 1999, he wrote a landmark paper charting the history of the scientific knowledge of the harmful effects of smoking which had been accumulating since the late eighteenth century.[2] The catastrophic impact of tobacco on health led him to a remarkable observation. "That so many diseases—major and minor—

---

* Dan Zegart's book, *Civil Warriors: the Legal Siege on the Tobacco Industry* (Delacorte Press/Random House, 2000) tells the heroic account of the class action led by the lawyer Ron Motley against the tobacco industry. With the help of Jeffrey Wigand (the film, *The Insider*, directed by Michael Mann, was based on his whistle-blowing story) and the anonymous and cryptically named informer "Deep Cough", a new era of tobacco litigation was brought to the US courts.

should be related to smoking is one of the most astonishing findings of medical research in this century."

Paralleling his scientific observations on the impact of smoking on the global population, Doll was willing to testify in court cases against Big Tobacco.* The great wealth of the tobacco industry ensures that it has the finest legal counsel, who, with their intimidating presence, create an exacting environment in which expert witnesses are required to give their evidence. Doll, however, a natural patrician, was not intimidated, and even in his 90th year was still willing to engage in the adversarial inquisition because, as Christopher his brother said, "It was important to him, that's why he did it."[3]

In the summer of 2002 Doll appeared in the case of Betty Bullock v Philip Morris in the superior court of the state of California. The plaintiff's lawyer, Michael J Piuze, assisted by the renowned trial consultant Ray Goldstein, argued that Philip Morris had concealed the dangers of cigarettes from his 64-year-old client who had contracted lung cancer. The jury awarded Betty Bullock a famous victory and $28 billion in punitive damages against the tobacco giant, which was subsequently reduced to $28 million.

On 25 August 2002 the *Los Angeles Times* gave an insight into Doll's standing as an expert witness.

> Dignified, affable and decorated with honours, Doll is a tobacco lawyer's worst nightmare. He sits there with noble countenance and solid science, his virtue unimpeachable, and wins the day. For him science speaks for itself and adding ego or politics is not a gentleman's way. By the time he has done answering questions from the plaintiff's lawyer, the Philip Morris attorney might as well have been representing Genghis Khan.

---

* Doll's first sworn testimony in the US was at the Palm Beach courthouse, 17-20 January 1997 in the Florida attorney general case v Big Tobacco. The plaintiff's lawyer was Ron Motley.

Doll respected the right of Big Tobacco to sell cigarettes but he did not think they should be allowed to advertise, particularly if the marketing was aimed at teenagers. It was the industry's policy to spread doubt about the harmful effects of smoking—which Doll believed was motivated by greed—that compelled him to confront Big Tobacco's dishonesty in the courts.

Doll's announcement that he was going to stop driving after seventy years behind the wheel was greeted with relief by many who shared Green College's car park with him. His vivid green Audi had suffered the bumps and scratches of too many tight manoeuvres that were now beyond his ability to control. It was another inevitable consequence of his physical decline; mentally, however, he was still incisive.

His productive Indian summer of scientific study reached its apogee with the publication on 26 June 2004 of the fifty years' observation on male British doctors.[4] Never before in the history of non-infectious epidemiology had so much been learned by so many from so few. It marked an astonishing example of the medical application of statistics and a memorable anniversary in time: being published in the *British Medical Journal* on exactly the same date—26 June—fifty years after the original study into the smoking habits of the nation's doctors. The paper represented far more than a celebratory milestone in public health. It provided decisive new information and convincingly showed that the risks of persistent cigarette smoking were significantly larger than had previously been suspected.

Doll and Peto estimated that during the fifty-year follow-up about six million British people were killed by tobacco use. They found that for those men born between 1900-30, who smoked only cigarettes and continued smoking, they died on average about ten years younger than life-long non-smokers. One discovery of deliverance for smokers was that if they quit the habit at age sixty, fifty, forty, or thirty they gained respectively, three, six, nine, or almost the full ten years of healthy life expectancy.

The *British Medical Journal* editorial noted: "Had the British doctors' study ceased, even after a long run of two decades, much valuable information would not have become available."[5] Using, and inventing, reliable statistical methods to analyse the patterns of disease in large populations, Doll and Peto were the world leaders in the study of the health effects of smoking. Doll's career had led to the emergence of epidemiology as one of medical science's great successes over the previous sixty years. Prophetically, for Doll was part of the prospective study, one unanticipated finding was the substantial decrease in the mortality rates among non-smokers due to prevention and the improved treatment of disease. This led him to observe, "The probability that a 70-year-old would survive to 90 was only 12 per cent at our 1950s non-smoker death rates, but it was 33 per cent at our 1990s non-smoker death rates. Still, however, few would survive to 100."[6]

Doll was 92 on 28 October 2004. But he did not mark the event with a celebratory lunch and a glass of Madeira. Instead, he gave a talk with Richard Peto on the fifty year study to a packed meeting of mainly white-coated doctors in the lecture theatre of the John Radcliffe Hospital, Oxford. Both men were relaxed, and comfortable with an audience that had come to recognise the power and necessity of statistics to clinical research and hence to clinical practice. It was a bravura performance of scientific enlightenment.

Doll's work had changed the health of the nation, yet there are two surprising features of his life in medicine. Firstly, from 1969 he did not practise the art of medicine, and he rarely saw individual patients; as a physician he had taken medical research out of the hospital ward and laboratory and put it into society. Secondly, as a society we glorify celebrities; but the man who made one of the most significant contributions to the health of the international community remains virtually unknown.

Marna Buckatzch, one of the social workers on Doll and Hill's 1950 case-control study, feels that while Doll saved millions from premature death "no one knows about him, except in the profession."[7] In an obscurantist-leaning society this may be inevitable, but Marie Kidd, who helped compile statistics on the British doctors' study, is less pessimistic about his legacy. "He lived through a remarkable period that saw a complete reversal of attitude. From a time when smoking was accepted as part of the cultural life, to a point where whole countries banned it, and where it has become a minority pursuit in the country where it was most practised."[8]

The dangers of tobacco have even penetrated the last bastion of recidivist Stalinism, North Korea. The regime's leader, Kim Jong-Il, who reportedly gave up smoking in 2003, banned students from smoking inside university buildings. He famously described the smoker as one of the "three main fools of the twenty-first century" along with people who know nothing about music or computers.

Generally the contribution of scientists to human wellbeing over the last hundred years has received little recognition in the collective consciousness. Some, like Doll, realised that their greatest achievement was not in who they were, or even what they had done, but rather how they had done it. What was permanent was the delineation of the method rather than the individual.

In November 2004 Doll wound up the project that many regarded as his masterpiece and which effectively announced the beginning of the modern era of cancer epidemiology. Of the 40,564 doctors who took part in the original study only 6,000 were still alive for Doll to write to. He thanked them for their assistance, which had enabled him to publish scientific papers on smoking, alcohol and aspirin, but added that he had taken the experiment as far as it could go. Over the fifty years of the study 17 doctors had been struck off, two had died of conflagration in their beds (probably smoking related) and two had changed their sex.

Socrates' declaration that "the unexamined life is not worth living" might well stand as Doll's epitaph. Certainly, while it is true that he went to great lengths examining how others lived their lives, he also scrutinised his own with equal intellectual self-discipline. He did not live with illusions. Doll was not a naturally warm person and genetically he was well suited to epidemiology, which of all the medical disciplines is perhaps the most dispassionate. He loved gardening and escaping into literature, yet he knew he was driven by a compulsion to work, which he found irresistible.

Doll did not switch off very much; and even in his 93rd year he was still working late into the night accompanied by his Bang and Olufsen radiogram pulsing out the music of concentration. Crucially, the world still wanted him. Jointly with Richard Peto, he was awarded the King Faisal international prize for medicine in 2005, which gave him the chance to fulfil an ambition: to ride a camel in the Arabian desert. He was regularly invited to address conferences, and in the last year of his life he gave lectures on the causes of cancer in seven countries on five continents. Although he told his GP, Ann McPherson, that he felt he was ageing "two months every one", he still believed that for him the only way to live was to the full.

Another aspect of Doll's personality that was obvious to all who knew him was his punctuality and aversion to "letting people down". His papers were invariably delivered on time, and his lectures rarely postponed: Doll's word was his bond. This obligation to duty was tested in May 2005 when a long-standing series of lectures in Canada clashed with an award ceremony at the Karolinska Institute in Stockholm. Doll had received more than enough honorary doctorates, but if he could make it to Sweden he would share an award with Nelson Mandela, a man he admired but had never met. Earlier in the year Doll had read *A Long Walk to Freedom*, the South African leader's autobiography, and had stood in the cell on Robben Island where Mandela had been incarcerated for much of his 27-year jail term. Such an opportunity comes but once in a lifetime, and Doll knew he was approaching the end of his.

It was a schedule that a far younger person would have found punishing, but Doll flew overnight from his lecture tour of Canada to arrive in London on the morning of Friday 12 May. He returned to Oxford, collected his formal dinner jacket, repacked his suitcase and returned to Heathrow for a flight to Stockholm that evening. After some late night beer in the piano bar of the Grand Hotel, Doll went to bed looking forward to Saturday's award ceremony. Unfortunately Mandela had been ill and was too frail to make the journey to Stockholm's architecturally stunning City Hall. Fortuitously for Doll, however, Professor Reijo Vihko and Margareta Wallenius-Kleberg, who were also being honoured with a doctorate, were in attendance. The day-long ceremony involved arduous hikes up vertiginous stairways and around long internal balconies; Doll held his place in the honoured formation—just. With kindness and formidable strength, Vihko took hold of Doll by the arm and semi-levitated him around the gilded building.

The following day, in a warm breeze that promised summer, Doll walked past the National Museum on Blasieholm peninsula. From a distance he looked more fragile than before; seemingly eroded by time, he appeared almost translucent. His creative surge was over—and he would be dead within two months. His ambition in life was to be a "valuable member of society". No one with a compassionate heart would deny him that accolade.

On 10 June 2005 the formal move was made into the Richard Doll Building in Headington. Costing more than £20 million, from one of its elevations the building resembles the prow of an ocean liner, perhaps not unlike that of the *Mauretania* that had taken Doll to New York in 1934. This spacious architectural tabernacle immortalises his contribution to medical research and the empire whose construction he had overseen. It houses the cancer epidemiology unit he had founded, as well as Peto's brainchild the clinical trials service unit, and the department of public health perinatal epidemiology unit. Doll admired its design and was honoured by the eponymous tribute, but its situation, two miles up the hill in Headington, signalled an end to the days when he could take a gentle walk to work along the garden path.

In the final months of his life Doll still enjoyed an enviable social life. If it was not dinner with Lalla Ward in one of their favourite restaurants, he was being taken to the cinema or having drinks with Richard Peto while inevitably discussing work. Also a new tradition had been started. Sunday lunch was normally spent in a pub somewhere in the Oxford countryside with Steve. Since living separately they had built a friendship around these weekly excursions. His longevity continued to attract journalists who wanted to interview him and write about how his science had changed the course of medical history[9]—and had entered the national bloodstream.

Early in July 2005 Doll had a silent heart attack and was put under the care of consultant cardiologist and family friend Oliver Ormerod in the John Radcliffe Hospital. For two weeks, under a tidal wave of visits and goodwill, Richard Doll was optimistic about recovering, but when his blood pressure fell irreversibly his rage against death ebbed away. In 1989 under cross-examination from Steven Sedley QC, Doll spoke philosophically about his mortality, "I cannot believe that my life is as valuable as the life of a twenty-year-old. I think it should not be given the same weight." This was not a self-effacing view; Doll thought every reasonable person should think the same way.

Resurrecting the logic that had caused a furore in 1973 when he called for those over 65 to "live dangerously", he knew that a disproportionate part of the health budget was spent on the last year of an individual's life. He strongly believed that it was wrong to spend large sums of money trying to keep an old person alive for a few months when by spending less money a young person could be kept alive for fifty years. At last Richard Doll had come to a point in his life when he was not "frightened of something". Perhaps unfairly, he asked both Ann McPherson and Oliver Ormerod to suspend their Hippocratic oath and expedite his death. When no such help was given he resigned himself to his biological fate. The fortitude and intellect that had guided him in life remained intact until his death, on Sunday 24 July.

Two months later, on 8 September, some of the world's leading epidemiologists gathered for the official opening ceremony of the Richard Doll Building. Many had been trained by Doll and they were there to pay homage to his contribution to the health of the global community. For medical historians, 8 September is an historic date in the evolution of epidemiological science since it was the day in 1854 that John Snow persuaded the board of guardians of St James's parish to remove the handle from the Broad Street pump. Snow was the greatest epidemiologist of the nineteenth century and Doll the greatest of the twentieth century. Both men's scientific findings met with widespread disbelief among scientists, politicians and the masses but their shared concern for public health forms a great chapter in the history of medicine.

One thing the assembled dignitaries did not know was that on 8 September 2005 Richard Doll's death certificate arrived from Southport in his own building. He was part of the fifty-year follow-up of British doctors. His death certificate—death due to heart failure—was his final contribution to its lasting testament.

Doll was a true hero of the National Health Service and his death produced a genuine sense of a loss for he was part of an idealistic generation who helped to build a better, fairer world. His work led to two incontrovertible achievements: the reduction of human suffering; and the advancement of human wellbeing. Most people will never have heard of his name, but by demonstrating how smokers could avoid premature death he deserves to be remembered with respect and gratitude. William Richard Shaboe Doll represented the ultimate in dedication, perseverance and integrity—not the last of his kind, but the only one of his kind.

NOTES

INTRODUCTION

1 Peto, Richard, personal communication.
2 Austoker, Joan, *History of the Imperial Cancer Research Fund, 1902–86* (Oxford University Press, 1988).
3 Doll, R and Hill, AB, 'Smoking and Carcinoma of the Lung', *British Medical Journal*, 1950, vol. 2, p. 739.
4 Doll, R, Peto, R, Wheatley, K, Gray, R and Sutherland, I, 'Mortality in Relation to Smoking: 40 years' observations on male British doctors', *British Medical Journal*, 1994, vol. 309, pp. 901–11.
5 May, Robert, letter in support of Sir Richard Doll for the Nathan Davis International Award, 15 February 2001.
6 Nurse, Paul, letter in support of Sir Richard Doll for the Nathan Davis International Award, 20 February 2001.
7 Doll, Richard, 'Tobacco: A Medical History', *Journal of Urban Health: Bulletin of the New York Academy of Medicine*, 1999, vol. 76, no. 3, p. 300.
8 Fisher, RA, 'Alleged Dangers of Cigarette Smoking', letter, *British Medical Journal*, 1957, vol. 2, p. 1518.
9 Bodmer, Walter, personal communication.
10 Doll, Richard, 'An Epidemiological Perspective of the Biology of Cancer', *Cancer Research*, 1978, vol. 38, pp. 3573–83.
11 Halsey, AH, personal communication.
12 Tudor Hart, Julian, personal communication.
13 Donaldson, Liam, personal communication.

CHAPTER 1

1 Doll, Christopher, personal communication.
2 Cooper, George, *And Hitler Stopped Play: Cricket and War at Lyminster House, West Sussex (1931–1946)* (Vanguard, 2001).
3 Field, John, *The King's Nurseries: The Story of Westminster School*, 2nd edn (James & James, 1987), p. 602.
4 Doll, Richard, personal communication.
5 Morgan, Kenneth O (ed.), *The Oxford History of Britain. The Twentieth Century* (Oxford University Press, 1983).
6 Field, John, op. cit.
7 Doll, Richard, op. cit.
8 Ibid.
9 Ibid.
10 Ibid.
11 Ibid.
12 Ibid.
13 Ibid.

14 Ibid.
15 Ibid.
16 Ibid.
17 Ibid.
18 Ibid.
19 Cook, Christopher, *The Journal of Public Health Medicine*, oral history project, interview with Sir Richard Doll, 30 July 2003.
20 Cheetham, Juliet, personal communication.
21 Doll, Christopher, personal communication.
22 Doll, Richard.

CHAPTER 2
1   Crofton, John, personal communication.
2   Doll, Richard, personal communication.
3   Crofton, John, op. cit.
4   Ledingham, John, personal communication.
5   Dornhorst, Tony, personal communication.
6   Crofton, John, op. cit.
7   Doll, Richard, op. cit.
8   Ibid.
9   Pemberton, John, 'Social Medicine Comes on the Scene in the United Kingdom, 1936–1960', *Journal of Public Health Medicine*, 1998, vol. 20, no. 2, pp. 149–53.
10 British Medical Association, report of committee on nutrition, *British Medical Journal Supplement*, 25 November 1933, pp. 1–16.
11 Pemberton, John, 'Malnutrition in England', *University College Magazine*, 1934 (July–August), pp. 153–9 (reprinted in *International Journal of Epidemiology*, 2003, vol. 32, pp. 493–5).
12 Doll, Richard, op. cit.
13 Crofton, John, op. cit.
14 Doll, Richard, op. cit.
15 Faulkner, Joan, personal communication.
16 Pemberton, John, op. cit.
17 Doll, Richard, op. cit.
18 Ibid.
19 Ibid.
20 Ibid.
21 Boyd Orr, John, *Food, Health and Income* (Macmillan, 1936).
22 Doll, Richard, op. cit.
23 Ibid.
24 Pemberton, John, op. cit.
25 Cooper, George, *And Hitler Stopped Play: Cricket and War at Lyminster House, West Sussex (1931–46)* (Vanguard, 2001).

26 Bayliss, Richard, personal communication.
27 Doll, Richard, op. cit.
28 Ibid.
29 Ibid.
30 Skegg, David, personal communication.
31 Doll, Richard, 'Notes on the Berger Rhythm and the Electroencephalogram', *St Thomas's Hospital Gazette*, 1937, pp. 294–7.
32 D'Arcy Hart, Philip, personal communication.
33 Dornhorst, Tony, op. cit.
34 Doll, Richard, personal communication.

CHAPTER 3
1 Doll, Richard, personal communication.
2 Ibid.
3 Ibid.
4 Ibid.
5 Ibid.
6 Ibid.
7 Ibid.
8 Ibid.
9 Ibid.
10 Allenbrooke, Field Marshall Lord, *War Diaries 1939–1945* (Weidenfeld & Nicolson, 2001), p. 67.
11 Doll, Richard, op.cit.
12 Ibid.
13 Doll, Richard, 'Dunkirk Diary. Experiences of a Battalion Medical Officer in the Retreat to Dunkirk: 1', *British Medical Journal*, 1990, vol. 300, pp. 1183–6.
14 Moss, Norman, *Britain, America and the Fateful Summer of 1940, Nineteen Weeks* (Arum Press, 1998), p. 94.
15 Doll, Richard, personal communication.
16 Doll, Richard, *Dunkirk Diary*, op. cit.
17 Doll, Richard, personal communication.
18 Ibid.
19 Ibid.
20 Ibid.
21 Ibid.
22 Ibid.
23 Ibid.
24 Ibid.
25 Kisch R, *Days of the Good Soldiers: Communists in the Armed Forces, World War II* (Journeyman Press, 1985).
26 Doll, Richard, op. cit.
27 Ibid.

28 Ibid.
29 Ibid.
30 Ibid.
31 Ibid.
32 Ibid.
33 Ibid.

CHAPTER 4

1   Beveridge, William, *The Pillars of Security* (Allen & Unwin, 1943), p. 109.
2   Doll, Richard, personal communication.
3   Dornhorst, Tony, personal communication.
4   D'Arcy Hart, Philip, personal communication.
5   Stewart, John, *The Battle for Health: A Political History of the Socialist Medical Association, 1930–51* (Ashgate Publishing, 1999), p. 132.
6   Avery Jones, Francis, foreword in Vessey, MP and Gray, M (eds.), *Cancer: Risks and Prevention* (Oxford University Press, 1985).
7   Hockaday, Derek, personal communication.
8   Bockus, Henry L, *Gastroenterology* (Saunders, 1944).
9   Hill, AB, foreword in Vessey, MP and Gray, M (eds.), *Cancer: Risks and Prevention* (Oxford University Press, 1985).
10 Armitage, Peter, personal communication.
11 Bull, Rosemary, personal communication.
12 Doll, R and Jones, FA, 'Environmental Factors in the Aetiology of Peptic Ulcer', *The Practitioner*, 1949, vol. 162, pp. 44–50.
13 Doll, Richard, personal communication.

CHAPTER 5

1   Le Fanu, James, *The Rise and Fall of Modern Medicine* (Little, Brown, 1999), p. 30.
2   Doll, Richard, *Austin Bradford Hill, Biographical Memoirs of the Royal Society* (The Royal Society, 1994).
3   Ibid.
4   Hill, AB, 'The Aim of the Statistical Method, editorial, *Lancet*, 1937, vol. 3, p. 37.
5   Doll, Richard, op. cit.
6   Bull, Rosemary, personal communication.
7   Doll, Richard, 'Voices of Epidemiology', A conversation with Doll conducted by Sarah Darby at the John Radcliffe Hospital, 9 August 2002.
8   Le Fanu, James, op. cit.
9   Doll, Richard, op. cit.
10 Armitage, P, 'The Role of Randomization in Clinical Trials', *Statistics in Medicine*, 1992, vol. 1, pp. 345–52.
11 Fisher, RA, 'The Arrangement of Field Experiments', *Journal of the Ministry of*

Agriculture of Great Britain, 1926, vol. 33, pp. 503–13.

12 Bradford Hill, A, *Controlled Clinical Trials, A Symposium* (Blackwell Scientific Publishing, 1960), p. 3.

13 Ibid.

14 Hill, AB, interview with Max Blythe, the Royal College of Physicians and Oxford Brookes University, 26 March 1990.

15 Medical Research Council, Streptomycin in Tuberculosis trials committee, 'Streptomycin Treatment for Pulmonary Tuberculosis', *British Medical Journal*, 1948, vol. 2, pp. 769–82.

16 Doll, Richard, op. cit.

17 Hill, AB, 'Suspended Judgement: memories of the British streptomycin trial in tuberculosis', *Controlled Clinical Trials*, 1990, vol. 11, pp. 77–9.

18 Daniels, M and Hill, AB, 'Chemotherapy of Pulmonary Tuberculosis in Young Adults; an analysis of the combined results of three Medical Research Council trials', *British Medical Journal*, 1952, vol. 1, pp. 1162–8.

19 Medical Research Council, 'Treatment of Pulmonary Tuberculosis with Streptomycin and Para-aminosalicylic Acid', *British Medical Journal*, 1950, vol. 2, pp.1074-85ff.

20 Doll, Richard, personal communication.

CHAPTER 6

1 Stocks, P in Massey, A (ed.), *Modern Trends in Public Health* (Butterworth, 1949), p. 591.

2 Austoker, Joan, *History of the Imperial Cancer Research Fund, 1902–86* (Oxford University Press, 1988).

3 Stocks, P, 'Regional and Local Differences in Cancer Death Rates', *General Register Office: Studies on Medical and Population Subjects*, No. 1 (HMSO, 1947).

4 Webster, Charles, 'Tobacco Smoking Addiction: a challenge to the National Health Service', *British Journal of Addiction*, 1984, vol. 79, pp. 7–16.

5 Kennaway, Ernest, 'Cancer of the Lung and Larynx', British Empire Cancer Campaign, 24th annual report, 1947, p. 190.

6 Passey, RD, 'Cancer of the Lung', British Empire Cancer Research Campaign, 6th annual report, 1929.

7 Roffo, AH, 'Durch Tabak beim Kaninchen entwickeltes Carcinom', *Zeitschrift für Krebsforschung*, 1931, vol. 33, pp. 321–32.

8 Tudor Edwards, A, 'Carcinoma of the Bronchus', *Thorax*, 1946, vol. 1, pp. 1–25.

9 Stewart, Alice, personal communication.

10 Bull, Rosemary, personal communication.

11 Pollock, D, *Denial and Delay: The Political History of Smoking and Health, 1951–1964* (Action on Smoking and Health, 1999), p. 5.

12 Milton T, 'The Contributions of Henry E. Sigerist to Health Service Organisation', *Journal of Public Health Policy*, 1995, vol. 16, pp. 152–93.

13 Pollock, D, op. cit, p. 3.
14 Doll, R, 'Tobacco: a medical history', *Journal of Urban Health: Bulletin of the New York Academy of Medicine,* 1999, vol. 76, pp. 289–313.
15 Austoker Joan, op. cit, p. 194.
16 Conversation with Richard Doll, *British Journal of Addiction,* 1991, vol. 86, pp. 365–77.
17 Hill, AB, 'Observation and Experiment', *The New England Journal of Medicine,* 1953, vol. 248, pp. 995–1001.
18 Pollock, D, op. cit, p. 8.
19 Bull, Rosemary, op. cit.
20 Hill, AB, interview with Max Blythe, the Royal College of Physicians and Oxford Brookes University, 26 March 1990.
21 Wynder, EL and Graham, EA, *Journal of the American Medical Association,* 1950, vol. 143, p. 329.
22 Doll, Richard, personal communication.
23 Doll, R and Hill, AB, 'Smoking and Carcinoma of the Lung, preliminary report', *British Medical Journal,* 1950, vol. 2, pp. 739–48.
24 Austoker, Joan and Bryder, Linda (eds.), *Historical Perspectives on the Role of the MRC* (Oxford University Press, 1989), pp. 52–3.
25 Gilliam, AG, 'A paper read to the 61st annual convention of the Association of Military Surgeons of the United States, November 1954' in *Advances in Cancer Research,* Greenstein, Jesse P. and Haddow, Alexander (eds.), vol. 3 (Academic Press, 1955).
26 Doll, R and Hill, AB, op. cit.
27 Box, Joan Fisher, *The Life of a Scientist* (John Wiley & Sons, New York, 1978).
28 Armitage, P and Berry, G, *Statistical Methods in Medical Research,* 3rd edn (Blackwell Science, 1996), p. 41.
29 Doll, R and Hill, AB, op. cit.
30 Doll, R, *Prevention of Cancer: Pointers from Epidemiology* (Nuffield Provincial Hospitals Trust, 1967).
31 Hill, AB in Vessey, MP and Gray, M (eds.), *Cancer—Risks and Prevention* (Oxford University Press, 1985).
32 Ibid.
33 Buckatzsch, Marna, personal communication.
34 Doll, R and Hill, AB, op. cit.
35 Ibid.
36 Pelling, M, *Cholera, Fever and English Medicine 1825–1865* (Oxford University Press, 1978).

CHAPTER 7
1 Hutt, Avis, personal communication.
2 Tudor Hart, Julian, personal communication.
3 Rae, Nick, personal communication.

4 Hutt, Avis, op. cit.
5 Churchill, Winston, 'Rejoice' speech, VE Day 1945.
6 Faulkner, Joan, personal communication.
7 Ibid.
8 Ibid.
9 *Humanise the Hospitals*, broadsheet issued by the Communist Party (Farleigh Press, 1947).
10 Roth, Martin, personal communication.
11 Doll, Richard, personal communication.
12 Webster, C, *The Health Service since the War, vol. 1, Problems of Health Care: The NHS before 1957* (HMSO, 1988).
13 Morris, Jerry, personal communication.
14 Ibid.
15 Backett, Maurice, personal communication.
16 Ibid.
17 Shuster, Sam, personal communication.
18 Doll, Richard, op. cit.
19 Faulkner, Marian, personal communication.

CHAPTER 8
1 Godber, George, personal communication.
2 Doll, Richard, personal communication.
3 National Health Service Act (1946) Section 1.
4 *Daily Mail*, 5 October 1950.
5 Bull, Rosemary, personal communication.
6 Kidd, Marie, personal communication.
7 Chisholm, Anne and Davie, Michael, *Beaverbrook: A Life* (Hutchinson, 1992).
8 Pollock, David, *Denial and Delay: The Political History of Smoking and Health, 1951–1964* (Action on Smoking and Health, 1999), p. 11.
9 Webster, Charles, 'Tobacco Smoking Addiction: a challenge to the National Health Service', *British Journal of Addiction*, 1984, vol. 79, pp. 7–16.
10 Godber, George, op. cit.
11 Ibid.
12 Avery Jones, Joan, personal communication.
13 Doll, Richard, op. cit.
14 Morris, Jerry, personal communication.
15 Webster, Charles, op. cit.
16 Hill, AB, 'Observation and Experiment' (Cutter lecture in preventive medicine), *New England Journal of Medicine*, 1953, vol. 248, pp. 995–1001.
17 Doll, Richard, op. cit.
18 Doll, R, Peto, R, Boreham, J and Sutherland, I, 'Mortality in Relation to Smoking: 50 years' observation on male British doctors', *British Medical Journal*, 2004, vol. 328, pp. 1519–33.

19 Peto, R, 'Smoking and Death: the past 40 years and the next 40', *British Medical Journal*, 1944, vol. 309, pp. 937–9.
20 Hill, AB, 'Do you Smoke?' letter, *British Medical Journal*, 1951, vol. 2, p. 1157.
21 Doll, R and Hill, AB, 'The Mortality of Doctors in Relation to their Smoking Habits', a preliminary report, *British Medical Journal*, 1954, vol. 1, pp. 1451–55.
22 Bull, Rosemary, op. cit.
23 Gilliland, Jean, personal communication.
24 *Daily Mail*, 2 June 1954.
25 Hill, AB foreword in Vessey, MP and Gray, M (eds.), *Cancer—Risks and Prevention* (Oxford University Press, 1985).
26 Hill, AB, interview with Max Blythe, 1990, Medical sciences video archive of the Royal College of Physicians, Oxford Brookes University.
27 Hammond, EC and Horn, D, 'The Relationship between Human Smoking Habits and Death Rates: a follow-up study of 187,766 men', *Journal of the American Medical Association*, 1954, vol. 155, pp. 1316–28.
28 Doll, R and Hill, AB, 'A study of the Aetiology of Carcinoma of the Lung', *British Medical Journal*, 1952, vol. 2, pp. 1271–86.
29 Proctor, RN, *The Nazi War on Cancer* (Princeton University Press, 1999).
30 Wassink, WF, 'Onstaansvoorwarden voor Longkanker', *Ned Tijdschr Geneeskd*, 1948, vol. 92, pp. 3732–47.
31 Davey Smith, G, Ströbele, SA and Egger, M, 'Smoking and Health Promotion in Nazi Germany', *Journal of Epidemiology and Community Health*, 1994, vol. 48, pp. 220–23.
32 Pearl, R, 'Tobacco Smoking and Longevity', *Science*, 1938, vol. 87, pp. 216–17.
33 Proctor, RN, op. cit.
34 Ibid.
35 Proctor, RN, personal communication.
36 Ibid.
37 Doll, R, 'Commentary: Lung Cancer and Tobacco Consumption', *International Journal of Epidemiology*, 2001, vol. 30, pp. 30–37.
38 Pollock, David, op. cit.
39 Pollock, David, op. cit, p. 15.
40 Doll, Richard, personal communication.
41 Elson, LA, Obituary of Richard Passey, *Journal of Pathology*, 1973, vol. 111, pp. 139–44.
42 Passey, R, 'Smoking and Lung Cancer', letter, *British Medical Journal*, 1953, vol. 1, pp. 1362–63.
43 Webster, C, 'Tobacco Smoking Addiction: a challenge to the National Health Service', *British Journal of Addiction*, 1984, vol. 79, pp. 7–16.
44 Pollock, David, op. cit., p. 25.
45 Godber, George, personal communication.
46 Berridge, Virginia, 'The Policy Response to the Smoking and Lung Cancer Connection in the 1950s and 60s', *Historian Journal*, 2006, 49 (4), pp. 1185–

1209.

47 Doll, R and Hill, AB, op. cit.

48 Hammond, EC and Horn, D, op. cit.

49 *Daily Mail*, 24 June 1954.

CHAPTER 9

1   Doll, R, 'The Scientific Approach', *Annals of Physical Medicine, 1954*, vol. 2, pp. 85–9.

2   Gilliland, Jean, personal communication.

3   Arnold, Lorna, *Britain and the H-Bomb* (Palgrave Publishers, 2001).

4   Aldridge, Richard, *The Hidden Hand* (John Murray, 2001).

5   Doll, R, 'Causes of Death among Gas-workers with Special Reference to Cancer of the Lung', *British Journal of Industrial Medicine*, 1952, vol. 9, p. 180.

6   Nordling, CO, 'A New Theory of Cancer-induction Mechanism', *British Journal of Cancer*, 1942, vol. 7, pp. 68–72.

7   Willis, RA, *Pathology of Tumours* (Butterworth, 1948).

8   Armitage, Peter, personal communication.

9   Nordling, CO, op. cit.

10 Armitage, P and Doll, R, 'The Age Distribution of Cancer and a Multi-stage Theory of Carcinogenesis', *British Journal of Cancer*, 1954, vol. 8, pp. 1–12.

11 Armitage, Peter, personal communication.

12 Doll, R, op. cit.

13 Armitage, P and Doll, R, op. cit.

14 Hill, AB, interview with Max Blythe, 1990, Medical sciences video archive of the Royal College of Physicians, Oxford Brookes University.

15 Doll, R, 'Major Epidemics of the 20th century from Coronary Thrombosis to AIDS', *Journal of the Royal Statistical Society*, Series A, 1987, vol. 150, pp. 373–95.

16 Doll, R, 'The Age Distribution of Cancer and a Multistage Theory of Carcinogenesis', *International Journal of Epidemiology*, 2004, vol. 33, pp. 1183–84.

17 Frank, SA, *Dynamics of Cancer Incidence, Inheritance, and Evolution* (Princeton University Press, 2007).

18 Doll, R, 'A Tentative Estimate of the Leukaemogenic Effect of Test Thermonuclear Explosions', *Journal of Radiological Protection*, 1996, vol. 16, pp. 3–5.

19 Ibid.

20 Ibid.

21 Armitage, Peter, op. cit.

22 Pike, Malcolm, personal communication.

23 Kidd, Marie, personal communication.

24 Godfrey, Malcolm, personal communication.

CHAPTER 10

1   Doll, R, 'Mortality from Lung Cancer in Asbestos Workers', *British Journal of Industrial Medicine*, 1955, vol. 12, pp. 81–6.

2   Cooke, WE, 'Pulmonary Asbestosis', *British Medical Journal*, 1927, vol. 2, pp. 1024–25.

3   Merewether, ERA and Price, CW, *Report on Effects of Asbestos Dust on the Lungs and Dust Suppression in the Asbestos Industry* (HMSO, 1930).

4   Doll, Richard, 'Epidemiological Discovery of Occupational Cancers', *Annals of Academic Medicine Singapore*, 1984, vol. 13, p. 331.

5   Wood, W Burton and Gloyne, SR, 'Pulmonary Asbestosis', *Lancet*, 1934, vol. 2, pp. 1383–85.

6   Gloyne, SR, 'Pneumoconiosis: a histological survey of necropsy material in 205 cases', *Lancet*, 1951, vol. 260, pp. 810–14.

7   Doll, Richard, personal papers at the Wellcome Library for the History and Understanding of Medicine.

8   Doll, Richard, personal communication.

9   Peto, Julian *et al.*, 'Relationship of Mortality to Measure of Environmental Asbestos Pollution in an Asbestos Textile Factory', *Annals of Occupational Hygiene*, 1985, vol. 29, no. 3, pp. 305–55.

10 Doll, Richard, 'Causes of Death among Gas-workers with Special Reference to Cancer of the Lung', *British Journal of Industrial Medicine*, 1952, vol. 9, pp. 180–85.

11 Doll, Richard, 'Mortality from Lung Cancer in Asbestos Workers', op. cit.

12 Doll, Richard, personal communication.

13 Ibid.

14 Tweedale, Geoffrey, *Magic Mineral to Killer Dust. Turner & Newall and the Asbestos Hazard* (Oxford University Press, 2000), p. 149.

15 Ibid.

16 Tweedale, Geoffrey, personal communication.

17 Doll, Richard, op. cit.

18 Castleman, Barry I., *Asbestos: Medical and Legal Aspects* (Aspen Publishers, 1996).

19 Doll, Richard, 'Mortality from Lung Cancer in Asbestos Workers', op. cit.

20 Peto, J, 'The Establishment of Industrial Hygiene Standards: an example', in Whittmore, A. (ed.), *Environmental Health Quantitative Methods for Industrial and Applied Mathematics* (Society for Applied Mathematics, 1977), pp. 104–14.

21 Tweedale, Geoffrey, op. cit.

22 Acheson, Donald, Introduction to Doll's paper, 'Mortality from Lung Cancer in Asbestos Workers', in Ashton, John (ed.), *The Epidemiological Imagination: A Reader* (Oxford University Press, 1994), p. 12.

23 Acheson, ED and Gardner, MJ, 'The Ill Effects of Asbestos on Health', *Asbestos: Final Report of Advisory Committee*, vol. 2 (HMSO, 1979).

24 Acheson, Donald, personal communication.

25 Doll, Richard, personal communication.
26 Knox, JF, Doll, R and Hill, ID, 'Cohort Analysis of Changes in Incidence of Bronchial Carcinoma in a Textile Asbestos Factory', *Annals of the New York Academy of Sciences*, 1965, vol. 132, pp. 526–35.
27 Hill, ID, personal communication.
28 Tweedale, Geoffrey, *Magic Mineral to Killer Dust*, op. cit., p. 181.
29 Newhouse, ML and Thompson, H, 'Mesothelioma of Pleura and Peritoneum Following Exposure to Asbestos in the London Area', *British Journal of Industrial Medicine*, 1965, vol. 22, pp. 261–69.
30 Knox, JF, Holmes, S, Doll, R and Hill, ID, 'Mortality from Lung Cancer and Other Causes among Workers in an Asbestos Textile Factory', *British Journal of Industrial Medicine*, 1968, vol. 25, pp. 293–303.
31 Doll, Richard, op. cit.
32 Standing medical advisory committee: sub-committee on cancer, Department of Health and Social Security, 1968–71.
33 Doll, Richard, personal communication.
34 'Control the Asbestos Hazard', leader, *Lancet*, 1967, vol. 1, pp. 1311–12.
35 Tudor Hart, Julian, personal communication.
36 Doll, Richard, 'Controlled trials: the 1948 watershed', *British Medical Journal*, 1998, vol. 317, pp. 1217–20.
37 Peto, Julian, personal communication.
38 Ibid.
39 Peto J, Doll, R, Howard, SV, Kinlen L and Lewinsohn, HC, 'A Mortality Study among Workers in an English Asbestos Factory', *British Journal of Industrial Medicine*, 1977, vol. 34, pp. 169–73.
40 Peto J, 'The Establishment of Industrial Hygiene Standards: an example', op. cit.
41 Peto, Julian, personal communication.
42 *Oxford Mail*, 31 January 1977.
43 Peto, Julian, op. cit.
44 Ibid.
45 Wagner, JC, Sleggs, CA and Marchand, P, 'Diffuse Pleural Mesothelioma and Asbestos Exposure in the North Western Cape Province', *British Journal of Industrial Medicine*, 1960, vol. 17, pp. 260–71.
46 Seidman, H, Selikoff, IJ and Hammond, EC, 'Short Term Asbestos Work Exposure and Long Term Observation', *Annals of the New York Academy of Sciences*, 1979, vol. 330, pp. 61–90.
47 Doll, Richard and Peto, Julian, 'Asbestos. Effects on Health of Exposure to Asbestos' (Health & Safety Commission, HMSO, 1985), pp. 1–62.
48 Peto, Julian, op. cit.
49 Doll, Richard, personal communication.
50 Acheson, ED and Gardner, MJ, *Asbestos: The Control Limit for Asbestos* (Health and Safety Commission, HMSO, 1983).

51 Acheson, Donald, personal communication.
52 *Hansard,* Asbestos Power Stations, 1983–84, vol. 46, p. 1412.
53 Peto, Julian, personal communication.
54 Doll, Richard, personal communication.
55 *Wall Street Journal,* 5 March 2001.
56 Peto J, Hodgson, JT, Matthews, FE and Jones, JR, 'Continuing Increase in Mesothelioma Mortality in Britain', *Lancet,* 1994, vol. 345, pp. 535–39.
57 Ibid.
58 Doll, Richard, op. cit.
59 Doll, Richard, 'The Challenge of Asbestos' (unpublished, 1984).
60 Peto, Julian, op. cit.
61 *Sunday Telegraph,* 17 March 2002.

CHAPTER 11
1   Doll, Richard, foreword in Cleave, TL and Campbell, GD, *Diabetes Coronary Thrombosis and the Saccharine Disease* (John Wright and Sons, 1966).
2   Doll, R, 'Bronchial Carcinoma: incidence and aetiology', *British Medical Journal,* 1953, vol. 2, pp. 521–27 and 585–90.
3   Hill, AB, foreword in Vessey, MP and Gray, M (eds.), *Cancer: Risks and Prevention* (Oxford University Press, 1985).
4   Doll, R and Hill, AB, 'Lung Cancer and Other Causes of Death in Relation to Smoking. A second report on the mortality of British doctors', *British Medical Journal,* 1956, vol. 2, pp. 1071–76.
5   Doll, R and Hill, AB, 'Lung Cancer and Tobacco', *British Medical Journal,* 1956, vol. 1, pp. 1160–63.
6   Doll R, 'Bronchial Carcinoma: incidence and aetiology', op. cit.
7   Hammond, EC and Horn, D, 'The Relationship between Human Smoking Habits and Death Rates: a follow-up study of 187,766 men', *Journal of the American Medical Association,* 1954, vol. 155, pp. 1316–28.
8   Berridge, Virginia, *Marketing Health: smoking and the discourse of public health in Britain, 1945–2000* (Oxford University Press, 2007), p. 45.
9   Doll, Richard, personal communication.
10 Peto, R, 'Smoking and Death: the past 40 years and the next 40', *British Medical Journal,* 1994, vol. 309, pp. 337–9.
11 Ibid.
12 Webster, C, 'Tobacco Smoking Addiction: a challenge to the National Health Service', *British Journal of Addiction,* 1984, vol. 79, pp. 7–16.
13 'The Dangers of Cigarette Smoking', editorial, *British Medical Journal,* 1957, vol. 1, pp. 1518–20.
14 Kidd, Marie, personal communication.
15 Holland, Walter, personal communication.
16 Fisher Box, J, *R. A. Fisher: The Life of a Scientist* (John Wiley & Sons, 1978).
17 Bodmer, W, 'R. A. Fisher, Statistician and Geneticist Extraordinary: a personal

view', *International Journal of Epidemiology*, 2003, vol. 32, pp. 938–43.

18 Fisher Box, J, op. cit., p. 430.

19 Fisher, RA, *Smoking: the Cancer Controversy* (Oliver and Boyd, 1959), p. 10.

20 Doll, R and Hill, AB, 'Smoking and Carcinoma of the Lung, preliminary report', *British Medical Journal*, 1950, vol. 2, pp. 739–48.

21 Fisher Box, J, op. cit., p. 474.

22 Fisher RA, 'Dangers of Cigarette Smoking', letter, *British Medical Journal*, 1957, vol. 2, p. 43.

23 Doll, R, 'Proof of Causality: deduction from epidemiological observation', *Perspectives in Biology and Medicine*, 2002, vol. 46, pp. 499–515.

24 Doll, R., 'Bronchial Carcinoma: incidence and aetiology', *British Medical Journal*, 1953, vol. 2, pp. 521–7 and 585–90.

25 Hill, AB, An interview with Max Blythe, 1990, Medical sciences video archive of the Royal College of Physicians, Oxford Brookes University.

26 Doll, Richard, personal communication.

27 Doll, R and Hill, AB, 'A Study of the Aetiology of Carcinoma of the Lung', *British Medical Journal*, 1952, vol. 2, pp. 1271–86.

28 Doll, Richard, op. cit.

29 Fisher Box, J, op. cit.

30 Ibid.

31 Doll Richard, op cit.

32 Hill AB, an interview with Max Blythe, op cit.

33 Armitage P, Fisher RA and Hill AB: 'A discussion', *International Journal of Epidemiology*, 2003; volume 32, pp. 945-948.

34 Bodmer, W, op. cit.

35 Fisher, RA, *Smoking: the Cancer Controversy*, op. cit.

36 Armitage, Peter *et al.*, op. cit.

37 Fisher Box, J, op. cit., p. 475.

38 Doll, Richard, op. cit.

39 Doll, R and Peto, R, 'Mortality in Relation to Smoking: 20 years' observations on male British doctors', *British Medical Journal*, 1976, vol. 2, pp. 1525–36.

40 Doll, Richard, op. cit.

41 Floderus, B, Cederlöf, R and Friberg, L, 'A 21-year Follow-up Based on the Swedish Twin Register', *International Journal of Epidemiology*, 1988, vol. 17, pp. 332–40.

42 Fisher Box, J, op cit.

43 Hill, AB, an interview with Max Blythe, op. cit.

44 Fisher Box, J, op. cit.

45 Yates, F and Mather, K, 'Ronald Aylmer Fisher 1890–1962', *Biographical Memoirs of the Royal Society of London*, 1963, vol. 9, pp. 91–120.

46 Fisher, RA, op. cit., p. 15.

47 Ibid., p. 38.

48 Bodmer, W, op. cit.

49 Webster, C, op. cit.
50 Bodmer, W, Fisher, RA, and Hill, AB: 'A discussion', *International Journal of Epidemiology*, 2003, vol. 32, pp. 945–8.
51 Fisher Box, J, op. cit., p. 475.
52 Bodmer, W, personal communication.
53 Doll, Richard, personal communication.
54 Wynder, EL, 'When Genius Errs: R. A. Fisher and the lung cancer controversy', *American Journal of Epidemiology*, 1991, vol.134, pp. 1467–8.

CHAPTER 12
1 Doll, Richard, personal communication.

CHAPTER 13
1 Shuster, Sam, personal communication.
2 Doll, Richard, personal communication.
3 Cox, David, personal communication.
4 Tudor Hart, Julian, personal communication.
5 Ibid.
6 Birch, Chris, letter, *The Guardian*, 27 July 2005.
7 Kidd, Marie, personal communication.
8 Doll, Richard, op. cit.
9 Ibid.
10 Morgan, Kenneth O (ed.), *The People's Peace: British History 1945–1989* (Oxford University Press, 1990), p. 203.
11 D'Arcy Hart, Philip, personal communication.
12 Tudor Hart, Julian, op. cit.
13 Shuster, Sam, op. cit.

CHAPTER 14
1 Doll, R, 'A Tentative Estimate of the Leukaemogenic Effect of Test Thermonuclear Explosions', *Journal of Radiological Protection*, 1966, vol. 16, pp. 3–5.
2 Doll, R, 'Hazards of Ionising Radiation: 100 years of observations on man', *British Journal of Cancer*, 1995, vol. 72, pp. 1339–49.
3 Court-Brown, WM and Doll, R, 'Leukaemia and Aplastic Anaemia in Patients Irradiated for Ankylosing Spondylitis', *Medical Research Council Special Report*, series no. 295 (HMSO, 1957).
4 'The Hazards to Man of Nuclear and Allied Radiations', *Medical Research Council Special Report*, command 9780 (HMSO, 1956).
5 Ibid.
6 Smith, P, Review: 'The 1957 MRC Report on Leukaemia and Aplastic Anaemia in Patients Irradiated for Ankylosing Spondylitis', *Journal of Radiological Protection*, 2007, vol. 27, pp. B3–B14.

7   Doll, Richard, personal communication.
8   Ibid.
9   Ibid.
10 Smith, P, op. cit.
11 Court-Brown, WM and Doll, R, op. cit.
12 Ibid.
13 Smith, P, op. cit.
14 'The Hazards to Man of Nuclear and Allied Radiations', op. cit.
15 Hafner, Barbara, personal communication.
16 Ashley-Miller, Michael, personal communication.
17 Arnold, Lorna, personal communication.
18 Smith, Peter, personal communication.
19 Doll, R and Jacobs, P, 'Court-Brown, William Michael, 1918–68', *Dictionary of National Biography* (Oxford University Press, 1969).
20 Hafner, Barbara, op. cit.
21 Jacobs, Patricia, personal communication.
22 Doll, Richard, op.cit.
23 Court-Brown, WM and Doll, R, 'Expectation of Life and Mortality from Cancer among British Radiologists', *British Medical Journal*, 1958, vol. 2, pp. 181–7.
24 Doll, R and Jacobs, P, op. cit.
25 Jacobs, Patricia, op. cit.
26 Doll, R and Jacobs, P, op. cit.
27 Ibid.
28 Darby, Sarah, 'A conversation with Richard Doll', *Epidemiology*, 2003, vol. 14, pp. 375–9.

CHAPTER 15
1   Avery Jones, F, foreword in Vessey, MP and Gray, M (eds.), *Cancer— Risks and Prevention* (Oxford University Press, 1985).
2   Godfrey, Malcolm, personal communication.
3   Doll, Richard, personal communication.
4   Faulkner, Joan, personal communication.
5   Sutherland, Isabelle, personal communication.
6   Godfrey, Malcolm, op. cit.
7   Faulkner, Joan, op. cit.
8   Sutherland, Isabelle, op. cit.
9   Hill, AB, foreword, in *Cancer: Risks and Prevention*, op. cit.
10 Wald, NJ, 'Smoking', in *Cancer: Risks and Prevention*, op. cit., p. 45.
11 Godber, George, personal communication.
12 Ibid.
13 Gray, M and Fletcher, C, 'Prevention through Legislation' in *Cancer: Risks and Prevention*, op. cit., p. 243.
14 Morris, Jerry, personal communication

15 Peto, R, 'Smoking and Death: the past 40 years and the next 40', *British Medical Journal*, 1994, vol. 309, pp. 937–9.
16 *Times*, 20 June 1962.
17 *Guardian*, 14 February 2007.
18 Doll, R and Hill, AB, 'Mortality in Relation to Smoking: ten years' observations on male British doctors', *British Medical Journal*, 1964, vol. 1, pp. 1399–1410 and 1460–67.
19 Ibid.
20 Ibid.
21 'Deaths from Smoking', *British Medical Journal*, leader, 1964, vol. 1, pp. 1451–2.
22 Morris, Jerry, op. cit.
23 Pollock, David, *Denial and Delay. The Political History of Smoking and Health, 1951–64* (Action on Smoking and Health, 1999), p. 132.

CHAPTER 16
1 Doll, R, 'Proof of Causality: deduction from epidemiological observation', *Perspectives in Biology and Medicine*, 2002, vol. 46, pp. 499–515.
2 Doll, R, 'Discovery Deposition', January 1997, Florida, USA.
3 World Health Organisation, Prevention of Cancer, technical report series 276 (WHO, 1964).
4 Pike, Malcolm, personal communication.
5 Pike, MC, Williams, EH and Wright, B, 'Burkitt's Tumour in the West Nile District of Uganda', *British Medical Journal*, 1967, vol. 2, pp. 395–9.
6 Doll, R, Payne, P and Waterhouse, J, *Cancer Incidence in Five Continents* (Springer-Verlag, Berlin, 1966), p. 1.
7 Ibid.
8 Samet, JM and Speizer, FE, Obituary of Sir Richard Doll 1912–2005, *American Journal of Epidemiology*, 2006, vol. 164, pp. 95–100.
9 Cook-Mozaffari, Paula, personal communication.
10 Pike, Malcolm, op. cit.
11 Doll, R, *Prevention of Cancer: Pointers from Epidemiology* (Nuffield Provincial Hospitals Trust, 1967).
12 Ibid.
13 Peto, R, editorial, *European Journal of Cancer*, 1999, vol. 35, p. 11.
14 Doll, R, op. cit.
15 Hill, AB, 'The Environment and Disease: association or causation?', *Proceedings of the Royal Society of Medicine*, 1965, vol. 58, pp. 295–300.
16 Doll, R, op. cit.
17 Ibid.
18 Court-Brown, W, book reviews, *Annals of Human Genetics*, 1968, vol. 32, p. 97.
19 Doll, R, 'Prospects for Prevention', *World Health Forum*, 1983, vol. 4, pp. 219–27.

Notes

CHAPTER 17

1   Advisory committee on obstetrics and gynaecology, studies in family planning, *Report on Intrauterine Devices* (Food and Drug Administration, 1966).

2   Medical Research Council subcommittee, 'Risk of Thromboembolic Disease in Women Taking Oral Contraceptives: a preliminary communication to the Medical Research Council by a subcommittee', *British Medical Journal*, 1967, vol. 2, pp. 335–59.

3   Ibid.

4   Vessey, MP and Doll, R, 'Investigation of Relation Between Use of Oral Contraceptives and Thromboembolic Disease', *British Medical Journal*, 1968, vol. 2, pp. 199–205.

5   Ibid.

6   'Oral Contraceptives and Thromboembolism', editorial, *British Medical Journal*, 1968, vol. 2, pp. 187–8.

7   *Oxford Mail*, 21 December 1971.

8   Ibid.

9   Peto, Richard, personal communication.

10 Day, Martyn, personal communication.

11 Cairns, John, personal communication.

12 Peto, Richard, op. cit.

13 Foreman, David, personal communication.

14 Faulkner, Joan, personal communication.

15 Ibid.

16 Sutherland, Isabelle, personal communication.

17 Ibid.

18 Speizer, FE, Doll, R and Heaf, P, 'Observations on Recent Increase in Mortality from Asthma', *British Medical Journal*, 1968, vol. 1, pp. 335–9.

19 Samet, JM and Speizer, FE, Obituary of Sir Richard Doll 1912–2005, *American Journal of Epidemiology*, 2006, vol. 164, pp. 95–100.

20 Tudor Hart, Julian, personal communication.

21 Peto, Richard, personal communication.

22 Kinlen, L, Obituary of Sir Richard Doll, *Nature*, 2005, vol. 438, p. 41.

23 Obituary of John Squire, *Lancet*, 1966, vol. 1, p. 157.

24 Booth, CC, 'Clinical Research', in Austoker, J and Bryder, L (eds.), *Historical Perspectives on the Role of the MRC* (Oxford University Press, 1989).

25 Doll, Richard, personal communication.

CHAPTER 18

1   Habakkuk, John, personal communication.

2   Smith, Joe, personal communication.

3   Till, 'Tim', personal communication.

4   Holt, Jim, personal communication.

5   Dunnill, Michael, personal communication.

6   Habbakkuk, John, op. cit.
7   Holt, Jim, op. cit.
8   Doll, Richard, personal communication.
9   Garnham, Peter, personal communication.
10 Ledingham, John, personal communication.
11 Kinlen, Leo, personal communication.
12 Hafner, Barbara, personal communication.
13 Faulkner, Joan, personal communication.
14 Rue, Rosemary, personal communication.
15 *Oxford University Gazette*, 2 May 1974.
16 Ledingham, John, op. cit.
17 Doll, Richard, op. cit.
18 Pike, Malcolm, personal communication.
19 Day, Martyn, personal communication.
20 Peto, Julian, personal communication.
21 *Daily Telegraph*, 28 June 1973.
22 *Daily Telegraph*, 3 July 1973.
23 *Daily Telegraph*, 29 June 1973.
24 *Daily Telegraph*, 30 June 1973.
25 Doll, R, Peto, R, Wheatley, K, Gray, R and Sutherland, I, *British Medical Journal*, 1994, vol. 309, pp. 901–11.
26 Morris, Peter, personal communication.
27 Dunnill, Michael, op. cit.
28 Ledingham, John, op. cit.
29 Weatherall, David, personal communication.
30 Ibid.
31 Ibid.
32 Doll, R, 'Introduction to DNA', in 'The Double Helix: Perspective and Prospective at Forty Years', Donald A Chambers (ed.), *Annals of the New York Academy of Sciences*, 1993, vol. 758, pp. 329–30.
33 Ibid.
34 Brittan, Julian, personal communication.
35 Peto, Julian, op. cit.
36 Weatherall, David, op. cit.
37 Draper, Gerald, personal communication.
38 Ledingham, John, op. cit.

CHAPTER 19
1   Greene, Gayle, *The Woman Who Knew Too Much. Alice Stewart and the Secrets of Radiation* (University of Michigan Press, 1999), p. 46.
2   Alice Stewart, personal communication.
3   Ibid.
4   Greene, Gayle, op. cit., p. 56.

Notes

5   Pemberton, John, 'Possible Developments in Social Medicine', *British Medical Journal*, 1943, vol. 2, pp. 754–5.
6   Oxford University Archive, folder MD/13/10.
7   Ibid.
8   Ibid.
9   Cooke, AM, *My First 75 Years in Medicine* (Royal College of Physicians of London, 1994).
10 *Daily Express*, 16 July 1942.
11 *Times*, 16 July 1942.
12 Greene, Gayle, op. cit., p. 70.
13 Ryle, J, 'Social Medicine: its meaning and its scope', *British Medical Journal*, 1943, vol. 2, pp. 633–6.
14 Bodleian Library, 6 February 1947, addendum 8, Ref. No MD/13/10.
15 Stewart, Alice, personal communication.
16 Holland, Walter W, 'Changing Names', *Scandinavian Journal of Social Medicine*, 1994, vol. 22, pp. 1–6.
17 Stewart, Alice, op. cit.
18 Greene, Gayle, op. cit., p. 83.
19 Ibid., p. 84.
20 *Oxford University Gazette*, 24 October 1952.
21 Greene, Gayle, op. cit.
22 Oxford University Archive, folder MD/13/10.
23 Greene, Gayle, op. cit.
24 Ibid.
25 Stewart, Alice, Webb, JW, Giles, D and Hewitt, David, 'Preliminary Communication: malignant disease in childhood and diagnostic irradiation *in utero*', *Lancet*, 1956, vol. 2, p. 447.
26 Stewart, Alice, op.cit.
27 Ibid.
28 Doll, Richard, personal communication.
29 Stewart, Alice, Webb JW and Hewitt, David, 'A Survey of Childhood Malignancies', *British Medical Journal*, 1958, vol. 1, pp. 1495–1508.
30 Greene, Gayle, op. cit., p. 86.
31 Court-Brown, WM, Doll, R and Hill, AB, 'The Incidence of Leukaemia following Exposure to Diagnostic Radiation *in utero*', *British Medical Journal*, 1960, vol. 2, pp. 1539–45.
32 Lewis, TLT, 'Leukaemia in Childhood after Ante-natal Exposure to X-rays, a survey at Queen Charlotte's Hospital', *British Medical Journal*, 1960, vol. 2, p. 1551.
33 'Foetal Irradiation and Leukaemia', editorial, *British Medical Journal*, 1960, vol. 2, p. 1581.
34 MacMahon, Brian, 'Prenatal X-ray Exposure and Childhood Cancer', *Journal of National Cancer Institute*, 1962, vol. 28, p. 1172.

35 Doll, R and Wakeford, Richard, *British Journal of Radiology*, 1997, vol. 70, pp. 130–39.

36 *Oxford Mail*, 20 January 1961.

37 Acheson, Donald, personal communication.

38 Bithell, John, personal communication.

39 Greene, Gayle, op. cit., p. 98.

40 Doll, Richard, 'The Rise of Epidemiology in Oxford' (unpublished, 2003).

41 Bodleian Library, MD/13/10/1 DV/JDG/22/10/1949.

42 Doll, Richard, personal communication.

43 Smith, Peter, personal communication.

44 Greene, Gayle, op. cit., p. 97.

45 Stewart, Alice, personal communication.

46 Jablon, S and Kato, H, 'Childhood Cancer in Relation to Pre-Natal Exposure to Atomic Bomb Radiation', *Lancet*, 1970, vol. 2, pp. 1000–03.

47 Greene, Gayle, op. cit., p. 92.

48 Smith, Peter, op. cit.

49 Greene, Gayle, op. cit., p. 99.

50 Pike, Malcolm, personal communication.

51 Peto, Julian, personal communication.

52 Doll, Richard, personal communication.

53 Draper, Gerald, personal communication.

54 Doll, Richard, *Dictionary of National Biography* entry for Alice Stewart, read prior to acceptance and publication.

55 Greene, Gayle, op. cit., p. 228.

56 Holland, Walter, personal communication.

57 Wakeford, Richard, book review, *Journal of Radiological Protection*, 2000, vol. 20, pp. 475–9.

58 Doll, Richard, personal communication.

59 Stewart, Alice, op. cit.

60 Doll, Richard, op. cit.

61 Greene, Gayle, op. cit., p. 61.

62 Stewart, Alice, op. cit.

63 Gilbert, ES, Cragle, DL and Wiggs, LD, 'Updated Analyses of Combined Mortality Data for Workers at the Hanford Site, Oak Ridge National Laboratory, and Rocky Falls Weapons Plant', *Radiation Research*, 1993, vol. 136, pp. 408–21.

64 Greene Gayle, op. cit., p. 164.

65 Ibid.

66 *The Windscale Inquiry*, report by Mr Justice Parker, presented to the Secretary of State for the Environment, 26 January 1978, vol. 1, report and annexes 3–5, pp. 48–9 (HMSO).

67 Greene, Gayle, op. cit.

68 Tucker, Anthony, Obituary of Alice Stewart, *Guardian*, 28 June 2002.

Notes

69 Mr Justice Gatehouse, judgement, in Christopher Merlin and Christine Ann
    Merlin v British Nuclear Fuels plc, 2 April 1990, from the notes of J. L.
    Harpham Ltd, official shorthand writers to the court.
70 Ibid.
71 Sedley, Stephen, personal communication.
72 Wakeford, Richard, op. cit.
73 Bithell, John, op. cit.
74 Doll, Richard, op. cit.
75 Dunnill, Michael, personal communication.
76 Greene, Gayle, op. cit.
77 Bithell, John, Obituary of Professor Alice Stewart, *Journal of Radiological
    Protection*, 2002, vol. 22, pp. 425–8.
78 Doll, Richard, *Dictionary of National Biography* entry for Alice Stewart, op. cit.
79 Stewart, Alice, op. cit.

CHAPTER 20
1   Doll, Richard, Radcliffe College, *Oxford Medical School Gazette*, 1977, vol. 29,
    no. 1.
2   Halsey, AH, personal communication.
3   *The Development of the Clinical School*, Report of a Working Party (Oxford
    University Press, 1971).
4   Dunnill, Michael, personal communication.
5   Doll, Richard, op. cit.
6   Doll, Richard, 'Green College, Oxford: its contribution to clinical medicine',
    British Medical Journal, 1982, vol. 285, pp. 1805–6.
7   Holt, JM and Aston, T, 'Annex B to Entitlements: memorandum by Mr Aston',
    Hebdomadal Council Papers, 1971, vol. 269, pp. 624–5.
8   Hockaday, TDR to Aston, T, 'Annex B to Entitlements: memorandum by Mr
    Aston', *Hebdomadal Council Papers*, 1971, vol. 269, p. 625.
9   *The Development of the Clinical School*, op. cit.
10 Holt, Jim, personal communication.
11 *Hebdomadal Council Papers*, 1975, vol. 282, p. 69.
12 Habakkuk, John, personal communication.
13 Garnham, Peter, personal communication.
14 Doll, Richard, personal communication.
15 Green College Record, 1987.
16 Hales, Kris to Richard Doll, Green College archive, 1976.
17 Holt, Jim, op. cit.
18 Millar, Andrew, personal communication.
19 Doll, Richard, op. cit.
20 Doll, Richard, to Paul Beeson, Green College archive, 1976.
21 Doll, Richard, *Oxford Times*, 26 October 1979.
22 Green, Cecil to Richard Doll, Green College archive, 1976.

23 Doll, Richard, 'Green College, Oxford: its contribution to clinical medicine', op. cit.

24 Gibson, William C., *No Time to Slow Down* (University of British Columbia, 1996), p. 373.

25 *Green College Record*, 1987.

26 Gibson, William C., op. cit., p. 374.

27 Doll, Richard, personal communication.

28 Sutherland, Isabelle, personal communication.

29 Lankester, Jack, personal communication.

30 Richards, Rex, personal communication.

31 Green College Record, op. cit.

32 Minutes of the General Committee, 13 Norham Gardens, 8 June 1978.

33 Doll, Richard, op. cit.

34 Report of committee on Radcliffe College, *Hebdomadal Council Papers*, 1977, vol. 287, pp. 641–4.

35 Doll, Richard, 'The Origin of Green College', 2004.

36 *Oxford Medical School Gazette*, 1977, vol. 2, p. 3.

37 Millar, Andrew, personal communication.

38 Ibid.

39 *Oxford Medical School Gazette*, op. cit.

40 Buchan, Alastair, personal communication.

41 *Oxford Medical School Gazette*, op. cit.

42 Ledingham, John, personal communication.

43 Millar, Andrew, op. cit.

44 Ibid.

45 Doll, Richard, personal communication.

46 Garnham, Peter, op. cit.

47 Hughes, Trevor, personal communication.

48 Millar, Andrew, op. cit.

49 Ibid.

50 Hughes, Trevor, op. cit.

51 Buchan, Alastair, op. cit.

52 Ibid.

53 Kettlewell, Michael, personal communication.

54 Garnham, Peter, op. cit.

55 Bower, Brian, communication to all members of the governing body of Green College, Green College archive.

56 Buchan, Alastair, op. cit.

57 Hughes, Trevor, op. cit.

58 Buchan, Alastair, op. cit.

59 Doll, Richard, op. cit.

60 Ibid.

61 Halsey, AH, personal communication.

62 Fletcher, EWL, Obituary of Lady Doll 1914–2001, *Green College Record*, 2003.

63 Lankester, Jack, personal communication.

64 Doll, Richard, op. cit.

65 Richards, Rex, op. cit.

66 Loudon, I, 'The First Twenty Years', *Green College Record 1979–1999*.

67 Ledingham, John, op. cit.

68 Millard, David, personal communication.

69 Buchan, Alastair, op. cit.

CHAPTER 21

1 National Program for the Conquest of Cancer, *Report of the National Panel of Consultants on the Conquest of Cancer* (US Government Printing Office, 1970).

2 Himsworth, H, *The Development and Organisation of Scientific Knowledge* (William Heinemann, 1970).

3 Armstrong, B and Doll, R, 'Environmental Factors and Cancer Incidence and Mortality in Different Countries, with Special Reference to Dietary Practices', *International Journal of Cancer*, 1975, vol. 14, pp. 617–31.

4 Kinlen, L, Obituary of Sir Richard Doll, Epidemiologist—a personal reminiscence with a select bibliography, *British Journal of Cancer*, 2005, vol. 93, pp. 963–6.

5 Armstrong, Bruce, personal communication.

6 Armstrong, B and Doll, R, op. cit.

7 Armstrong, Bruce, op. cit.

8 Peto, Richard, 'The Preventability of Cancer in Vessey, MP and Gray, M (eds.), *Cancer—Risks and Prevention* (Oxford University Press, 1985), p. 14.

9 Peto, Richard, personal communication.

10 Doll, R and Peto, R, 'Mortality in Relation to Smoking: 20 years' observations on male British doctors', *British Medical Journal*, 1976, vol. 2, pp. 1525–36.

11 Editorial, *British Medical Journal*, 1976, vol. 2, p. 1522.

12 Doll, R and Peto, R, op. cit.

13 Passey, RD, 'Carcinogens in Cigarette Smoke', *British Medical Journal*, 1954, vol. 2, p. 1485.

14 Pike, MC and Doll, R, 'Age at Onset of Lung Cancer: significance in relation to effect of smoking', *Lancet*, 1965, vol. 1, pp. 665–8.

15 Mathews, John, personal communication.

16 Foreman, D, personal communication.

17 Smith, P, personal communication.

18 Day, Martyn, personal communication.

19 'That Lethal Weed', leader, *British Medical Journal*, 1976, vol. 2, p. 1522.

20 Ibid.

21 Berridge, V, 'The Policy Response to the Smoking and Lung Cancer Connection in the 1950s and 1960s', *Historical Journal*, 2006, vol. 46, p. 4.

22 Flowers, Brian, personal communication.

23 Cairns, John, personal communication.
24 Doll, R, 'Strategy for Detection of Cancer Hazards to Man', *Nature*, 1977, vol. 265, pp. 589–96.
25 Doll, R, 'Possibilities for the Prevention of Cancer', Royal Society Lecture, 13 November 1986.
26 Doll, R, 'Strategy for Detection of Cancer Hazards to Man', op. cit.
27 Peto, Richard, personal communication.
28 Peto, R, 'Distorting the Epidemiology of Cancer: the need for a more balanced overview', *Nature*, 1980, vol. 284, pp. 297–300.
29 Doll, R, 'The effect of changes in the environment on the health of the community – an epidemiologist's view', *Journal of the Royal College of General Practitioners*, 1975, vol. 25, pp. 326–34.
30 Peto, Richard, op. cit.
31 Doll, R, 'Strategy for Detection of Cancer Hazards to Man', op. cit.
32 Peto, Richard, personal communication.
33 Ibid.

CHAPTER 22
1   Peto, Richard, personal communication.
2   Samet, JM and Speizer, FE, Obituary of Sir Richard Doll 1912–2005, *American Journal of Epidemiology*, 2006, vol. 164, pp. 95–100.
3   Foreman, David, personal communication.
4   Le Fanu, James, *The Rise and Fall of Modern Medicine* (Little Brown, 1999), p. 355.
5   Doll, Richard, personal communication.
6   Doll, R and Peto, R, 'The Causes of Cancer: Quantitative Estimates of Avoidable Risks of Cancer in the United States Today', *Journal of the National Cancer Institute*, 1981, vol. 66, pp. 1195–1308.
7   Key, Timothy, personal communication.
8   Key, J, Allen, NE, Spencer, EA and Travis, RC, 'The Effect of Diet on Risk of Cancer', *Lancet*, 2002, vol. 360, pp. 861–8.
9   Doll, R, Muir, CS and Waterhouse, JAH (eds.), *Cancer Incidence in Five Continents*, vol. 11 (Springer-Verlag, 1970).
10 Doll, R, 'Strategy for Detection of Cancer Hazards to Man', *Nature*, 1977, vol. 265, pp. 589–96.
11 Key, J, Allen, NE, Spencer, EA and Travis, RC, op. cit.
12 International Agency for Research on Cancer, 'Cancer: causes, occurrence and control' (IARC Scientific Publications, no. 100, 1990).
13 Epstein, SS and Joel B Swarts, 'Fallacies of Lifestyle Cancer Theories', *Nature*, 1981, vol. 289, p127–9.
14 Peto, Richard, personal communication.
15 Ibid.
16 Peto, R, 'Distorting the Epidemiology of Cancer: the need for a more balanced

overview', *Nature*, 1980, vol. 284, pp. 277–300.

17 Greenberg, DS, 'The Dark Side of Cancer Research', Review, *Nature*, 2007, vol. 449, pp. 660–61.

18 Hill, AB, 'The Environment and Disease: Association or Causation?', *Proceedings of the Royal College of Medicine*, 1965, vol. 58, pp. 295–300.

19 Doll, Richard, personal communication.

20 'Fluoride, Teeth and Health', report of Royal College of Physicians (Pitman, 1976).

21 Lock, Stephen, 'Priorities: some personal views', *British Medical Journal*, 1976, vol. 2, pp. 1548–51.

22 Burk, D and Yiamouyiannis, J, *Congressional Record*, 1975, vol. 191, H7172–7176.

23 Doll, R and Kinlen, LJ, *Lancet*, 1977, vol. 1, pp. 1300–02.

24 Ibid.

25 Cook-Mozaffari, Paula, personal communication.

26 *Guardian*, Obituary of Lord Jauncey of Tullichettle, 25 July 2007.

27 Opinion of Lord Jauncey *in causa* Mrs Catherine McColl against Strathclyde Regional Council. Judgement given 29 June 1983.

28 *Daily Telegraph*, Obituary of Lord Jauncey of Tullichettle, 23 July 2007.

29 Opinion of Lord Jauncey, op. cit.

30 Ibid.

31 Ibid.

32 Ibid.

33 *Independent*, Obituary of Lord Jauncey of Tullichettle, 25 July 2007.

34 Opinion of Lord Jauncey, op. cit.

35 Ashley Miller, Michael, personal communication.

36 Yiamouyiannis, J, 'Fluoridation and Cancer', *Lancet*, 1977, vol. 2, p. 296.

37 Lord Jauncey of Tullichettle, personal communication.

38 Epstein, S, Comments in Peto, R and Schneiderman, M (eds.), *The Quantification of Occupational Cancer*, Banbury Report 9, 1981, p. 572.

39 Epstein, SS, *The Politics of Cancer Revisited* (East Ridge Press, 1998).

40 Peto, R, 'Why Cancer? The causes of cancer in developed countries', *Times Health Supplement*, 1981, pp. 12–14.

CHAPTER 23

1 Gilliland, Jean, personal communication.

2 Cheetham, Julia, personal communication.

3 Doll, Richard, personal communication.

4 Royal Commission, 'The Use and Effects of Chemical Agents on Australian Personnel in Vietnam', 9 vols. (Australian Government Publishing Service, 1985).

5 Ellis, Graham, personal communication.

6 Royal Commission, 'The Use and Effects of Chemical Agents on Australian

Personnel in Vietnam', op. cit., vol. 8, p. 103.

7   Ibid., vol. 9, p. 126.

8   Ibid., vol. 8, p. 137.

9   Ellis, Graham, op. cit.

10   Royal Commission, 'The Use and Effects of Chemical Agents on Australian Personnel in Vietnam', op. cit., vol. 8, p. 135.

11   Ibid., vol. 8, p. 177.

12   Coombs, John, 'The Agent Orange Phenomenon: the Report of the Australian Royal Commission', in Young, A. L. and Reggiani, G. M. (eds.), *Agent Orange and its Associated Dioxins: assessment of a controversy* (Elsevier Science Publishers, 1988), pp. 282–317.

13   Royal Commission, 'The Use and Effects of Chemical Agents on Australian Personnel in Vietnam', op. cit., vol. 8, p. 180.

14   Mathews, John, personal communication.

15   Axelson, O, 'Rebuttals of the Final Report on Cancer by the Royal Commission on the Use and Effects of Chemical Agents on Australian Personnel in Vietnam', report number Liu-YMED-R-6 (University of Linköping, 1986).

16   Young AL, letter, *American Journal of Industrial Medicine*, 1991, vol. 19, pp. 399–402.

17   Armstrong, BK, 'Storm in a cup of 2,4,5-T', *Medical Journal of Australia*, 1986, vol. 144, pp. 284–5.

18   International Agency for Research on Cancer, Monograph Series on the Evaluation of the Carcinogenic Risk of Chemicals to Humans, 'Some halogenated hydrocarbons and pesticides exposures', International Agency for Research on Cancer, 1986, vol. 41.

19   Doll, R, 'Effects of Exposure to Vinyl Chloride: an assessment of the evidence', *Scandinavian Journal of Work and Environmental Health*, 1988, vol. 14, pp. 61–78.

20   Hardell L, Walker, MJ, Walhjalt, B, Friedman, LS and Richter, ED, 'Secret Ties to Industry and Conflicting Interests in Cancer Research', *American Journal of Industrial Medicine*, 2007, vol. 50, pp. 227–33.

21   Doll, R, 'Effects of Exposure to Vinyl Chloride', op. cit.

22   McLaughlin, JK, Boice, JD, Tarone, RE and Blot, WJ, letter, *American Journal of Industrial Medicine*, 2007, vol. 40, pp. 699–700.

23   Mastrangelo, G, Fedeli, U, Fadda, E et al., 'Increased Risk of Hepatocellular Carcinoma and Liver Cirrhosis in Vinyl Chloride Workers: synergistic effect of occupational exposure with alcohol intake', *Environmental Health Perspectives*, 2007, vol. 112, pp. 1188–92.

24   International Agency for Research on Cancer, Monograph on the Evaluation of Carcinogenic Risks to Humans, '1,3-Butadiene, ethylene oxide, and vinyl halides (vinyl fluoride, vinyl chloride and vinyl bromide)', *Lancet*, 2007, vol. 97.

25   Leet, Terry, personal communication.

26   Young, AL, op. cit.

27   Wakeford, R, letter, *American Journal of Industrial Medicine*, 2007, vol. 50, pp. 239–40.
28   Atterstam, Inger, personal communication.
29   Hughes, Trevor, personal communication.
30   Sutherland, Isabelle, personal communication.

CHAPTER 24
1   Slack, P, *The Impact of Plague in Tudor and Stuart England* (Routledge and Kegan Paul, 1985).
2   Porter, R, 'History Says No to the Policeman's Response to AIDS', *British Medical Journal*, 1986, vol. 293, pp. 1589–90.
3   Doll, R, 'Major Epidemics of the 20th Century: from coronary thrombosis to AIDS', *Journal of the Royal Statistical Society*, 1987, series A, vol. 150, pp. 373–95.
4   Gowans, James, personal communication.
5   Ibid.
6   Peto, J, 'AIDS and Promiscuity', *Lancet*, 1986, vol. 2, p. 979.
7   Letter from Sir James Gowans to Sir Richard Doll, 20 November 1986.
8   Ibid., 6 January 1987.
9   Black, D, Bodmer, W, Cox, D, Doll, R, Durbin, J, Hoffenberg, R, Kingman, J, Peto, J and Weiss, R, letter, *Lancet*, 1987, vol. 2, p. 1277.
10   Simpson, D, Obituary of Sir Richard Doll, *Tobacco Control*, 2005, vol. 14, pp. 289–90.
11   *Observer*, 24 April 2005.
12   Arnold, Lorna, *Britain and the H-Bomb* (Palgrave, 2001), p. 131.
13   McGinley, K with O'Neill, EP, *No Risk Involved* (Mainstream Publishing Company, 1991).
14   Edwards R, 'Written out of History', *New Scientist*, 1996, issue 2030, pp. 14–15.
15   Gardner, M, editorial, 'Cancer among Participants in Tests of British Nuclear Weapons', *British Medical Journal*, 1988, vol. 295, pp. 309–10.
16   Notes and News, *Lancet*, 1988, vol. 1, p. 313.
17   Darby, SC, Kendall, GM, Fell, TP, O'Hagan, JA, Muirhead, CR, Enis, JR, Ball, AM, Dennis, JA and Doll, R, 'Mortality and Cancer Incidence in UK Participants in UK Atmospheric Nuclear Weapon Tests and Experimental Programmes', National Radiological Protection Board, R214 (HMSO, 1988), and 'A Summary of Mortality and Incidence of Cancer in Men from the United Kingdom who Participated in the United Kingdom's Atmospheric Nuclear Weapon Tests and Experimental Programmes', *British Medical Journal*, 1988, vol. 296, pp. 332–8.
18   Darby, Sarah, personal communication.
19   Hadlington, S, 'Cancer Risk "Slightly Higher" of UK Nuclear Test Participants', *Nature*, 1988, vol. 331, p. 383.
20   Darby, SC, Kendall, GM, Fell, TP, Doll, R, Goodill, AA, Conquest, AJ, Jackson,

DA and Haylock, RGE, 'Further Follow-up of Mortality and Incidence of Cancer in Men from the United Kingdom who Participated in the United Kingdom's Atmospheric Nuclear Weapon Tests and Experimental Programmes', *British Medical Journal*, 1993, vol. 307, pp.1530–35.

21 Edwards, R, op. cit.

22 Ibid.

23 Beral, Valerie, personal communication.

24 Smith, AFM, 'Mad Cows and Ecstasy: chance and choice in the evidence-based society', *Journal of the Royal Statistical Society*, Series A, 1996, vol. 159, pp. 367–83.

25 Wakeford, R, 'Epidemiology and Litigation—the Sellafield Childhood Leukaemia Cases', *Journal of the Royal Statistical Society*, Series A, 1998, vol. 161, pp. 313–25.

26 Mole, RH, 'Ionizing Radiations and Human Leukemia', in *William Dameshek and Frederick Gunz's Leukemia* (Harcourt Brace Jovanovich, 1990).

27 Beral, V, Roman, E and Bobrow, M, *Childhood Cancer and Nuclear Installations* (British Medical Journal Publishing Group, 1993).

28 Wakeford, R, op. cit.

29 Arnold, Lorna, personal communication.

30 Gardner, MJ, Snee, MP, Hall, AJ, Powell, CA, Downes, S and Terrell, JD, 'Results of Case-control Study of Leukaemia and Lymphoma among Young People near Sellafield Nuclear Plant in West Cumbria', *British Medical Journal*, 1990, vol. 300, pp. 423–9.

31 Snee, Michael, personal communication.

32 Mr Justice Gatehouse, judgement, in Christopher Merlin and Christine Ann Merlin v British Nuclear Fuels plc, 2 April 1990, from the notes of J. L. Harpham Ltd, official shorthand writers to the court.

33 Ibid.

34 Day, Martyn, personal communication.

35 Radford, Edward, personal communication.

36 Bowden, Paul, personal communication.

37 Mr Justice Gatehouse, judgement, op. cit.

38 Hytner, Ben, personal communication.

39 Wakeford, R., op. cit.

40 Darby, Sarah, personal communication.

41 Rokison, Ken, personal communication.

42 Day, Martyn, op. cit.

43 Bowden, Paul, op. cit.

44 Kinlen, Leo, personal communication.

45 Day, Martyn, op. cit.

46 Wakeford, Richard, op. cit.

47 Wakeford, Richard, personal communication.

48 Day, Martyn, op. cit.

49 Bowden, Paul, op. cit.

50 Hytner, Ben, op. cit.

51 Bowden, Paul, op. cit.

52 Day, Martyn, op. cit.

53 Snee, Michael, op. cit.

54 Parker L, Craft, AW, Smith, J, Dickinson, H, Wakeford, R, Binks, K, McElvenny, D, Scott, L and Slovak, A, 'Geographical Distribution of Preconceptional Radiation Doses to Fathers Employed at the Sellafield Nuclear Installation, West Cumbria', *British Medical Journal*, 1993, vol. 307, pp. 966–71.

55 Boulton, F, Obituary of Richard Doll, *Medicine Conflict and Survival*, 2006, vol. 22(1), pp. 78–82.

56 Kinlen, LJ, 'The Relevance of Population Mixing to the Aetiology of Childhood Leukaemia', in Crosbie, W. A. and Gittus, J. H. (eds.), *Medical Response to Effects of Ionising Radiation* (Elsevier, 1989), pp. 272–7.

57 Bowden, Paul, op. cit.

58 Day, Martyn, op. cit.

59 Hytner, Ben, op. cit.

60 Bowden, Paul, op. cit.

61 Doll, R, Evans, HJ and Darby, SC, 'Paternal Exposure Not to Blame', *Nature*, 1994, vol. 367, pp. 634–46.

62 Osmond C, Obituary of Professor Martin Gardner, *Journal of the Royal Statistical Society*, 1993, vol. 156, part 3, pp. 498–500.

CHAPTER 25

1 Cross-examination of Sir Richard Doll by Mr S. Sedley QC before Mr Justice Gatehouse, Christopher Peter Merlin and Christine Ann Merlin v British Nuclear Fuels plc, Royal Court of Justice, The Strand, London, 1 December 1989.

2 Doll, R, Peto, R, Wheatley, K, Gray, R and Sutherland, I, 'Mortality in Relation to Smoking: 40 years' observations on male British doctors', *British Medical Journal*, 1994, vol. 309, pp. 901–11.

3 Smee, C, Parsonage, M, Anderson, R and Duckworth, S, 'Effect of Tobacco Advertising on Tobacco Consumption', a discussion document reviewing the evidence (Department of Health, 1992).

4 Beecham, L, 'Medicopolitical Digest CCSC sets up Working Party on the New NHS', *British Medical Journal*, 1994, vol. 308, p. 140.

5 Doll, R and Peto, R *et al.*, op. cit.

6 Doll, R, 'Lung Cancer: observed and expected changes in incidence from active and passive smoking', 14th International Cancer Congress, Budapest, August 1986.

7 Wald, NJ, Boreham, J, Bailey, A, Ritchie, C, Haddow, JE and Knight, G, 'Urinary Cotinine as Marker of Breathing Other People's Tobacco Smoke', *Lancet*, 1984, vol. 1, pp. 230–31.

8   Doll, R and Peto, J, guest editorial, 'Passive Smoking', *British Journal of Cancer*, 1986, vol. 54, pp. 381–3.
9   Weiss, Robin, personal communication.
10 Ibid.
11 Doll, R and Peto, R, 'There is No Such Thing as Ageing', *British Medical Journal*, 1997, vol. 315, pp. 1030–32.
12 Smith, Richard, 'Richard Doll at 85', *British Medical Journal*, 1997, vol. 315, p. 315.
13 Doll, R, Peto, R, Hall, E, Wheatley, K and Gray, R, 'Mortality in Relation to Consumption of Alcohol: 13 years' observations on male British doctors', *British Medical Journal*, 1994, vol. 309, pp. 911–18.
14 Doll, R, 'One for the Heart', *British Medical Journal*, 1997, vol. 315, pp. 1664–8.
15 Shaw, GB, *The Doctor's Dilemma* (Bodley Head, 1931).
16 Holland, Walter, personal communication.
17 Weatherall, David, personal communication.
18 Keen, Harry, personal communication.
19 Mosley, Celia, personal communication.
20 Ibid.

CHAPTER 26
1   Doll, R, 'Uncovering the Effects of Smoking: historical perspective', *Statistical Methods in Medical Research*, 1998, vol. 7, pp. 87–117.
2   Doll, R, 'Tobacco: a medical history', *Journal of Urban Health*, 1999, vol. 76, pp. 289–313.
3   Doll, Christopher, personal communication.
4   Doll, R, Peto, R, Boreham, J and Sutherland, I, 'Mortality in Relation to Smoking: 50 years' observation on male British doctors', *British Medical Journal*, 2004, vol. 328, pp. 519–28.
5   Stampfer, M, 'New Insights from the British Doctors', *British Medical Journal*, 2004, vol. 328, p. 1507.
6   Doll, R, 'Sir Richard Doll 1912–2005. Half a Century of Cancer Epidemiology' (Cancer Research UK Scientific Yearbook, 2004/2005).
7   Buckatzch, Marna, personal communication.
8   Kidd, Marie, personal communication.
9   Garfield, S, 'The Man who Saved a Million Lives', *Observer Magazine*, 24 April 2005.

Further Reading

Richard Doll was the author, often in collaboration with others, of over 500 scientific papers, articles and reviews. His collection of written work can be accessed at the Wellcome Library in Euston Road, London. The main Archives and Manuscripts catalogue can be reached at http://archives.wellcome.ac.uk. The Doll papers are located by searching on PP/DOL.

Other works referenced in this book include:

Allenbrooke, Field Marshall Lord, *War Diaries 1939–1945* (London: Weidenfeld & Nicolson, 2001)

Armitage, P and Berry, G, *Statistical Methods in Medical Research*, 3rd edn (Oxford: Blackwell Science, 1996)

Arnold, Lorna, *Britain and the H-Bomb* (London: Palgrave Publishers, 2001)

Austoker, J and Bryder, L (eds.), *Historical Perspectives on the Role of the MRC* (Oxford: Oxford University Press, 1989)

Austoker, Joan, *History of the Imperial Cancer Research Fund, 1902–86* (Oxford: Oxford University Press, 1988)

Beral, V, Roman, E and Bobrow, M, *Childhood Cancer and Nuclear Installations* (London: British Medical Journal Publishing Group, 1993)

Berridge, Virginia, *Marketing Health: smoking and the discourse of public health in Britain, 1945–2000* (Oxford: Oxford University Press, 2007)

Beveridge, William, *The Pillars of Security* (London: Allen & Unwin, 1943)

Boyd Orr, John, *Food, Health and Income* (London: Macmillan, 1936)

Bradford Hill, A, *Controlled Clinical Trials, A Symposium* (Oxford: Blackwell Scientific Publishing, 1960)

Bradford Hill, A, *Principles of Medical Statistics* (London: The Lancet, 1937)

Castleman, Barry I, *Asbestos: Medical and Legal Aspects* (New York: Aspen Publishers, 1996)

Chisholm, Anne and Davie, Michael, *Beaverbrook: A Life* (London: Hutchinson, 1992)

Cleave, TL and Campbell, GD, *Diabetes Coronary Thrombosis and the Saccharine Disease* (Bristol: John Wright and Sons, 1966)

Cooke, AM, *My First 75 Years in Medicine* (Royal College of Physicians of London, 1994)

Cooper, George, *And Hitler Stopped Play: Cricket and War at Lyminster House, West Sussex (1931–1946)* (Cambridge: Vanguard, 2001)

Crosbie, WA and Gittus, JH (eds.), *Medical Response to Effects of Ionising Radiation* (Amsterdam: Elsevier, 1989)

Doll, R, Muir, CS and Waterhouse, JAH (eds.), *Cancer Incidence in Five Continents*, vol. 11 (Berlin: Springer-Verlag, 1970)

Doll, R, *Prevention of Cancer: Pointers from Epidemiology* (London: Nuffield Provincial Hospitals Trust, 1967)

Epstein, SS, *The Politics of Cancer Revisited* (Fremont Center, NY: East Ridge Press, 1998)

Field, John, *The King's Nurseries: The Story of Westminster School*, 2nd edn (London: James & James, 1987)

Fisher Box, J, *R. A. Fisher: The Life of a Scientist* (London: John Wiley & Sons, 1978)

Fisher, RA, *Smoking: the Cancer Controversy* (London: Oliver and Boyd, 1959)

Frank, SA, *Dynamics of Cancer Incidence, Inheritance, and Evolution* (Princeton, NJ: Princeton University Press, 2007)

Gibson, William C, *No Time to Slow Down* (Vancouver: University of British Columbia, 1996)

Greene, Gayle, *The Woman Who Knew Too Much. Alice Stewart and the Secrets of Radiation* (Ann Arbor, MI: University of Michigan Press, 1999)

Himsworth, H, *The Development and Organisation of Scientific Knowledge* (London: William Heinemann, 1970)

Humanise the Hospitals, broadsheet issued by the Communist Party

(Watford: Farleigh Press, 1947)

Kisch R, *Days of the Good Soldiers: Communists in the Armed Forces, World War II* (London: Journeyman Press, 1985)

Le Fanu, James, *The Rise and Fall of Modern Medicine* (London: Little Brown, 1999)

McGinley, K with O'Neill, EP, *No Risk Involved* (Edinburgh: Mainstream Publishing Company, 1991)

Morgan, Kenneth O (ed.), *The People's Peace: British History 1945–1989* (Oxford: Oxford University Press, 1990)

Pelling, M, *Cholera, Fever and English Medicine 1825–1865* (Oxford: Oxford University Press, 1978)

Pollock, D, *Denial and Delay: The Political History of Smoking and Health, 1951–1964* (London: Action on Smoking and Health, 1999)

Proctor, RN, *The Nazi War on Cancer* (Princeton, NJ: Princeton University Press, 1999)

Shaw, GB, *The Doctor's Dilemma* (London: Bodley Head, 1931)

Slack, P, *The Impact of Plague in Tudor and Stuart England* (London: Routledge and Kegan Paul, 1985)

Stewart, John, *The Battle for Health: A Political History of the Socialist Medical Association, 1930–51* (Aldershot: Ashgate Publishing, 1999)

Massey, A (ed.), *Modern Trends in Public Health* (London: Butterworth, 1949)

Tweedale, Geoffrey, *Magic Mineral to Killer Dust. Turner & Newall and the Asbestos Hazard* (Oxford: Oxford University Press, 2000)

Vessey, MP and Gray, M (eds.), *Cancer: Risks and Prevention* (Oxford: Oxford University Press, 1985)

Webster, C, *The Health Services Since the War, vol. 1, Problems of Health Care: The NHS before 1957* (London: HMSO, 1988)

Young, AL and Reggiani, GM (eds.), *Agent Orange and its Associated Dioxins: assessment of a controversy* (Amsterdam: Elsevier Science Publishers, 1988)

Index

Index

Index

Index